INCREASING SMALL RUMINANT PRODUCTIVITY IN SEMI-ARID AREAS

Current Topics in Veterinary Medicine and Animal Science

Recent publications

1984

26. Manipulation of Growth in Farm Animals, edited by J.F. Roche and D. O'Callaghan. ISBN 0-89838-617-8
27. Latent Herpes Virus Infections in Veterinary Medicine, edited by G. Wittmann, R.M. Gaskell and H.-J. Rziha. ISBN 0-89838-622-5
28. Grassland Beef Production, edited by W. Holmes. ISBN 0-89838-650-0
29. Recent Advances in Virus Diagnosis, edited by M.S. McNulty and J.B. McFerran. ISBN 0-89838-674-8
30. The Male in Farm Animal Reproduction, edited by M. Courot. ISBN 0-89838-682-9

1985

31. Endocrine Causes of Seasonal and Lactational Anestrus in Farm Animals, edited by F. Ellendorff and F. Elsaesser. ISBN 0-89838-738-8
32. Brucella Melitensis, edited by J.M. Verger and M. Plommet. ISBN 0-89838-742-6

1986

33. Diagnosis of Mycotoxicoses, edited by J.L. Richard and J.R. Thurston. ISBN 0-89838-751-5
34. Embryonic Mortality in Farm Animals, edited by J.M. Sreenan and M.G. Diskin. ISBN 0-89838-772-8
35. Social Space for Domestic Animals, edited by R. Zayan. ISBN 0-89838-773-6
36. The Present State of Leptospirosis Diagnosis and Control, edited by W.A. Ellis and T.W.A. Little. ISBN 0-89838-777-9
37. Acute Virus Infections of Poultry, edited by J.B. McFerran and M.S. McNulty. ISBN 0-89838-809-0

1987

38. Evaluation and Control of Meat Quality in Pigs, edited by P.V. Tarrant, G. Eikelenboom and G. Monin. ISBN 0-89838-854-6
39. Follicular Growth and Ovulation Rate in Farm Animals, edited by J.F. Roche and D. O'Callaghan. ISBN 0-89838-855-4
40. Cattle Housing Systems, Lameness and Behaviour, edited by H.K. Wierenga and D.J. Peterse. ISBN 0-89838-862-7
41. Physiological and Pharmacological Aspects of the Reticulo-rumen, edited by L.A.A. Ooms, A.D. Degryse and A.S.J.P.A.M. van Miert. ISBN 0-89838-878-3
42. Biology of Stress in Farm Animals: An Integrative Approach, edited by P.R. Wiepkema and P.W.M. van Adrichem. ISBN 0-89838-895-3
43. Helminth Zoonoses, edited by S. Geerts, V. Kumar and J. Brandt. ISBN 0-89838-896-1
44. Energy Metabolism in Farm Animals: Effects of Housing, Stress and Disease, edited by M.W.A. Verstegen and A.M. Henken. ISBN 0-89838-974-7
45. Summer Mastitis, edited by G. Thomas, H.J. Over, U. Vecht and P. Nansen. ISBN 0-89838-982-8

1988

46. Modelling of Livestock Production Systems, edited by S. Korver and J.A.M. van Arendonk. ISBN 0-89838-373-0
47. Increasing Small Ruminant Productivity in Semi-arid Areas, edited by E.F. Thomson and F.S. Thomson. ISBN 0-89838-386-2

Increasing Small Ruminant Productivity in Semi-arid Areas

Proceedings of a Workshop
held at the International Center for Agricultural Research in the Dry Areas,
Aleppo, Syria, 30 November to 3 December 1987

Edited by

E.F. THOMSON & F.S. THOMSON

International Center for Agricultural Research in the Dry Areas,
P.O. Box 5466, Aleppo, Syria

KLUWER ACADEMIC PUBLISHERS
DORDRECHT – BOSTON – LONDON

Library of Congress Cataloging in Publication Data
Increasing small ruminant productivity in semi-arid areas :
  proceedings of a workshop held at the International Center for
  Agricultural Research in the Dry Areas, Aleppo, Syria, November 30
  to December 3, 1987 / E.F. Thomson and F.S. Thomson [editors].
      p. cm. -- (Current topics in veterinary medicine and animal
  science ; v. 47)

    1. Sheep--Middle East--Congresses. 2. Sheep--Africa, North-
  -Congresses. 3. Ruminants--Middle East--Congresses. 4. Ruminants-
  -Africa, North--Congresses.   I. Thomson, E. F. (Euan F.)
  II. Thomson, F. S. III. International Center for Agricultural
  Research in the Dry Areas. IV. Series.
  SF375.5.M628I53 1988
  636.3'00953--dc19   88-15550
                                                           CIP

ISBN-13: 978-94-010-7086-7   e-ISBN-13: 978-94-009-1317-2
DOI: 10.1007/978-94-009-1317-2

Published by Kluwer Academic Publishers,
P.O. Box 17, 3300 AA Dordrecht, The Netherlands.

Kluwer Academic Publishers incorporates
the publishing programmes of
Martinus Nijhoff, Dr W. Junk, D. Reidel, and MTP Press.

Sold and distributed in the U.S.A. and Canada
by Kluwer Academic Publishers,
101 Philip Drive, Norwell, MA 02061, U.S.A.

In all other countries, sold and distributed
by Kluwer Academic Publishers Group,
P.O. Box 322, 3300 AH Dordrecht, The Netherlands

E.F. Thomson and F.S. Thomson (eds), Increasing Small Ruminant Productivity in Semi-arid Areas
© 1988 ICARDA . ISBN 978-94-010-7086-7

Table of Contents

E.F. Thomson and F.S. Thomson (eds), Increasing Small Ruminant Productivity in Semi-arid Areas
© *1988 ICARDA . ISBN 978-94-010-7086-7*

Foreword

Livestock production represents about 30% of the agricultural revenue of the countries of West Asia and North Africa and livestock products are the main output from areas receiving less than 300 mm annual rainfall. The 300 million small ruminants account for a large proportion of this output and represent a significant capital reserve for the small farmers who predominate in these countries. The wheat-based diet of the rural and urban population is balanced with milk products and meat which provide essential amino acids, minerals, and vitamins.

High population growth rates and rising incomes are together responsible for increasing demand for livestock products. But the countries of West Asia and North Africa are unable to meet these demands from domestic production. Imports of meat, dairy products, and coarse grains for livestock are already high and are projected to increase significantly by the year 2000. Thus there is an urgent need to promote domestic feed production and increase output of livestock products by using more efficient livestock, larger numbers, or both.

The International Center for Agricultural Research in the Dry Areas (ICARDA), one of 13 Centers of the Consultative Group for International Agricultural Research (CGIAR), was established in 1977. Its main aim is to increase food production using sustainable farming systems, with a focus on improved crop varieties and management, farm resource management, and pasture and forage production. Because of the important role of small ruminants in the agriculture of North Africa and West Asia and the increasing demands for livestock products and feeds, ICARDA wishes to strengthen its research on small ruminants. It therefore convened a workshop in late 1987 at which leading international and regional experts helped to identify priority areas for research on small ruminants. These proceedings are a result of that workshop.

Overview papers were presented to give a background to the workshop and disciplinary groups, which focused on the interactions between disciplines, formulated recommendations for future research. Hopefully this workshop will stimulate further multi-disciplinary planning meetings in the West Asian and North African region.

G. Jan Koopman
Deputy Director General
(International Cooperation)
ICARDA, Aleppo
March 1988

E.F. Thomson and F.S. Thomson (eds), Increasing Small Ruminant Productivity in Semi-arid Areas
© *1988 ICARDA . ISBN 978-94-010-7086-7*

Acknowledgements

The workshop organizer is indebted to the numerous colleagues who helped arrange the workshop and to the participants who contributed papers and made the discussions so lively and constructive. Aida Battikha and Christina Materon deserve special thanks for their help with the preparation of the manuscript and illustrations. Thanks are also due to ICARDA for allocating scarce funds to finance the workshop and the printing of the proceedings.

Euan F. Thomson
Workshop Organizer
March 1988

Part I

Livestock Systems and Nutrition

E.F. Thomson and F.S. Thomson (eds), Increasing Small Ruminant Productivity in Semi-arid Areas
© *1988 ICARDA . ISBN 978-94-010-7086-7*

The Contribution of Livestock Products to Human Dietary Needs with Special Reference to North Africa and West Asia

P.L. Pellet and V.R. Young

Global aspects

As wealth increases, more food is consumed and there are major changes in the pattern of the foods selected. These changes were tabulated by Perisse et al. (1969) who demonstrated that the proportion of dietary energy intake from fats rose steeply with income while that from total carbohydrates declined. Simultaneously, the proportion of the total protein intake from animal sources increased. Subsequent observations confirm and extend these earlier conclusions.

It is no longer appropriate to limit considerations of the factors determining nutritional status only to the food supply and nutrients (Pellett 1983a; 1987). Following the demonstration of the synergism between nutrition and infection in the 1960s (Scrimshaw et al. 1968) and the adoption of more consciously political approaches in the 1970s, nutritionists have realised that both the basic (socioeconomic and political) and the immediate (food intake and health) causes of hunger and malnutrition should be addressed.

Some of the health, wealth, and dietary data from 130 countries are summarized in Table 1. As wealth (indicated by gross national product (GNP)) increases, infant (IMR) and under-5 mortality rates (MR) decline, as does the prevalence of low birth weight (LBW) infants. The dietary changes accompanying these health changes are increases in the dietary energy availability in relation to requirement, the total and animal protein intake per day, the percentage of animal protein in relation to total protein, and the total fat and retinol intakes. Perisse and Polacchi (1980) proposed that retinol intake was one of the indicators most sensitive to changes in economic status but, from our analysis, animal protein seems to be equally sensitive. Other indicators associated with differences in economic status are access to clean drinking water, availability of health services, and adult literacy (Pellett 1987).

A further elaboration of these relationships is shown in Table 2 where a cross-country correlation matrix between selected health, economic, and dietary data is presented. These results are derived from data from the same 130 countries as in Table 1. As GNP increases, child and infant mortality rates and the percentage of low birth weight infants decline and life expectancy increases. Since total dietary energy, protein, animal protein, and fat availabilities are highly correlated with wealth, there are also significant correlations between infant and child mortality rates and protein, animal protein, and fat

Table 1. Health, wealth, and dietary data for 130 countries.

Group	No. of countries	Population (10⁶)	GNP (USD)	IMR[1]	Under five MR[1]	Life expectancy (years)	Children under 5 years (%)	LBW[2] (%)	Births attended by health personnel (%)	Drinking water access (%)	Kcal/ Kcal needs (%)	Protein per day (TP) (g)	Animal protein per day (AP)(g)	AP/TP (%)	Fat per day (g)	Retinol per day (µg)
1	32	462	295	137	227	46	18	16	22	31	91	53	11	21	38	140
2	32	1498	1623	87	130	56	17	13	50	52	101	62	15	25	51	190
3	30	1692	2207	43	58	66	14	11	82	68	111	70	27	37	63	260
4	36	1165	7817	13	15	74	8	6	99	>90	129	94	54	57	126	620
All	130	4817	2598	67	102	61	14	10	64	62	109	71	28	36	71	313

Source: Nutrient information mainly FAO (1984; 1986) supplemented from FAO (1980), all other data UNICEF (1987).
[1] infant mortality rate (IMR) and under five mortality rate are the annual numbers of deaths at less than 1 year and 5 years of age, respectively, per 1000 live births.
[2] Low birth weight.

Table 2. Cross-country correlation matrix between health and dietary data, 130 countries.

	No. of country pairs	GNP (USD)	IMR [1]	Protein (TP) (g/day)	Animal protein (AP) (g/day)	AP/TP (%)	Fat (g/day)
Child mortality rate	121–129	−0.59	0.99	−0.68	−0.73	−0.72	−0.67
Life expectancy (years)	121–130	0.63	−0.97	0.72	0.76	0.75	0.72
Low birth weight (%)	113–120	−0.49	0.55	−0.64	−0.61	−0.58	−0.61
Children under 5 years (%)	121–130	−0.59	0.78	−0.67	−0.74	−0.69	−0.74
GNP (USD)	120–121	–	−0.61	0.68	0.78	0.73	0.78
IMR [1]	121–129	−0.61	–	−0.70	−0.75	−0.75	−0.70
Protein (g/day)	120–129	0.68	−0.70	–	0.88	0.74	0.85
Animal protein (g/day)	120–129	0.78	−0.75	0.88	–	0.95	0.91
AP/TP (%)	120–129	0.73	−0.75	0.74	0.95	–	0.83
Fat (g/day)	121–129	0.78	−0.70	0.85	0.91	0.83	–

Source: Protein, animal protein and fat (FAO 1984; 1986) supplemented by FAO (1980), all other data UNICEF (1987).
Note: All correlation coefficients P < 0.001.
[1] Annual deaths at less than 1 year per 1000 live births.

consumption. These dietary factors are also significantly correlated with life expectancy since the largest component determining life expectancy values is infant mortality. However, such significant statistical relationships between dietary factors and measures of the health of a population must not be considered causal, since all have direct or indirect relationships with poverty indicators. The relationships between health, economic status, and dietary data and the percentages of children under 5 years are also interesting and emphasize the fundamental importance of population growth as a determinant of nutritional status.

Regional and national considerations

In this paper regions are as defined by FAO (1984; 1985). Thus, "Near East" includes many of the countries of North Africa and West Asia but excludes *inter alia* Algeria, Morocco, Tunisia, and Pakistan. These countries are, however, included when national data are tabulated.

The proportions of the dietary energy from protein, fat, and carbohydrate in several regions of the world and the changes that have occurred over the past 2 decades are shown in Table 3. The absolute amounts of protein and fat available for total consumption are significantly greater in North America and developed countries than in the other regions shown. However, for the Near East region in particular, although the food energy supply has increased significantly, the proportion of animal protein in relation to total protein and of energy from fat in relation to total energy have not changed to the same extent. The most recent estimate of the percentage of animal protein (24%) has increased only slightly from the 21% estimated in 1961–63 and it is still far

6

Table 3. Supplies of the major nutrients by region, 1961–63, 1969–71, and 1979–81.

Region[1]	Dietary energy supply (% from CHO)						Protein (% from animal protein)						Fat (% of Kcal from fat)					
	1961–63		1969–71		1979–81		1961–63		1969–71		1979–81		1961–63		1969–71		1979–81	
	Kcal	%	Kcal	%	Kcal	%	g	%	g	%	g	%	g	%	g	%	g	%
Near East	2230	72	2400	71	2840	69	67	21	68	21	78	24	43	17	48	18	64	20
Africa	2120	72	2170	72	2260	72	53	19	54	20	56	20	38	18	40	18	43	19
Far East	1940	77	2020	78	2160	77	47	13	48	15	51	16	28	13	28	13	33	14
Latin America	2370	70	2500	70	2620	69	62	39	65	38	67	42	52	20	56	20	60	21
LDCs[2]	1980	75	2060	75	2070	75	54	19	54	19	53	19	29	14	30	15	30	15
North America	3263	48	3490	47	3578	47	100	67	105	69	105	68	145	40	159	41	167	42
Developed countries	3110	59	3280	57	3390	55	90	50	95	54	99	57	101	29	114	32	126	33

Source: Adapted from data presented by FAO (1985).

Note: Total dietary energy supply (DES) values in 1981–83 for some of the regions are: Developed countries 3390; Africa 2230; Far East 2190; Latin America 2620; Near East 2900; and LDCs 2080. Average annual rate of increase in DES for the Near East has been 1.3% since 1961–63.

[1] Regions are those as defined by FAO. Near East region includes 20 countries of North Africa and West Asia but excludes Pakistan, Algeria, Morocco, and Tunisia.

[2] LDCs = Least Developed Countries.

below the 68% for North America and 57% for developed countries. For the African region, neither the absolute amounts of dietary energy supply, protein, or fat nor their proportions have changed significantly over the past 2 decades.

The nutritional value of the diet in the Near East and North Africa has been reviewed in more detail elsewhere (Pellett 1983b; Miladi and Pellett 1986) but the contributions of the various food groups to the total food energy supply between 1961 and 1981 are shown in Table 4. In the Near East region, animal products supply only about 11% of the total dietary energy supply (DES) compared to 32% in developed market economies, while more than twice the proportion of food energy originates from cereal products than is the case for developed market economies. The share of the DES from the various food groups is shown in Table 5 for selected countries in the Near East region. Data for developed countries are also shown for comparison. Only the United Arab Emirates approaches the dietary pattern typical for developed market economies but it is probably the most wealthy country in the world in terms of per capita GNP. The other wealthy countries in the region (Cyprus, Kuwait, Libya, and Saudi Arabia) have considerably larger proportions of their DES from animal products than the regional average but are still well below the average for developed countries. Mauritania and Somalia seem to be exceptions to the general relationship between wealth and the amount of animal products in the dietary. In these countries many of the population are nomadic and highly dependent on their herds for food so animal products are widely consumed despite relatively poor economic conditions in the countries as a whole. The other countries of the region have dietaries based on cereals and generally receive less than 12% of their energy from animal products, compared to about 32% for developed countries as a group.

Table 4. Share (%) of dietary energy supply (DES) from various food groups in the Near East region and in developed countries.

Food group	Near East Region			Developed Countries		
	1961–63	1969–71	1979–81	1961–63	1969–71	1979–81
Vegetable products	90	90	89	69	68	68
Cereals	65	62	58	31	27	26
Pulses, nuts	5	4	4	3	2	2
Roots, tubers	2	2	2	5	4	4
Sugar	7	9	10	.13	14	13
Vegetables, fruits	7	7	6	5	5	5
Vegetable oil	5	7	8	8	10	11
Animal products	10	10	11	31	32	32
Meat, offal	4	4	4	13	14	15
Milk	4	3	4	9	9	9
Animal fats	2	2	2	6	6	5
Eggs	<1	<1	<1	2	2	2
Fish	<1	<1	<1	1	1	2
Total food energy (Kcal)	2230	2400	2840	3110	3280	3390

Source: FAO (1985).

Table 5. Share (%) of the dietary energy supply (DES) from various food groups for selected countries of North Africa and West Asia compared with developed countries.

	Annual increase per caput DES (%) 1969–81	Share of DES (%), 1979–81					
		cereals	roots tubers	pulses nuts	animal products	sugar	other foods
Afghanistan [1]	−0.8	81.5	1.4	2.4	7.9	2.0	4.8
Algeria	3.6	56.8	2.2	2.2	10.6	11.7	16.5
Cyprus [1]	1.6	40.0	2.5	6.9	23.1	7.9	19.6
Egypt	2.2	62.1	1.5	2.7	6.4	9.8	17.5
Iran [1]	3.7	64.1	1.2	2.6	8.8	11.8	11.5
Iraq [1]	0.3	60.6	0.5	3.0	9.1	15.5	11.3
Jordan [1]	−0.2	61.8	1.6	2.2	9.9	12.7	11.8
Kuwait	1.6	52.3	0.8	2.3	20.1	11.0	13.5
Libya	4.7	40.3	1.5	4.2	15.3	11.2	27.5
Mauritania	0.5	57.2	0.5	5.9	22.3	7.4	6.7
Morocco	0.7	63.0	1.3	2.6	7.0	12.6	13.5
Pakistan	0.7	75.5	0.4	1.7	7.0	8.6	6.8
Saudi Arabia	4.3	45.3	0.7	3.4	18.0	9.5	23.1
Somalia	−0.8	56.9	0.9	1.8	26.2	5.8	8.4
Sudan	1.0	51.7	1.8	4.6	12.5	10.5	18.9
Syria	2.3	68.6	1.0	3.8	8.0	5.9	12.7
Tunisia	2.0	54.9	1.2	4.1	8.5	9.0	22.3
Turkey	0.8	72.8	1.4	3.3	6.2	4.9	11.4
UAE	0.4	31.3	0.9	3.4	30.0	12.4	22.0
Yemen AR	1.4	65.1	1.3	5.5	10.2	5.9	12.0
Yemen PDR	0.7	69.8	0.1	1.7	11.2	7.4	9.8
Developed countries	0.3	26.4	3.7	2.4	3`.7	13.0	22.8

Source: FAO (1985).

[1] Data for 1977 (FAO 1980), annual percentage increase in DES from 1961–65 to 1977.

It was illustrated in Table 3 that the DES in the Near East region has changed significantly since the early 1960s and that by 1979–81, 2840 calories were available per head, an increase of some 30%. Data in Table 6 show that for the Near East region, this increase in food energy supply is reflected not only by a similar decrease in the absolute numbers of those estimated as malnourished (calculated from the basal metabolic rate (BMR) $\times$ 1.2), but that the proportion of the population so affected declined from 15% in 1970 to only 8% in 1980. The definition of malnutrition using BMR $\times$ 1.2 is very stringent and somewhat controversial and in the Fifth World Food Survey (FAO 1985) a higher estimate for minimal daily needs (BMR $\times$ 1.4) was also used. Using the higher estimate, the proportion of the population estimated to be malnourished would be approximately 50% higher for developing countries.

Total population, annual population growth rate, GNP, IMR, and dietary data for 20 countries of North Africa and West Asia compared with developed countries are shown in Table 7. With the exception of Somalia and Mauritania,

Table 6. Undernourished population in regions of developing market economies based on DES availability of less than $1.2 \times$ BMR.

Regions or economic groups	Population with DES availability $< 1.2 \times$ BMR (10^6)		% of population with DES availability $< 1.2 \times$ BMR	
	1969–71	1979–81	1969–71	1979–81
Africa	57	70	20	19
Far East	208	210	21	17
Latin America	36	38	13	11
Near East	23	16	15	8
LDCs	55	77	26	28
MHICs [1]	126	98	16	10

Source: FAO (1985).
[1] Middle-high income countries.

the same broad relationships occur between diet and measures of overall health as were discussed on a world basis. The economically poor countries mostly consume 25% or less of their protein as animal protein with the energy from fat being generally below 30%; the richer countries have higher values inclining towards, but never reaching those of the United States. Again, with the exceptions of Mauritania and Somalia, as dietary supplies of food energy, protein, and fat increase there is a corresponding decline in IMR. No causal relationship is implied between these dietary data and health but as wealth increases, so also do the proportions of animal products, and hence fat, in the diet. In addition, there are improvements in general hygiene and the availability of health services (Pellett 1987).

Data for the agricultural population and livestock and food production in selected countries of the Near East region are shown in Table 8. Although those engaged in agriculture remain a large proportion of the total population in many countries of the region, with an average of almost 50% for the region as a whole, this population is either declining or increasing at a considerably lower rate than the increase in total population. Sheep and goats predominate and there have been reasonable annual increases in livestock production (total cattle, sheep, and goats) from 1971 to 1984. The FAO publication Agriculture Towards 2000 (FAO 1981) indicates that, with development, the demand for meat, dairy products, and eggs rises faster than the demand for crops. Thus, FAO projections for agricultural development in the next 20 years call for livestock production to increase faster than crop production. Two scenarios are used: the first involves a doubling of agricultural production between 1980 and 2000 while the second and less ambitious scenario is built around an 80% rise in output. Using these scenarios, annual livestock production should increase by 4.5 or 3.7%, respectively, while crop production is projected to rise by only 3.5 or 3.0% between 1980 and 2000. Few countries have achieved anything like this increase in production (Table 8). The median increase for the 20 countries listed is less than 1% per annum, although meat and milk

Table 7. Population, annual population growth rate, GNP, IMR, and macronutrient availability for countries of North Africa and West Asia compared to the United Kingdom and the United States.

Country	Population (10⁶)	Annual population growth rate (1971–84)	GNP per caput 1982–83 (USD)	IMR (deaths per 1000 live births)	Energy (Kcal)	Protein (g)	Fat (g)	Calories cereals (%)	protein (%)	fat (%)	Animal protein (%)
Afghanistan	14.6	1.0	230 [1]	200	2310	71	36	81.5	12.2	14.0	14.5
Algeria	22.0	3.2	2350	110	2585	66	57	56.8	10.2	19.7	21.3
Cyprus	0.7	0.5	3720	18	3390	106	123	40.0	12.5	32.6	43.5
Egypt	46.8	2.4	690	110	3175	81	65	64.0	10.2	18.5	15.9
Iran	45.1	3.2	2160	100	3085	82	66	64.0	10.7	19.1	19.0
Iraq	15.7	3.5	3020	70	2920	76	49	60.6	10.4	15.1	22.6
Jordan	3.5	2.7	1690	60	3075	76	76	62.0	10.0	22.3	24.6
Kuwait	1.8	6.0	19870	31	3345	102	103	37.8	12.2	27.6	54.3
Libya	3.6	4.0	8510	90	3810	98	135	40.3	10.3	31.8	37.8
Mauritania	1.9	2.8	470	140	2075	71	55	50.7	13.7	24.0	48.0
Morocco	23.6	2.9	870	100	2605	68	50	63.0	10.4	17.3	17.0
Pakistan	101.7	3.0	380	120	2180	56	43	63.1	10.3	17.8	23.8
Saudi Arabia	11.2	4.6	16000	100	2940	82	80	44.7	11.1	24.3	42.6
Somalia	5.6	5.1	250	140	1985	65	62	50.9	13.0	28.2	53.7
Sudan	21.5	3.0	440	120	2315	65	72	51.7	11.3	28.0	28.4
Syria	10.6	3.6	1680	60	3005	85	81	50.4	11.2	24.2	25.6
Tunisia	7.2	2.3	1390	90	2765	76	69	55.8	11.0	22.5	21.8
Turkey	50.0	2.3	1370	110	3000	83	71	53.7	11.0	21.4	24.5
Yemen AR	6.5	2.0	500	160	2475	77	43	67.3	12.4	15.7	21.6
Yemen PDR	2.1	2.3	470	140	2275	61	46	60.3	10.8	18.3	30.6
UK	56.5	0.4	9660	11	3225	85	142	21.0	10.5	39.5	59.8
USA	238.8	1.0	13160	11	3640	106	168	18.2	11.6	41.6	67.7

Source: FAO (1980; 1984; 1986); UNICEF (1985).
[1] Data for 1980.

Table 8. Agricultural population, livestock, and food production increases for selected countries of the Near East.

Country	Agricultural population			Livestock (million)			Annual rate of change 1971–84 (%)			
	million	% of total population	annual increase 1971–84 (%)	cattle	sheep	goats	live-stock [1]	food	meat	milk
Afghanistan	11.1	76	0.5	3.8	20.0	3.0	1.5	1.7	4.0	2.0
Algeria	9.6	44	0.9	1.8	19.0	3.1	4.7	1.7	4.4	5.3
Cyprus	0.2	29	− 0.7	< 0.1	0.5	0.4	0.7	0.5	2.4	4.2
Egypt	22.6	48	1.6	1.9	1.5	1.7	− 0.6	1.5	2.5	1.5
Iran	15.3	34	1.2	8.3	34.0	13.6	0.4	2.3	5.0	3.6
Iraq	5.8	37	1.9	1.5	8.5	2.4	− 2.6	− 0.2	5.8	0.5
Jordan	0.8	23	− 0.1	< 0.1	1.0	0.5	0.2	3.8	5.3	− 1.7
Kuwait	< 0.1	2	5.4	0.2	0.6	0.3	22.1	–	12.2	12.6
Libya	0.4	11	− 3.4	0.2	4.9	1.5	6.2	6.9	9.2	6.6
Mauritania	1.5	79	2.2	1.4	5.2	3.3	0.7	0.3	2.0	1.3
Morocco	11.4	48	1.7	2.6	12.0	4.5	− 3.2	2.2	3.3	4.3
Pakistan	51.7	51	1.9	16.5	25.0	29.7	4.8	3.2	5.7	2.0
Saudi Arabia	6.4	57	3.6	0.5	3.8	2.4	9.4	11.7	13.5	10.5
Somalia	4.3	77	4.5	3.6	9.7	15.7	0.2	0.5	0.5	0.6
Sudan	15.9	74	2.3	20.0	19.0	13.5	3.9	1.1	3.0	6.5
Syria	4.8	45	2.8	0.8	13.0	1.1	4.1	6.4	7.3	6.3
Tunisia	2.6	36	0.2	0.6	5.3	0.9	0.7	1.9	3.1	3.7
Turkey	23.7	47	− 0.1	17.3	48.7	17.5	0.6	2.9	2.5	1.4
Yemen AR	4.8	74	1.4	1.0	1.9	2.2	0.9	− 0.2	2.7	0.9
Yemen PDR	1.2	57	1.3	0.1	0.9	1.4	2.4	1.2	0.4	− 0.3
UK	0.9	2	− 3.1	13.1	35.5	< 0.1	0.1	2.3	1.5	1.7
USA	4.1	2	− 3.9	110.0	10.0	1.5	− 2.7	1.2	1.4	0.8

Source: FAO (1986).
[1] Combined annual increases for cattle, sheep, and goats.

production have increased at somewhat higher rates and are above the rates for population increases in many countries. However, as indicated earlier, the amounts of animal protein and energy from fat in the dietary of the Near East region have increased only slightly.

Protein and amino acid allowances

The most important function of dietary protein is to provide the substrate necessary to maintain tissue and organ protein synthesis in the adult, support an acceptable rate of net protein gain in growing infants and children, and for milk production in lactating women. Protein requirements are highly correlated with whole body protein synthesis and turnover, which change with normal growth and development (Young and Pellett 1987). Protein synthesis rates are high in the newborn and, per unit of body weight, they decline with progressive growth and development. The rate of protein synthesis in the

Table 9. Daily average energy and protein requirements for men and women, 18–30 years.

Weight (kg)	Daily energy allowance (Kcal) at various activity levels			Daily protein allowance (g) at two levels of digestibility	
	1.4× BMR	1.8× BMR	2.2× BMR	0.95	0.85
Men					
50	2050	2600	3200	39	44
65	2350	3000	3700	52	58
80	2650	3400	4200	63	71
Women					
40	1500	1950	2350	32	35
55	1850	2350	2850	43	48
70	2150	2750	3350	55	62

Source: FAO/WHO/UNU (1985).
Note: Order of magnitude values for activity levels as multiples of BMR are: light 1.5–1.6; moderate 1.6–1.8; and heavy 1.8–2.2 with female values generally lower than those for males. Digestibility values of 0.95 are appropriate for diets based on refined cereals and animal products, while values of 0.85 apply to diets heavily based on coarse whole grain cereals and vegetables. Food energy allowances would decline by 10–20% as age increases to above 60 years but protein allowances remain unchanged.

young is higher than that in adults even when the net protein deposition associated with growth is deducted. At all ages, rates of whole body protein synthesis and breakdown are considerably greater than the intake of dietary protein estimated to meet the need for maintenance of nitrogen and for growth. In fact, there is extensive utilization within the body of the amino acids liberated during protein breakdown. This recycling of amino acids and the rates of synthesis and breakdown of body proteins change in response to various stimuli, including alterations in the level and adequacy of protein and amino acid intakes (Young et al. 1981).

Daily average food energy and protein requirements for young adults are shown in Table 9. In the past, food energy allowances were conventionally considered as single values for reference males and females, but this is no longer acceptable since individual activity levels can vary enormously (FAO/WHO/UNU 1985). Daily energy allowances are not only dependent on estimated activity but also on body weight. Allowances are now tabulated in terms of multiples of BMR, which is an indication of minimal daily needs (FAO/WHO/UNU 1985). Daily intakes of less than 1.4 × BMR are one of the indicators of malnutrition, as proposed by FAO (FAO 1985). There are several countries where average food energy intakes appear to be marginal (Table 7). These tend to be the poorest countries with high infant mortality rates. The situation in relation to protein supply is broadly similar. While the values for energy from protein, expressed as a percentage of total energy supply, are similar for all countries of the region and do not differ greatly from the values in developed countries, the percentage of animal protein in

Table 10. Essential amino acid composition (mg/g protein) of some animal protein foods compared to wheat, chickpeas, lentils, and faba beans.

Foods	Lysine	Total sulphur amino acids	Threonine	Tryptophan
Beef	89	40	46	12
Cows milk	78	33	44	14
Egg	70	57	47	17
Wheat	25	36	30	10
Chickpeas	74	29	40	14
Lentils	83	10	34	7
Faba beans	65	15	34	9

Source: Pellett and Shadarevian (1970); FAO/WHO/UNU (1985).
Note: The other essential amino acids for the human (isoleucine, leucine, valine, histidine, and phenylalanine) are unlikely to be limiting in real dietaries.

relation to total protein varies considerably. This may have important implications in relation to the overall protein value of the diet.

A major proportion of the food energy for the region is supplied by cereals, of which more than 60% is represented by wheat. In Table 10, the indispensable amino acid compositions of some animal protein foods are shown in comparison to wheat, chickpeas, lentils, and faba beans. Lysine and threonine levels are considerably higher in animal products than they are in wheat and thus relatively small amounts of animal foods can improve the overall protein quality of cereal diets low in these amino acids. Legumes, while low in sulfur amino acids, are also high in lysine. This is well known and food protein complementation was, until recently, an important component of dietary advice for all age groups. However, a recent report on protein and energy requirements (FAO/WHO/UNU 1985) tabulated human amino acid requirements at various ages including the adult (Table 11) and thus implied that protein complementation is only important in the nutrition of the young child.

Amino acid patterns (mg amino acids/g protein) of the average diets in several regions and economic groups are shown in Table 11 in relation to reference patterns of amino acid requirement. These data were calculated using information from the FAO (FAO 1985) on representative foods from various food groups in different regions. By combining these data with the distribution of cereals typical for the regions it is possible to calculate amino acid patterns for the diet as a whole. The amino acid levels in the regional diets shown are reasonable and compare well with calculations made from individual dietaries in North America and in developing countries (FAO/WHO/UNU 1985; Pellett and Young 1988). When the dietary amino acid pattern of Africa and the Near East is compared with the earlier FAO/WHO (1973) reference amino acid pattern, lysine, sulfur amino acids, and threonine are either limiting or marginal for all age groups. However, when compared with the 1985 FAO/WHO/UNU amino acid requirement pattern for the adult, the dietary values are well in excess for all amino acids

Table 11. Amino acid patterns [1] (mg/g protein) in the diet of North America, developed countries, and some regional diets compared to reference patterns.

Amino acids	North America	Developed countries	Africa	Near East	Far East	Latin America	Least developed countries	Reference patterns FAO/WHO 1973	FAO/WHO/UNU 1985		Proposed [2]
									young child	adult	
Isoleucine	52	48	42	44	47	47	46	40	28	13	35
Leucine	77	77	75	73	81	82	81	70	66	19	65
Lysine	68	65	47	42	46	56	47	54	58	16	50
Total SAA	35	36	34	36	40	34	37	35	25	17	25
Total aromatic	78	81	72	79	86	79	83	61	63	19	65
Threonine	39	40	35	34	39	39	38	40	34	9	25
Tryptophan	12	12	12	12	12	11	12	10	11	5	10
Valine	54	53	48	49	57	53	55	50	35	13	35

[1] Calculated from dietary patterns as presented by FAO (1985) using the Massachusetts Nutrient Data Bank and FAO (1970) values for protein and essential amino acids of representative foods.

[2] For theoretical arguments behind these recommendations see Young et al. (1988).

and consideration of the intake of indispensable amino acids would appear to be important only for the young child.

There is, however, increasing evidence (see Young et al. 1988) that this conclusion is unjustified. Data from a series of MIT studies of whole body amino acid kinetics indicate that, at least for leucine (Meguid et al. 1985a), valine (Meguid 1986b), lysine (Meredith et al. 1986), and threonine (Zhao et al. 1986), the relatively low amino acid requirements indicated by FAO/WHO/UNU (1985) for adults are probably erroneous, being considerably below true requirements. Based on a more extensive evaluation, Young and Pellett (1987) concluded that the actual amino acid requirement for indispensable amino acids in the adult is likely to be similar to that proposed by FAO/WHO/UNU (1985) for the 2–5 year old age group. We now believe (Young et al. 1988) that a more appropriate recommendation for the adult would be the pattern shown in Table 11, where lysine and threonine values are somewhat below those for the young child but are well above the proposed 1985 FAO/WHO/UNU adult values. If this is so, then for average diets in Africa and the Near East the supply of dietary lysine appears to be marginal, even for the adult. This amino acid is in good supply in animal foods and legumes so with cereal-based diets, food protein complementation remains important for all age groups. If our present conclusions (Young et al. 1988; Pellett and Young 1988) are confirmed, both nutrition policies and international agricultural research activities require re-evaluation of the changes made in priorities following the FAO/WHO/UNU report (FAO/WHO/UNU 1985).

Minerals and vitamins in animal foods

There are marked differences in the content and availability of essential minerals and vitamins among various food protein sources. Some compositional data are illustrated in Table 12; vitamins A and B_{12}, calcium, and iron are particularly significant. For iron, the extent to which this element is available in foods depends not only on the amount of iron supplied but also on its chemical nature and the composition of the foods with which it is consumed (Beaton 1974; Bothwell et al. 1979). Furthermore, there are marked differences in the form of iron in animal and plant protein foods, with the former providing a substantial proportion of the total iron as heme iron. This form of iron is usually absorbed relatively efficiently and is largely unaffected by dietary factors. On the other hand, plant food proteins contain non-heme iron, the availability of which is less than that of heme iron and is modified markedly by various factors such as the nutritional status of the consumer with regard to iron, the level of ascorbic acid in the dietary, and the level of calcium, phosphorus, and binding materials such as tannic acid and phytate. A diet based on plant protein foods may not meet iron requirements, especially in premenopausal women, so red meat may help to meet requirements more easily than plant protein foods, despite the fact that they might otherwise supply equivalent levels of utilizable protein.

The percentage contributions of the various food groups in relation to requirements for vitamin B_{12} and selected minerals are shown in Table 13 for the dietary in the United Kingdom, where 37% of the DES and 60% of the protein are of animal origin. These data indicate the future trends likely to be seen in the Near East. While milk and cheese provide only 10% of the food energy, they supply 60% of the calcium, and more than 20% of daily vitamin B_{12} and zinc needs. Although meat supplies about 16% of the food energy, it is a negligible source of calcium but provides 55% of the vitamin B_{12}, 36% of the zinc, 24% of the iron, and 28% of selenium.

Also shown in Table 13 are data for Syria, where cereals provide a much larger 69% of the food energy while animal products (milk and meat groups) supply only 8%. Despite this, these animal foods supply very significant proportions of the calcium (milk only), vitamin B_{12}, and retinol. It should be noted however that while the proportions are high, the absolute amounts provided are much lower than in the UK since total daily intakes are also much less. For the Syrian diet, fruits and vegetables are relatively more important sources of micronutrients. Despite the fact than plant foods do not supply preformed retinol they make an important contribution of various carotenoids which can be converted to retinol (vitamin A) in the body. The total iron values for Syria may be somewhat misleading since the iron availability is likely to be low.

Table 12. Representative values of macro and micro nutrients in 100g portions of animal and plant foods in relation to daily requirements.

Food	Energy (Kcal)	Pro-tein (g)	Fat (g)	Cal-cium (mg)	Iron (mg)	Vitamin A (μgRE)	Thiamine (mg)	Ribo-flavin (mg)	Vitamin B_{12} (μg)
Chicken [1]	220	29.0	10.9	15	1.14	32	0.06	0.12	0.30–1.30 [2]
Beef [3]	420	22.4	36.0	13	3.30	0	0.08	0.10	1.20
Lamb [4]	240	20.6	14.5	6	3.10	0	0.16	0.22	1.36
Goat [5]	165	18.7	9.4	11	2.20	0	0.17	0.32	–
Milk (whole)	60	3.3	3.4	120	0.05	31	0.04	0.16	0.36
Cheese (hard)	400	24.9	33.1	512	0.68	303	0.03	0.38	0.83
Egg (whole)	160	12.2	11.2	56	2.08	520	0.08	0.28	1.32
Wheat	355	11.5	2.2	36	3.1	–	0.57	0.12	–
Barley	360	9.7	1.9	50	4.0	–	0.38	0.20	–
Lentils	350	23.7	1.3	68	7.0	8	0.46	0.30	–
Chickpeas	376	19.2	6.2	134	7.3	3	0.46	0.16	–
Faba beans (dry)	354	25.0	1.8	77	6.0	8	0.53	0.30	–
Daily requirement									
Male adult	–	56	–	800	10	1000	1.4	1.6	3.0
Female adult	–	44	–	800	18	800	1.0	1.2	3.0

Source: Pellett and Shadarevian (1970); Pennington and Church (1985).
Requirement values NAS-NRC 1980.
[1] cooked whole; [2] dark meat has higher vitamin B_{12};
[3] raw chuck steak with fat; [4] leg roast; [5] raw, vitamin B_{12} data not available.

Table 13. Percentage contributions of the various food groups to daily availability of selected mineral and vitamins in the United Kingdom and Syria.

Nutrient	Country	Daily availa-bility	Percentage nutrients supplied by					
			cereals	milk products	meat	roots tubers	vege-tables	fruit
Food energy	UK	3250	21	10	16	6	2	2
(kcal)	Syria	3010	69	4	4	1	4	5
Calcium	UK	956	23	60	3	2	4	2
(mg)	Syria	575	14	39	<1	<1	16	9
Iron	UK	11.3	30	3	24	7	11	5
(mg)	Syria	20.4	44	1	6	1	17	7
Zinc	UK	9.1	22	22	36	3	7	1
(mg)	Syria	5.7	53	8	15	1	19	<1
Selenium	UK	60	50	7	28	1	2	2
(mg)	Syria	48	81	2	9	1	4	1
Vit. B_{12}	UK	7.1	–	20	55	–	–	–
(mg)	Syria	1.3	–	41	42	–	–	–
Retinol	UK	725	–	29	37	–	–	–
(mg)	Syria	311	–	23	46	–	–	–
Retinol Eq.	UK	1448	–	16	19	–	22	1
(mg)	Syria	944	–	8	16	–	44	20.

Source: All values for United Kingdom except food energy and retinol data are from Hazell (1985). Remaining values calculated from FAO (1980; 1984; 1985) using food composition data of Pellett and Shadarevian (1970) and Pennington and Church (1985).

The mineral content of foods has been a significant area of study for many years but it is only relatively recently that the bioavailability of mineral elements has been emphasized together with studies on the chemical forms in which various dietary minerals are found in foods. This subject has been extensively reviewed by Hazell (1985). The chemical forms of many dietary minerals have yet to be determined but in animal foods (especially meat) any essential mineral is most likely to occur as an organic complex, such as a metalloenzyme or some other metalloprotein. In plant foods, such functional forms are known to be present in far smaller amounts with the minerals mainly being non-specifically bound to structural (e.g., fiber) or storage (e.g., phytate) components which tend to adversely affect mineral availability. In animal foods the organic forms of minerals are usually well absorbed because they are readily dissolved during digestion and are protected from the inhibitors derived from plant foods which reduce the absorption of inorganic forms. Thus, not only are minerals generally present in higher levels in animal foods, but they are likely to be more available.

Animal foods and child nutrition

The importance of quite small quantities of milk and meat in the diet of children is illustrated in Table 14. Daily consumption of 200 ml milk would

Table 14. Estimated child requirements of protein and other nutrients in relation to intakes of milk and meat.

| Age group | Daily requirement | | | | | Approximate percentage of daily requirement supplied by | | | | | | | | | |
| | | | | | | 200 ml whole milk | | | | | 25 g cooked lamb | | | | |
	energy (Kcal)	protein (g)	lysine (mg)	calcium (mg)	vitamin B_{12} (µg)	energy (Kcal)	protein (g)	lysine (mg)	calcium (mg)	vitamin B_{12} (µg)	energy (Kcal)	protein (g)	lysine (mg)	calcium (mg)	vitamin B_{12} (µg)
9–12 months	950	14	900	600	0.5	14	46	59	40	>100	5	50	63	<1	80
1–2 years	1150	14	800	700	0.7	10	46	66	34	100	4	50	71	<1	57
2–4 years	1350	16	900	800	1.0	9	41	58	30	70	3	44	63	<1	40
4–6 years	1550	18	1000	800	1.0	8	37	53	30	70	3	39	56	<1	40

Source: Protein, food energy, and lysine requirements FAO/WHO/UNU (1985); calcium and vitamin B_{12} requirements NAS-NRC (1980); milk and lamb composition Pellett and Shadarevian (1970) and Pennington and Church (1985).

supply 8-14% of the daily food energy needs, depending on the age of the child, but could supply some 40% of the protein, over 50% of the lysine, 35% of the calcium, and more than 70% of the vitamin B_{12}. Similarly, while 25g of meat would supply less than 5% of the food energy it could provide 45% of the daily needs of protein, 60-70% of the lysine, and 40-80% of the vitamin B_{12}. Meat is a poor source of calcium but both milk and meat are of considerable importance in supplying lysine to complement predominantly cereal diets and in providing vitamin B_{12}. Milk in particular is also a significant source of vitamin A and riboflavin and its potential importance in diets of developing countries has been reviewed by Young and Pellett (1985).

It is recognized that in poor countries animal products are expensive and therefore availability is limited. However, nutrition education should emphasize that quite small quantities of animal protein foods can dramatically improve the overall nutritional value of diets that are based heavily on cereals. This is especially important for infants and for pregnant and lactating women. This should not however affect recommendations encouraging breast feeding of young infants in view of the presence in human milk of substances protecting against diarrheal disease, the potential contraceptive effects of breast feeding, and the psychological benefits to the mother/child dyad (Jelliffe and Jelliffe 1971; Hambraeus and Sjolin 1979). Nevertheless, in good environments, human infants grow and develop when they receive a wide variety of modified and synthetic diets based on cows' milk (Fomon 1974; Cockburn 1983).

Milk is also an important food for infants recovering from malnutrition. Questions have been raised about whether milk is a suitable food for this purpose because of its lactose content and the reductions in lactase activity subsequent to malnutrition (Torun et al. 1983). Low lactose milk has been proposed as an alternative to normal whole milk to avoid this risk, but recent studies (Torun et al. 1983; Solomons 1985) indicate that clinical recovery was identical whether whole milk or lactose hydrolyzed milk was used for the refeeding of malnourished infants. Similarly, modest intakes of milk can be well tolerated by adults with genetically caused, low-intestinal lactase activity (Newcomber 1984).

Nutritional implications of high animal food intake

The benefits of increased levels of animal protein products in the dietary are likely to be many and varied. However, not only are animal foods often expensive because of their low energy efficiency in production (Pimentel and Hall 1984), but there may also be potential risks to health when animal protein foods are consumed at high levels. Some positive and negative attributes of animal foods are summarized in Table 15. Potential risks occur not only in the economically developed nations where degenerative diseases are of major public health concern, but also among the more affluent individuals in poor

Table 15. Some positive and negative attributes of animal foods in the dietary.

Positive	Negative
Highly desirable	Low energy efficiency in production hence generally high cost
Highly digestible	
High levels of essential amino acids, especially lysine	Perishable
Excellent sources of many vitamins and minerals in highly available forms	High levels of saturated fats and cholesterol
	Low levels of complex carbohydrates and fiber
Small quantities can remedy deficiencies in high cereal diets	
	Possible effects on calcium balance of the body at high levels of intake

countries whose dietary patterns, and consequently morbidity and mortality, approach those of developed nations. Some of these relationships for the Near East region have been discussed by Pellett (1983b).

It has long been recognized that the amount and nature of ingested fat affects plasma cholesterol concentration and that hypercholesterolemia correlates strongly with the incidence of coronary artery disease. Other factors such as genetic background, smoking, hypertension, overweight, diabetes, and certain behavioral patterns also appear to increase susceptibility to coronary artery disease. Nevertheless, the important nutritional determinants of blood cholesterol levels remain the total fat and the saturated fat contents of the diet (Pyorala 1987). Typically, animal protein foods have significantly higher levels of saturated fatty acids in their triacylglycerols than do foods of vegetable origin. Many of the broad relationships between diet and health have been discussed in a recent symposium (Simopoulos 1987).

In a review of major intervention studies, Brisson (1981) concluded that increasing the consumption of fats rich in polyunsaturated fatty acids and decreasing the intake of cholesterol and fats of animal origin were ineffective in reducing coronary heart disease. On the other hand, a recent large-scale intervention study (see Roberts 1987) indicated that aggressive cholesterol lowering therapy combining drugs with diet and limiting fat intake to 22% of total calories could halt the growth of lesions in major blood vessels and in some cases shrink them. In contrast, some would conclude that sub-optimal intake of nutrients may be important in the pathogenesis of ischemic heart disease. In a 12-year study on nearly 1500 women in Sweden, food energy intake was inversely correlated to the incidence of myocardial infarction and was independent of the normally recognized major risk factors (Lapidus et al.

1986). The lipid theory of heart disease has been vigorously debated now for more than 4 decades and this will probably continue. However, it is reasonable to suggest that over-consumption of foods rich in fat is undesirable for long-term maintenance of health.

Finally, the interrelationships between body calcium homeostasis and dietary protein should be considered. From metabolic balance studies (Johnson et al. 1970; Allen et al. 1979) it appears that high-protein diets may cause a deterioration of body calcium balance. The major effect of a high-protein diet appears to be on the kidney and is associated with reduced reabsorption of filtered calcium. Although the public health significance of these observations is uncertain, it has been suggested that high-protein diets may contribute to the etiology of osteoporosis although other factors, such as calcium, phosphorus, and boron (Nielsen et al. 1987) intakes, estrogenic status, and exercise are likely to be more significant. The levels of protein intake that cause these effects are well above those generally consumed in North Africa and West Asia.

The consumption of high levels of animal protein foods over long periods has also been linked to a higher than normal incidence of certain forms of cancer (NAS-NRC 1982) but the cause is still unknown. However, at this time, there is no reason to suggest that an increase in animal protein in the diets of the Near East region would not have a desirable outcome.

Conclusions

As countries become richer, the consumption of animal protein and total food availability increase. Of all the FAO defined world regions, the largest increases in total food supply (up 27% since 1960) and decreases in the numbers malnourished (down 30%) have been in the Near East. Yet for the region as a whole, the percentage of the dietary energy supplied from animal products and the percentage of animal protein to total protein have increased less. For individual countries changes have been large, but even amongst the richer countries cereals are still important, indicating the desirability of maintaining the traditional dietary patterns of the region. The diets of the economically disadvantaged countries, however, have changed little and remain inadequate in both quantity and quality.

Because of the large differences in lysine content between animal products and cereals (Table 10), and as legumes rarely supply more than about 5% of the food energy in the Near East diet (FAO 1985), there is a high correlation between lysine content and the percentage of animal protein in the diet (R = 0.96, P < 0.001, see Tables 3 and 11). From this linear relation (Lys (mg/g protein) = 0.47 animal protein % + 36.4) it can be estimated that the requirement level of 50 mg lysine per gram protein (Table 11) should be met if diets containing at least 28% animal protein in relation to total protein are available. Thus, if allowance is made for less than perfect digestibility, it would appear that diets containing about one third of their protein from animal sources should meet estimated lysine needs. The present mean value for the region is 24% (FAO 1984) which agrees well with the median value of 25% for the countries listed in Table 7. With the exceptions of Mauritania and Somalia, the poorer countries are those with low levels of animal protein consumption and those where livestock production should be encouraged. If increased animal food consumption remains economically difficult, then more pulses in the dietary would improve the lysine concentration. A more detailed analysis elsewhere (Pellett and Young 1988) confirms these observations.

In addition to supplying indispensable amino acids and protein in a highly digestible form, animal protein foods are important sources of minerals and vitamins. Relatively small quantities of animal foods can transform cereal-based diets by virtue of both their protein and non-protein components. This is particularly obvious when milk is added to the diet of children (Young and Pellett 1985).

Despite these desirable attributes, large amounts of animal products can give cause for health concerns. Not only is the saturated fat content high in such diets, but the fiber content (unavailable carbohydrate) is also low. Such dietary consumption patterns are epidemiologically associated with ischemic heart disease, diabetes, obesity, and other diseases in rich countries and in rich individuals of poor countries. These problems are generally associated with lipid-derived food energy above 30%. The present median value for the countries listed in Table 7 is about 22% compared to 42% in North America and 33% in developed countries (Table 3), indicating that considerable increases in consumption of animal protein foods could occur before the major problems typical of developed regions become prominent.

At present, it would appear that the advantages of increasing animal food consumption considerably outweigh any possible disadvantages. Concern should, however, be expressed for those individuals and countries whose diets presently contain in excess of 30% of the food energy in the form of fat since further increases would be undesirable. The poorest countries (except Somalia and Mauritania which need other solutions) are those which would benefit most from modest increases in availability of animal foods arising from more efficient livestock production. Unfortunately, these countries are least likely to be able to afford such increases unless priority is given to assisting them to improve their livestock production capability. It is thus recommended that nutritional considerations should be included as a high priority in agricultural development plans in the region.

Acknowledgements

Grateful acknowledgement must be made of the important contributions of Mary Jane Laus and Ellen Sussman of the Massachusetts Nutrient Data Bank who tabulated and performed the cross-country correlations in Table 2 and the amino acid compositions of regional diets in Table 11.

References

Allen, L.H., Oddoye, E.A. and Margen, S. 1979. Protein-induced hypercalciuria: a long-term study. American Journal of Clinical Nutrition 32: 741–749.

Beaton, G.H. 1974. Epidemiology of iron deficiency anaemia. Pages 477–528 in Iron in Biochemistry and Medicine (Jacobs, A. and Worwood, M., eds). Academic Press, New York, USA.

Bothwell, T.H., Charlton, R.W., Cook, J.D. and Finch, C.A. 1979. Iron Metabolism in Man. Blackwell Scientific, Oxford, UK. 576 p.

Brisson, G.J. 1981. Lipids in Human Nutrition: An Appraisal of Some Dietary Concepts. J.K. Burgess Englewood, N.J., USA. 175 p.

Cockburn, F. 1983. Milk composition: the infant human diet. Proceedings of the Nutrition Society (GB) 42: 361–372.

FAO (Food and Agriculture Organization). 1970. Amino acid content of foods and biological data on proteins. FAO Nutritional Studies No. 24. FAO, Rome, Italy.

FAO (Food and Agriculture Organization). 1980. Food Balance Sheets, 1975–77. Average and per caput food supplies. FAO, Rome, Italy.

FAO (Food and Agriculture Organization). 1981. Agriculture: Toward 2000. FAO, Rome, Italy.

FAO (Food and Agriculture Organization). 1984. Food Balance Sheets 1979–81. FAO, Rome, Italy.

FAO (Food and Agriculture Organization). 1985. The Fifth World Food Survey. FAO, Rome, Italy.

FAO (Food and Agriculture Organization). 1986. Country Tables: Basic Data on the Agricultural Sector. Economic and Social Policy Department. FAO, Rome, Italy.

FAO/WHO (Food and Agriculture Organization/World Health Organization). 1973. Energy and Protein Requirements. Report of a Joint FAO/WHO Ad Hoc Expert Committee. WHO Technical Report Series No. 522. WHO, Geneva, Switzerland.

FAO/WHO/UNU (Food and Agriculture Organization/World Health Organization/Universidad de las Naciones Unidas). 1985. Energy and Protein Requirements. Report of a Joint FAO/WHO/UNU Expert Consultation. WHO Technical Report Series No. 724. WHO, Geneva, Switzerland.

Fomon, S.J. 1974. Infant Nutrition. Second edition. W.B. Saunders, Philadelphia, USA. 575 p.

Hambraeus, L. and Sjolin, E. 1979. The mother-child dyad-nutritional aspects. Almquist and Wiksell International, Stockholm, Sweden.

Hazell, T. 1985. Minerals in foods: dietary sources, chemical forms, interactions, bioavailability. World Review of Nutrition and Dietetics 46: 1–23.

Jelliffe, D.B. and Jelliffe, E.F.P. 1971. The uniqueness of human milk. American Journal of Clinical Nutrition 24: 968–1024.

Johnson, N.E., Alcantra, E.N. and Linkswiler, H. 1970. Effect of level of protein intake on urinary and fecal calcium retention of young adult males. Journal of Nutrition 100: 1425–1430.

Lapidus, L., Andersson, H., Bengtsson, C. and Bosaeus, I. 1986. Dietary habits in relation to incidence of cardiovascular disease and death in women: a 12-year follow–up of participants in the population study of women in Gothenburg, Sweden. American Journal of Clinical Nutrition 44: 444–448.

Meguid, M.M., Matthews, D.E., Bier, D.M., Meredith, C.N., Soeldner, J.S. and Young, V.R. 1986a. Leucine kinetics at graded leucine intakes in young men. American Journal of Clinical Nutrition 43: 370–380.

Meguid, M.M., Matthews, D.E., Bier, D.M., Meredith, C.N. and Young, V.R. 1986b. Valine kinetics at graded valine intakes in young men. American Journal of Clinical Nutrition 43: 781–786.

Meredith, C.M., Wen, Z-W., Bier, D.M., Matthews, D.E. and Young, V.R. 1986. Lysine kinetics at graded lysine intakes in young men. American Journal of Clinical Nutrition 43: 787–794.

Miladi, S. and Pellett, P.L. 1986. Food and nutrition in the Middle East and North Africa. Pages 133–158 in Dry Area Agriculture, Food Science and Human Nutrition (Nygaard, D.F. and Pellett, P.L., eds). Pergamon Press for the United Nations University, New York, USA.

NAS/NRC (National Academy of Sciences/National Research Council). 1980. Recommended dietary allowances. Ninth edition. National Academy of Sciences, Washington, D.C., USA. 185 p.

NAS/NRC (National Academy of Sciences/National Research Council). 1982. Diet Nutrition and Cancer. National Academy Press, Washington, D.C., USA.

Newcomber, A.D. 1984. Clinical consequences of lactase deficiency. Pages 53–58 in Clinical Nutrition Supplement (Paige, D.M., ed.). Vol. 3 (2). Nutrition Publications Inc., Pleasantville, New Jersey, USA.

Nielsen, F.H., Hunt, C.D., Mullen, L.M. and Hunt, J.R. 1987. Effect of dietary boron on mineral, estrogen and testosterone metabolism in post menopausal women. Faseb Journal 1: 394–397.

Pellett, P.L. 1983a. Changing concepts of world malnutrition. Ecology of Food and Nutrition 13: 115–125.

Pellett, P.L. 1983b. Food and Nutrition in the Near East Region: A Situation Analysis. International Food and Nutrition Program. INP Discussion Paper No. 20. Center for International Studies M.I.T., Cambridge, Massachusetts, USA.

Pellett, P.L. 1987. Determination of nutritional status. Food and Nutrition 13 (1). In press.

Pellett, P.L. and Shadarevian, S. 1970. Food Composition Tables for Use in the Middle East. Second edition. American University of Beirut, Beirut, Lebanon. 116 p.

Pellett, P.L. and Young, V.R. 1988. National and international implications of revised estimates of human adult needs for indispensable amino acids. American Journal of Clinical Nutrition. Submitted for publication.

Pennington, J.A.T. and Church, H.N. 1985. Bowes and Church's Food Values of Portions Commonly Used. Fourteenth edition. J.B. Pippincott Co., Philadelphia, USA. 257 p.

Perisse, J., Sizaret, F. and Francois, P. 1969. The effect of income on the structure of the diet. Nutrition Newsletter (FAO) 7 (3): 1–10.

Perisse, J. and Polacchi, W. 1980. Geographical distribution and recent changes in world supply of vitamin A. Food and Nutrition (FAO) 6 (1): 21–27.

Pimentel, D. and Hall, C.W. (eds). 1984. Food and Energy Resources. Academic Press, New York and London. 268 p.

Pyorala, K. 1987. Dietary cholesterol in relation to plasma cholesterol and coronary heart disease. American Journal of Clinical Nutrition 45: 1176–1184.

Roberts, L. 1987. Study bolsters case against cholesterol. Science 237: 28–29.

Scrimshaw, N.S., Taylor, C.E. and Gordon, J.E. 1968. Interactions of Nutrition and Infection. World Health Organization Monograph No. 57. WHO, Geneva, Switzerland.

Solomons, N.W. 1985. Rehabilitating the severely malnourished infant and child. Journal of the American Dietetic Association 85 (1): 26–36.

Simopoulos, A.P. 1987. Diet and Health: Scientific Concepts and Principles. Conference Proceedings. American Journal of Clinical Nutrition Supplement Vol. 45. International Life Sciences Institute Research Foundation, Washington, D.C., USA.

Torun, B., Solomons, N.W., Caballero, B., Flores-Hurta, S., Orozco, G. and Batres, R. 1983. Milk with intact and hydrolysed lactose in the treatment of severe malnutrition. Pages 109–115 in Milk Intolerance and Rejection. Karger, Basel, Switzerland.

UNICEF (United Nations International Children's Emergency Fund). 1985. The State of the World's Children 1985. UNICEF, New York, USA.

UNICEF (United Nations International Children's Emergency Fund). 1987. The State of the World's Children 1987. UNICEF, New York, USA.

Young, V.R., Meguid, M., Meredith, C., Matthews, D.E. and Bier, D.M. 1981. Recent developments in knowledge of human amino acid requirements. Pages 133–153 in Nitrogen Metabolism in Man (Waterlow, J.C. and Stephen, J.M.L., eds). Applied Science Publishers, London, UK.

Young, V.R. and Pellett, P.L. 1985. Milk proteins with reference to human needs and world food supply and nutritional situation. Pages 18–46 in Milk Proteins '84 (Galesloot, T.E. and Tinbergen, B.J., eds). Centre for Agricultural Publishing and Documentation (Puduc), Wageningen, The Netherlands.

Young, V.R. and Pellett, P.L. 1987. Protein intake and requirements with reference to diet and health. American Journal of Clinical Nutrition 45: 1323–1343.

Young, V.R., Bier, D.M. and Pellett, P.L. 1988. A theoretical basis for increasing substantially current estimates of the amino acid requirements in adult man. American Journal of Clinical Nutrition. Submitted for publication.

Zhao, X.L., Wen, Z-W., Meredith, C.M., Matthews, D.E., Bier, D.M. and Young, V.R. 1986. Threonine kinetics at graded threonine intakes in young men. American Journal of Clinical Nutrition 43: 795–802.

E.F. Thomson and F.S. Thomson (eds), Increasing Small Ruminant Productivity in Semi-arid Areas
© 1988 ICARDA . ISBN 978-94-010-7086-7

The Importance of Barley in Food Production and Demand in West Asia and North Africa

K. Somel

Introduction

Within West Asia and North Africa (WANA) [1] there is a wide spectrum of environmental conditions, from the areas of higher rainfall around the Mediterranean and of high elevation in central and eastern Turkey, Afghanistan, Pakistan, Ethiopia, and the Atlas mountains, to the drier steppe and desert areas. Irrigated agriculture is important along the principal rivers but most agricultural land is rainfed. Although there are land reserves in Sudan and Ethiopia, the limits of agricultural land have been reached in all the other countries of the region. Therefore, increases in agricultural production are possible only through increasing the intensity of crop production and yields. There is also a wide spectrum of social and economic conditions, with substantial differences within the region in incomes, urbanization, agricultural policies, and the degree of public control over production and resources.

There are certain similarities between the countries within WANA. One such similarity is in the crop-livestock systems observed in the region, particularly in the drier areas. Here, the dominant crop is barley as it is more adapted to dry conditions, with small ruminants, mainly sheep, making up the livestock component. Barley is used principally as feed for sheep with other feed sources complementing the barley-livestock production system. These include native pastures, the steppe, fallow lands, crop residues, and industrial by-products such as cottonseed cake.

The demand for barley is therefore a derived demand and as such its importance does not stem so much from its contribution to calorie intake but from its contribution to the production and consumption of high quality animal protein. It has been demonstrated that the price of meat relative to barley grain is a driving element in the production of barley (Mona 1986).

In this paper, which is based on the results of the Agriculture: Toward 2000 (AT2000) project conducted by the Global Perspectives Study Group of the FAO (FAO 1987), the production of and demand for barley will be presented within the context of current and projected levels of food demand and production in WANA.

---

[1] For the purposes of this study, WANA comprises Afghanistan, Algeria, Cyprus, Egypt, Ethiopia, Iran, Iraq, Jordan, Lebanon, Libya, Morocco, Pakistan, Saudi Arabia, Sudan, Syria, Tunisia, Turkey, Yemen Arab Republic, and People's Democratic Republic of Yemen.

Barley in agricultural production

The base year for the AT2000 study is 1983 which, depending on the availability of information, is based on the average of 1982–84 or 1981–85. Using this base, over three quarters of barley production and area in 93 developing countries (LDCs), excluding China, are in WANA (FAO 1987). Within WANA, barley accounts for nearly half of coarse grain production and area but less than a fifth of cereal production and area, mainly due to the dominance of wheat (Table 1).

Barley production is generally based on a minimum input technology. Nearly two thirds of barley production is in areas of low or uncertain rainfall (FAO 1987). Fertilizer use on barley is estimated to be around 35 kg/ha (NPK) and it accounts for only 8% of total fertilizer use in WANA. A third of the total seed used is improved seed (FAO 1987). Hence, at slightly over 1 t/ha, yields are low and highly variable over space and time. In the base year of 1983, yields in the main barley-producing countries ranged from less than 0.5 t/ha to 2 t/ha (FAO 1987). The dependence on rainfall has produced similar variation between years.

About 2 million tonnes of both beef and mutton are currently produced in WANA and together they comprise over two thirds of total meat production. Milk production is predominantly from cows, while ewes' milk is used mainly for cheese and yoghurt. Overall, cattle production is concentrated in the wetter areas and sheep production in the drier areas. Barley is used more for sheep whereas other coarse grains are used more for cattle and poultry. Use of barley as animal feed is nearly 3.5 times its direct food use. In general, due to the extensive nature of livestock production, a considerable portion of energy intake goes towards maintenance, which results in low productivity. Carcass weights are estimated to be around 110 kg for cattle and 15 kg for sheep and goats.

The production projections for the year 2000 in WANA are mainly based on productivity increases in both crop and livestock production. In crops, and to some extent in livestock, this is due to land limitations. Hence, for crops 72% of the production increases will be due to increases in yields, 21% to increases in crop yields, and only 7% to increases in area of land under crops. However, certain shifts are expected between crops, especially with wheat production shifting more to the wetter and irrigated areas and being replaced by barley in the lower rainfall areas. It is through these shifts that wheat is expected to maintain its recent growth rates in yield which imply high growth rates in input use, e.g., over 6% annual growth rate in total and per unit area fertilizer use and an increase in the share of improved seeds from one to nearly two thirds between 1983 and 2000.

Barley is expected to double its historical growth rate in yields to 2.4% per annum and production increases are also expected through increased area. Yield increases will be possible with improved technology. For example, quadrupling total fertilizer use, through an annual rate of increase in per unit

Table 1. Production of major food commodities in WANA (areas in million hectares, production in million metric tonnes, yields in kg/ha).

	Year			Growth rates (% per year)	
	1961/63	1981/85 [1]	2000	1961/85	1981/85–2000 [2]
Total Cereals [3]					
Area	54	64	70	0.8	1.0
Production	53	88	140	2.6	2.8
Yield	1.0	1.4	2.0	1.8	2.2
Wheat					
Area	28	33	34	0.8	0.1
Production	25	48	71	3.3	2.4
Yield	0.9	1.5	2.1	2.5	2.3
Barley					
Area	11	13	15	0.8	1.2
Production	10	14	26	2.1	3.6
Yield	0.9	1.1	1.7	1.2	2.4
Maize					
Area	3.7	4.0	4.9	0.5	1.1
Production	5.1	8.5	14.2	2.5	3.0
Yield	1.4	2.1	2.9	2.0	1.9
Coarse grains [4]					
Area	24	28	32	0.7	0.5
Production	23	31	53	1.6	3.3
Yield	1.0	1.1	1.7	0.9	2.3
Pulses [5]					
Area	4.5	5.3	6.0	0.8	0.8
Production	3.2	4.3	5.9	1.3	1.9
Yield	0.7	0.8	1.0	0.5	1.1
Cattle and buffalos					
Meat production	1.2	2.1	3.5	2.4	3.3
No. of animals (million)	88	121	150	1.4	1.4
Milk production	13	23	39	2.6	3.3
Sheep and goats					
Meat production	1.2	2.0	3.6	2.6	3.7
No. of animals	251	355	490	1.6	2.0
Milk production	4.1	6.3	9.2	2.2	2.3
Poultry					
Meat production	0.3	1.7	4.3	7.8	6.0

Source: AT2000 files (FAO 1987).
[1] For livestock, 1983–85.
[2] For livestock, 1983/85–2000.
[3] Total cereals include wheat, rice, and coarse grains.
[4] Coarse grains include barley, maize, sorghum, millet, and other cereals.
[5] Excluding soybeans, only food legumes.

area fertilizer use of 7.6%, is expected to be one critical factor in increasing yields. Research in the region and by ICARDA provides evidence for the technical and economic feasibility of such yield and production increases.

As principal sources of protein, pulses and livestock products are expected to surpass recent growth rates. For pulses, yields are virtually stagnant but are expected to increase slightly, and the associated technical changes will be small. For livestock products, however, substantial changes are projected with 44% of the increases in meat production expected to be attributed to gains in carcass weight and the rest equally divided between increases in the off-take rate and livestock numbers. The dependence on cereals for animal feed is expected to increase substantially.

Increasing livestock numbers implies that native pastures, including the steppe, will come under increasing pressure and result in serious degradation, mainly through soil erosion. Hence, increases in livestock productivity must be associated with intensified production, although the extent to which this can be achieved remains conjectural. However, production increases in barley, by far the most important feed resource in WANA, could relieve the pressures on the native pastures arising from increases in the livestock population.

Barley and livestock production in the drier regions of WANA are not only complementary but are usually observed in integrated enterprises, which allow management of the uncertainties arising from climatic variability and associated risks. In good years, when more feed is available, herds expand and provide a buffer for poor years i.e., surplus barley is transformed into a buffer stock of meat. In poor years, even though meat prices are low, this buffer stock is reduced and continues to provide security against the crisis.

Changes in barley production practices may radically alter long-term average yields but more stable crop yields cannot be guaranteed under the adverse climatic conditions. Thus larger buffer barley stocks, which are costly and need storage, may be required. This can be complemented with improved livestock management, e.g., higher feed conversion rates and higher productivity. Until these developments become fairly widespread, livestock production in WANA will continue to be cyclical and related to climatic variability.

Barley in food demand

In 1983 per capita incomes (at constant 1980 prices) in WANA were 1175 USD compared to 780 USD in the 93 LDCs of the AT2000 study (FAO 1987). There were also differences in consumption patterns: in 1983, per capita consumption of wheat as food was 131 and 51 kg for WANA and the 93 LDCs, respectively, for meat 17 and 12 kg, for milk 69 and 44 kg, and for pulses 7.6 and 9.2 kg. There is a striking contrast in the indirect feed use of cereals with 57 kg in WANA and 31 kg in the 93 LDCs. Hence, consumption patterns in WANA currently reflect the high average per capita income levels. High income elasticity commodities are consumed at rates above those of developing countries as a whole, along with wheat, the traditional staple in large parts of the region.

Table 2. Demand for major food commodities in WANA (million metric tonnes).

Commodity	Food demand		Feed demand		Total demand		Deficits (−)		SSR (%) [1]	
	1983	2000	1983	2000	1983	2000	1983	2000	1983	2000
Total cereals	75.4	116.6	23.1	53.4	116.6	193.9	− 32.6	− 58.9	71	70
Wheat	53.3	80.5	4.4	9.6	69.1	105.4	− 21.6	− 33.9	69	68
Coarse grains	15.3	24.7	18.6	43.8	40.2	76.3	− 10.3	− 22.9	73	70
Barley	3.4	5.3	11.5	27.6	19.3	37.4	− 5.5	− 11.2	71	70
Maize	6.2	9.6	5.7	13.4	13.2	25.2	− 4.8	− 11.0	64	56
Pulses	3.1	4.6	0.4	0.4	4.1	5.7	0.2	0.2	107	103
Total meat	6.9	12.9	–	–	6.9	12.9	− 1.3	− 1.5	81	88
Beef	2.6	4.4	–	–	2.6	4.4	− 0.6	− 0.9	77	80
Lamb	2.3	3.9	–	–	2.3	3.9	− 0.3	− 0.3	89	91
Poultry	2.0	4.5	–	–	2.0	4.5	− 0.5	− 0.3	77	94
Milk	28.0	47.2	3.9	6.6	35.5	59.8	− 6.5	− 11.4	82	81
Total calories per capita per day (kcal)	2550	2715	503	736	3526	3893	− 958	− 1172	73	70

Source: AT2000 files, based on actual 1983 supply utilization accounts and projections for 2000.
[1] SSR = self-sufficiency ratio.

The projections to 2000 consider that, at 2.6% per year, population growth will be a major influence on the growth of food demand. Moderate per capita income growth (1.1% per year) from a high base will influence growth of food demand with a continued bias towards high income elasticity commodities and indirect consumption of barley as feed for livestock (Tables 2 and 3).

The demand for barley as a significant component of coarse grain demand is expected to increase annually at 4.0%. However, the feed demand for barley is projected to increase at 5.3%, which is faster than the growth of feed demand for coarse grains and cereals. This growth in derived demand stems from the high projected growth rate in demand for meat (3.7%) and milk (3.1%). About a third of this meat demand will be for lamb but most of the milk demand is for cows' milk. However, dairy products made from ewes'

Table 3. Projected annual growth rates (%) of demand in WANA.

	Direct food demand	Feed demand	Total demand
Calories per capita per day (kcal)	0.4	2.3	0.6
Cereals	2.6	5.1	3.0
Wheat	2.5	4.6	2.5
Coarse grains	2.8	5.2	3.8
Barley	2.6	5.3	4.0
Pulses	2.3	− 0.4	2.0
Meat	3.7	–	3.7
Milk	3.1	3.1	3.1

Source: AT2000 files (FAO 1987).

milk, such as yoghurt and cheese, are a most important source of high quality protein in rural diets and must not be overlooked (Somel and Mokbel 1986; Thomson et al. 1986). Demand for pulses, as an important source of protein for the poor along with protein from cereals, is projected to grow at around the rate of population growth.

Policy implications

The WANA region is currently characterized by large food deficits which are met by imports. The deficit in wheat, which is the main staple in large parts of the region, is particularly important. There are large deficits in coarse grains and livestock products and even the apparent self-sufficiency in pulses is in fact due to high production and surpluses in Turkey.

The projections to 2000 show moderate advances and reverses in self-sufficiency ratios (Table 2). Attaining complete food self-sufficiency, while a common policy objective, remains difficult and perhaps impossible this century. While self-sufficiency ratios remain stable, the absolute magnitude of the deficits in wheat, coarse grains, and livestock products will increase substantially.

The projected deficits are comparable to those of other studies (Khaldi 1984; Paulino 1986; Sarma 1986; Sarma and Yeung 1985) and while the numbers may differ in different studies, the projected patterns are similar.

Research priorities must be linked to the pivotal areas of projections: wheat, feedstuffs, livestock production, and irrigation and water management. In very few places in the world are land constraints as binding as in WANA and major parts of the region have rainfed agriculture, while the major part of agricultural production is in irrigated areas.

Projected production increases are dependent upon using the scarce water resources (from irrigation or rainfall) more efficiently and in combination with other inputs such as fertilizer in order to raise both yields and cropping intensity. Hence, increasing water use efficiency should be a primary focus of research.

In WANA livestock are currently produced extensively and in drier areas production depends on large common grazing areas. Can the livestock production increases projected for WANA be achieved without radical changes in production technology and management?

It appears that current research efforts are predominantly based on the existing extensive livestock production systems. These systems cannot continue without drastic measures to protect the environment. Therefore research for the 21st century must consider intensive livestock production. Intensification is used here to mean less dependence on extensive grazing on common land and greater dependence on feedstuff production in viable areas of production. However, complete feedlot sheep production is neither implied nor envisaged in the foreseeable future in WANA. Even with this qualification, it would seem that the research problems associated with intensified livestock production are somewhat different from those of the current extensive systems. The change of focus would have implications for management research, changes in the quality and quantity of veterinary service inputs, and in the crops involved.

There is also the need for policies not to increase but preferably reduce the pressure of livestock production on marginal cropping areas and the steppes with tenuous environmental balances. Increased feed availability may result in increasing herd sizes rather than increasing intensification. Increased herds kept under the currently practiced systems would cause excessive damage to the environment in marginal areas and the steppes so the increased feed available should primarily be used as a substitute for such grazing areas in order to arrest environmental damage.

The crops that are used as feedstuffs, particularly for sheep in the dry areas, are few with barley being overwhelmingly dominant. The response of the current systems to increased feed demand has been to produce more barley by continuous cropping or expanding into marginal areas, both with serious effects on soils. Research should be able to increase the crop mix by introducing new forage legumes as feed crops and as elements in crop rotations. Finally, wheat, which is in a class by itself, should be supported both by maintenance research and by efforts to improve production.

The question remains on the opportunity costs of meeting demand through domestic production increases rather than imports, mainly from outside the region. Currently, agricultural prices are depressed in international markets due to the surpluses created by developed market economies, particularly in the EEC and North America, and due to the limits imposed on LDC exports by protectionist measures and market saturation. Production subsidies in developed countries have distorted international prices to such low levels that the lowest cost producers of some commodities, e.g., dairy products in New Zealand, may be driven out of the market and become importers. Under these conditions, the general tendency in the developing countries is to import, provided there are resources which can generate the funds for imports.

The long-term prospects indicate the need for caution. There are increasing pressures in developed countries to reduce subsidies and surpluses and many studies clearly illustrate positive global economic and welfare effects if such protective measures were reduced in the developed countries (e.g., Valdes and Zietz 1980). Finally, while imports by LDCs may provide relief in the short term, they compete with domestic production and may adversely influence the development of domestic agriculture. This is invariably overlooked as priority is given to providing cheap food to urban consumers, not without due regard to the political pressures that these concentrated urban populations can generate.

If prices are depressed because of distortions in the market which are not expected to last, in the long term it may be desirable to invest in domestic agriculture. For WANA, even with the projected large deficits, substantial

Table 4. Agricultural investment requirements in WANA (1980 billion USD), 1983–2000.

	Net	Gross
Irrigation	57	78
Mechanization	29	36
Total crop investment	102	151
Herd increases	–	18
Production and processing of livestock products	1	40
Investment in primary agriculture [2]	103	178
Total agricultural investment	138	298

Source: AT2000 files (FAO 1987).

[1] Could not be estimated due to lack of information on depreciation.

[2] Includes crop and livestock production but excludes transportation, processing, and marketing.

investment in agriculture will be necessary in any case. A major portion of this investment will have to be in irrigation and associated infrastructure due to limits on land expansion. However, substantial investment is projected in livestock production and processing (Table 4).

WANA faces important challenges in reorganizing a dynamic agricultural sector beset by an uncertain climate and prices to one that will meet the demands of the growing economies. Solutions will come from a commitment to improve both the technological structure and economic conditions in the agricultural sector.

Acknowledgements

This paper is based on the results of the Agriculture: Toward 2000 (AT2000) project conducted by the Global Perspectives Study group in the Food and Agriculture Organization of the United Nations (FAO 1987). The author participated in this project during sabbatical leave in 1985/86. The project was directed by Dr. Nikos Alexandratos, and many contributed to it. The modeling activity was coordinated by Dr. Jelle Bruinsma. The views presented in this paper are not necessarily those of FAO, ICARDA, or their donors.

References

FAO (Food and Agriculture Organization). 1987. Agriculture: Toward 2000 (Revised 1987). FAO, Rome, Italy.

Khaldi, N. 1984. Evolving Food Gaps in the Middle East/North Africa: Prospects and Policy Implications. IFPRI Research Report 47. IFPRI, Washington, D.C., USA.

Mona, N.H. 1986. Structure and Responsiveness of Barley Production in Syria. PhD dissertation. Texas A&M University, Texas, USA.

Paulino, L. 1986. Food in the Third World: Past Trends and Projections to 2000. IFPRI Research Report 52. IFPRI, Washington, D.C., USA.

Sarma, J.S. 1986. Cereal Feed Use in the Third World: Past Trends and Projections to 2000. IFPRI Research Report 57. IFPRI, Washington, D.C., USA.

Sarma, J.S. and Yeung, P. 1985. Livestock Products in the Third World: Past Trends and Projections to 1990 and 2000. IFPRI Research Report 49. IFPRI, Washington, D.C., USA.

Somel, K. and Mokbel, M. 1986. The importance of Livestock in Rural Welfare. ICARDA Discussion Paper 19. ICARDA, Aleppo, Syria.

Thomson, E.F., Bahhady, F., Termanini, A., and Mokbel, M. 1986. Availability of home-produced wheat, milk products and meat to sheep-owning families at the cultivated margin of the NW Syrian steppe. Ecology of Food and Nutrition 19: 113–121.

Valdes, A. and Zietz, J. 1980. Agricultural Protection in OECD Countries: Its Cost to Less-Developed Countries. IFPRI Research Report 21. IFPRI, Washington, D.C., USA.

E.F. Thomson and F.S. Thomson (eds), Increasing Small Ruminant Productivity in Semi-arid Areas
© *1988 ICARDA . ISBN 978-94-010-7086-7*

Research Strategies for Development: Improving Sheep and Goat Production in Developing Countries

D.F. Nygaard and P. Amir

Introduction

The importance of animals to people and the role of small ruminants in farm families in developing countries is well documented. They "can obtain their nourishment from grasses and other fibrous forage which people cannot directly utilize. In turn, they provide humans with an adequate supply and proper balance of energy, minerals, vitamins, and essential amino acids which human metabolism cannot do without. The non-food contributions of ruminants – many of which cannot be precisely estimated – are also substantial" (Winrock International 1978). However, there are few projects that focus on livestock issues and financial support is meager.

Three impressions emerge from the literature. Firstly, ruminants play a crucial role in agricultural production, and they play that role in a number of ways. This is particularly true of sheep and goats in West Asia and North Africa. Secondly, there does not seem to be much happening in animal research; no breakthroughs, few new programs, and, in general, little excitement. Researchers appear to be conservative both in identifying potentially productive avenues of research and in integrating animal research into agricultural production and rural development activities. This is in contrast, for example, to the tremendous interest and financial support for research in agroforestry issues that has arisen in just the past 5 years.

Finally, there seems to be much potential for examining the linkages between ruminants and other agricultural and non-agricultural activities, i.e., the complementary way in which ruminants contribute to the productivity of a system, and for exploiting the opportunities that exist for collaborative research and development programs. While financial support may be difficult to muster for sustained research on animal production problems alone, there are a host of research and production activities in which animals are important components.

Therefore, it is the premise of this paper that animals contribute to agricultural systems and farm family incomes in developing countries in unique, numerous and complicated ways which make it difficult for researchers to capture research funds. The paper focuses on the role of small ruminants in agricultural systems. The second part of the paper explicitly explores the new research and development agenda of developing countries and of the donor community in search of the linkages and opportunities mentioned above.

The role of small ruminants in agricultural systems

The small ruminants of importance to ICARDA and the focus of this paper are sheep and goats. In rural areas in developing countries, ruminants are kept by farm families for milk, meat, fiber, traction, leather, manure, etc. (Table 1) and are generally an integral, but not dominant, component of the complex agricultural systems except in the driest areas. Therefore, an assessment of the status of sheep and goats and strategies for improving their productivity must consider their role within larger and more complex production systems (Winrock International 1983).

There are a number of advantages to having small ruminants in agricultural systems. They not only complement other parts of the agricultural system, but also add stability to a farmer's income and consumption and add liquidity to his cash flow, provide flexibility to a farmer's management options, have social value and serve religious purposes, and give status and serve as a store of wealth.

These advantages are due to a number of characteristics of sheep and goats including their small size which allows low investment costs, rapid maturity rates, and easy housing, reproductive efficiency (including short gestation and lactation periods and multiple births), feeding behavior (including feeding strategies complementary to larger ruminants and ability to travel further when grazing and graze on rougher terrain), adaptability to dry areas, socio-economic factors (sheep and goats are generally not associated with religious taboos), and heterogeneity in their genetic resources (Winrock International 1983).

There are also some disadvantages to small ruminants which are related to their small size and grazing habits. They are subject to theft, not useful for draft purposes, have low outputs relative to input costs, and can degrade grazing land when grazing is not controlled.

If small ruminants have these advantages, why have they not received more attention by the development community? A World Bank study (World Bank 1983) suggests that the current and potential role of small ruminants in many developing countries has not been recognized and so there is a lack of support within developing countries and international donor and lending agencies. While considerable attention has been given to mixed crop-animal systems, few projects have a primary emphasis on sheep and goats.

Ecological, biological, policy, and socioeconomic constraints are usually interrelated so research, training, and development programs require a balanced production system approach. A combination of support activities are needed including "regional and herd health programs, government assistance

Table 1. Ruminant products utilized by people.

Classification	Contribution	Main sources [1]
Meat	Food	All ruminants
Milk	Food	Cattle, buffalo, goats, sheep, camel, yak
Fiber	Wool	All ruminants
	Pelts	Sheep, camelids
Inedible products	Inedible fats	Cattle, buffalo, sheep
	Horns, hooves, bones	Cattle, buffalo
	Tankage	Cattle, buffalo, sheep
	Endocrine extracts	Cattle, buffalo, sheep
Traction	Agriculture	Cattle, buffalo, camel
	Cartage	Cattle, buffalo, yak, camel
	Packing	Camelid, yak, buffalo, cattle, reindeer
	Herding	Buffalo, camel
	Irrigation pumping	Buffalo, cattle, camel
	Threshing grains	Cattle, buffalo, camel
	Passenger conveyance	Buffalo, cattle, yak, camel
Waste	Fertilizer	Domestic ruminants
	Fuel (dung)	Cattle, buffalo, yak, camelids, sheep, goats
	Methane gas	Cattle, buffalo
	Construction (plaster)	Cattle, buffalo
	Feed (recycled)	Cattle
Storage	Capital	Domestic ruminants
	Grains	Cattle, buffalo, sheep
Conservation	Grazing	All ruminants
	Seed distribution	All ruminants
	Ecological	
	Maintenance	All ruminants
	Restoration	All ruminants
Pest Control	Plants in waterways	Buffalo
	Weeds	Domestic ruminants
	Snails (paddies, canals)	Buffalo
Cultural, including	Exhibitions, rodeos	Cattle, sheep, goat, buffalo
recreation	Sport fighting	Cattle, buffalo, sheep
	Hunting	Game ruminants
	Pet	Goat, sheep, deer
	Racing, riding	Buffalo, cattle, camel
	Religious	Goat, buffalo, sheep, cattle
	Bride price	Cattle, sheep, goat, camel

Source: World Bank (1983).

[1] Species listed in order of importance, where identified.

to research and extension programs, and formulation of favorable credit, marketing, and pricing policies for small ruminants and their products" (Winrock International 1983).

Potential for improving productivity

Johnson et al. (1986) suggest that there is an untapped potential for improving the productivity of sheep and goats in developing countries. They explain this potential by looking at current animal numbers, the productivity gap accrual and potential production levels, economic incentives, and possibilities to lower input costs.

Current animal numbers. In 1985, developing countries accounted for 56% of the world's estimated 1.2 billion sheep and 95% of the 523 million goats. Both absolute numbers and percent of world totals in developing countries have increased consistently since 1960 with numbers of small ruminants increasing greatly in the developing countries in the past 15 years but stagnating in the developed world (Table 2). The significance of small ruminants relative to cattle, particularly in the Middle East compared with Africa, is shown in Tables 2 and 3. Due to the current low level of meat production in these regions, there appears to be much potential for continued expansion of local production.

Productivity gap. Comparison of output per animal among regions, among controlled management situations, and among farms indicates that there is a sizeable gap between the actual and potential productivity of small ruminants in farming systems. The World Bank study (World Bank 1983) showed that there is a 17% lower yearly offtake and a 20% lower carcass yield in developing than in developed countries. For goats, differences are more striking with 61 and 35% offtake, 6.9 and 4.3 kg carcass yield, and 103 and 12.4 kg milk yield per head for developed and developing regions, respectively. Controlled experimental data are also available from several developing countries that demonstrate improved growth rate, reproduction, or lactation yields (Johnson et al. 1986). At ICARDA, one of the few places where this gap has been

Table 2. Plant and animal production in developed countries compared to developing countries.

	Developed Countries			Developing Countries		
	1970 (millions)	1985	% change	1970 (millions)	1985	% change
Cereals (t)	617.7	917.4	48.5	788.0	1263.1	60.3
Pulses (t)	12.6	15.2	20.8	38.8	39.9	2.8
Milk (t)	312.9	379.7	21.3	49.4	80.9	63.6
Cattle (head)	388.7	423.1	8.9	756.7	897.1	18.6
Sheep (head)	552.1	538.3	−2.5	598.5	678.9	13.4
Goats (head)	26.0	27.1	4.4	431.9	496.2	14.9
Meat (t)	69.7	95.2	36.5	35.5	73.8	107.9

Source: FAO.

Table 3. Plant and animal production in West Asia and North Africa compared to Sub-Saharan Africa.

	West Asia and North Africa			Sub-Saharan Africa		
	1970 (millions)	1985	% change	1970 (millions)	1985	% change
Cereals (t)	59.0	88.9	50.7	22.7	31.0	36.7
Pulses (t)	2.7	3.7	37.6	3.0	3.2	6.0
Milk (t)	9.0	14.1	55.8	2.4	3.2	30.2
Cattle (head)	61.2	78.2	27.7	57.4	73.2	27.4
Sheep (head)	172.9	213.5	23.4	38.4	52.3	36.3
Goats (head)	81.8	97.4	19.1	66.3	78.8	18.9
Meat (t)	3.2	6.1	90.6	2.1	2.9	38.1

Source: FAO.

measured in economic terms, research has shown dramatic income differences among different management regimes for sheep-based farming systems (Nordblom and Thomson 1987).

Economic incentives. While traditional farmers in developing countries have many reasons for including small ruminants in mixed farming systems, the most likely motivation is economic. Farmers are known to be economically efficient in their use of available technology and respond quickly to new market opportunities (Schultz 1964). In addition to population increases, rising incomes in the developing world generally, and West Asia and North Africa in particular, have led to substantial increases in consumer demand for meat so farmers benefit from higher prices for meat and other animal products. In addition, within such a dynamic system, there are wide annual swings in meat prices, presenting another opportunity for improving management decisions to increase financial returns.

Lower input costs. Sheep and goat production does not require costly inputs, and inputs (and outputs) are easily divisible. Furthermore, new technology can reduce input costs per unit of output. Johnson et al. (1986) note growing evidence "that significant productivity increases of small ruminants can be attained with low-cost inputs such as feed produced on marginal land with cheap labor. Also, the capital cost of the animals themselves is relatively small".

New technologies can also be cost effective. Motorized transport in the steppe areas in North Africa and West Asia has drastically altered production practices among nomadic sheep herders. While the effects of introducing this technology are not all positive, it does give farmers more control of, and more options in, their management portfolio.

Classification of production systems

In examining the role of small ruminants in agricultural systems in the developing world, it is useful to look at alternative production systems, particularly because research opportunities for animal scientists exist primarily within a systems context. Researchers at Winrock have classified production systems into three main categories and nine sub-categories (Table 4) (Winrock International 1982). Of most importance is the role that sheep and goats play in the three of the four mixed crop/animal systems. Systems in which animals have a major role can also be classified with respect to the relationship among producers. This can be independent (e.g., fattening operations), competitive (e.g., nomads vs landowners), or complementary (where seasonal requirement for labor, for example in a cropping activity, complements the labor demand of a livestock activity). In animal production, there are also conflicts between intensive and extensive systems, between private and public grazing lands, or between developers and conservationists on public lands or common property. It is these conflicts that get the attention of the development community because conflicts cause bottlenecks in the development process. It is the premise of this paper that it is the interface between the partners in such conflicts that are most complex, most interesting, and where most potential exists for increases in productivity if solutions can be found. To attack these problems, clearly a systems approach to research is required.

Priorities for research and development of small ruminant production

In order to attract more financial support for research and development on livestock and related programs, present and future priorities must focus on the interaction and linkages of the various components of the system. It will take a critical mass of scientific effort to make progress on increasing the contribution of small ruminants to mixed crop/animal production systems.

Table 4. Classification of production systems based on predominant agricultural activities.

Animal based (animal component major)
Pastoral immigration
Pastoral sedentary
Mixed crop and animal (animal component important, often essential)
Cattle, sheep, goats–millet and sorghum
Cattle, sheep, goats–wheat and clove
Cattle, sheep, goats, pigs, chicken–maize
Buffalo, cattle–rice, roots, and tubers
Crop based (animal component minor)
Large-scale plantation
Large-scale cash commercial
Small-scale food crops

Source: Winrock International (1982).

Five development themes are receiving increasing attention by the development community: diversification, sustainability, seasonability, employment generation, and human nutrition. The themes are likely to dominate development programs over the next 5 years and perhaps the next decade. No attempt has been made to list them in order of priority.

Diversification

As countries have approached self-sufficiency in one staple (for example, rice in Indonesia) alternate production activities become important. This is also true when economic plans aim to reduce food imports, and food security becomes a concern. Questions of forward and backward linkages in the food chain, intensification of agricultural production and complementarity in the use of factors of production become critical. Certainly, animal production and animal products are key factors in this process.

Part of the diversification process will pull land and labor out of agricultural use while increasing the demand for agricultural products in growing urban areas. Increasing incomes augment the demand for high value food such as meat. Ironically, diversification at the national level could lead to specialization at the farm level, which also has an impact on the role of animals in the system.

Sustainability

Sustainability of fragile systems and ecological degradation have become more important with increasing damage to our resource base. The answer lies in resource management and currently this is a major focus of development efforts by the World Bank and USAID. Large financial resources will be allocated to environmental studies and projects over the next 10 years to research such topics as agroforestry, range management, and watershed management.

Seasonability

As we have learned more about the temporal (and spatial) allocation problems caused by climatic and sociological factors, seasonability has been given increased emphasis. For example, human nutrition problems arise from seasonal variability on income streams, and this can be particularly profound in the poorer areas. Effective programs can alleviate the problems that arise from these seasonal conditions.

Employment

One result of studies on the distributional benefits (or costs) of development activities has been the increasing attention given to generating employment opportunities. The problems caused by rural-urban immigration, the opportunities to examine the role of women in agricultural production and decision making, the plight of landless laborers in rural areas, and intra-household decision processes all focus on employment for rural families. Creating new employment opportunities is one of the most pressing problems in countries with rapidly growing populations.

Human nutrition

Human nutrition, which has long been a goal of development programs, has recently received more attention due to a better understanding of the impact of macroeconomic policies affecting nutrition oriented intervention programs and the distributional effects of development activities.

Other constraints are of more immediate concern to producers of sheep and goats. In a recent survey, livestock specialists were asked to identify major constraints to sheep and goat production. There was general agreement that in West Asia and North Africa the most important constraints are feed supplies and feeding strategy, health, socioeconomic factors, and management of production systems. Surprisingly, the constraints are not very different from

Table 5. Major constraints affecting production by region (sheep and goats).

Region	Economic and social constraints (according to priority)								
	Domestic demand	Export demand	Import supply	Price & trade policy	Production system	Credit	Tenure	Environmental	Management
North America	1		4	6		8		7	8
Middle America	2			7		6	4		
South America	2	4		3	7	8			6
Western Europe	2			1	3				
Eastern Europe	2			1	2				
USSR	4			2	3	5			4
China	2			4	3				4
N Africa–Mid East	4			7	5	4			
Central Africa	6						2		
South Africa	3			6	5	6	4		
India	3			6	2		7		
S and SE Asia	2				4				
Japan	3		4		2				
Oceania	2	1		4					
Rest of world	1				4				

Source: Scoville and Sarhan (1978).

one region to another (Table 5); the USAID study suggests genetic improvement as another constraint (World Bank 1983). There is little doubt that feed is of most concern to the producers of sheep and goat produce as it affects rates of gain and fertility, and hence productivity (Winrock International 1978).

Nevertheless, losses of animals and animal productivity from health problems (particularly diseases and parasites) can be important and solutions are costly. A number of factors are covered in the rubric socioeconomic, e.g., marketing, credit, policy, land tenure, and human capital development. Production and management strategies include giving attention to the scale of operation, flock size and composition, timing of the reproduction cycle, and nutrition priorities for different animals in the herd. Finally, these come together in a systems context. Fitzhugh (1987) notes that, "Because sheep and goats are part of complex agricultural systems, setting priorities and implementing research and development projects should follow a systems approach. The systems approach provides a strategy for evaluating the target production system, identifying constraints and designing interventions that have a favorable net impact on the system's productivity and efficiency".

We will now look more carefully at the relationships between the topics discussed so far using a matrix tableau (Fig. 1). In this example, the matrix demonstrates the integration of livestock activities in most development programs. More importantly, it shows the opportunities for livestock researchers to participate in these programs.

There are 25 cells in which potential collaboration could take place. The cells do not provide equal opportunities for livestock research and develop-

Skills & Training	Market-ing	Roads & Trans.	Attitudes & Taboos	Wages	Physical constraints					
					Preda-tors	Feed supply	Water	Dis-ease	Breed-ing	Technical knowledge
			2	5	3					
5	3					1				
						1		5		
						3				
						3				
						1				
						1		5		
	3					1	6	2		
	4	7	5			1	6	3		
	5					1		2		
	7		4			1		5		
						1		3	4	
4						1				
		6				5	3			
5						2		3		

Source: Scoville and Sarhan (1978).

Opportunities

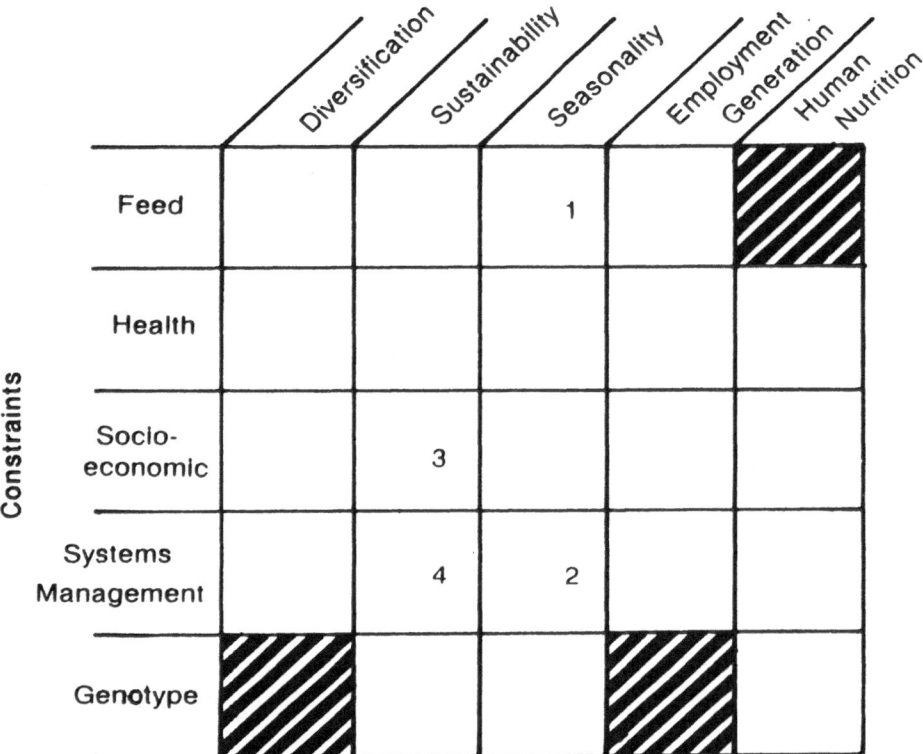

Fig. 1. Research opportunities/constraints matrix.

ment and three of them are shaded to suggest they are of marginal interest. However, most of the others offer attractive options. In the sustainability column, for example, a number of opportunities exist for research and development in any one of the five categories of constraints. To illustrate the value of the matrix, specific examples for four of the cells (numbered 1 - 4) in which development programs have embraced livestock's problems are briefly described in more detail.

The first example is drawn from a farming systems research project in Tunisia conducted by INRAT (the Tunisian Institute for Agricultural Research) in collaboration with ICARDA. The emphasis of the program is the integration of the livestock and cropping enterprises on mixed farming systems in Northern Tunisia. In an evaluation of the project after 3 years of research, livestock scientists documented the pervasive feed problem in the region, and in their own research they were giving particular priority to the seasonal shortfall in feed supplies. In an average year, feed supplies are balanced with

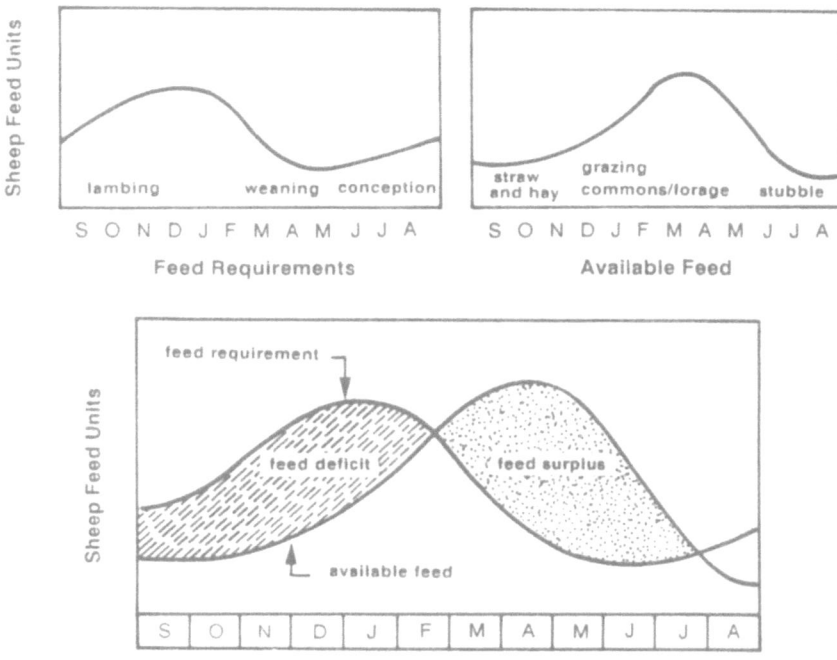

Fig. 2. Annual feed balance in northern Tunisia, estimate (Fresco et al. 1987).

feed demand but the feed is not always available when it is needed (Fig. 2). As a result of this focus on seasonal issues, plant scientists have revised their research to look more carefully at feed production during deficit periods and alternative storage possibilities for feed grown during the wet season. In addition, social scientists have begun to focus on questions relating to feed distribution and to follow seasonal cash flow patterns. The latter is done with a view to developing strategies for purchasing feed for or in the periods of deficit. The general thrust of the program has now shifted to a focus on seasonal issues.

A substantially more sophisticated approach to a similar development program has been conducted by Winrock International in Western Kenya. This program is looking at the possibility of introducing dual-purpose goats into a complex mixed cropping/animal system. The program focuses on whole farm modelling and management. Hart and Knipscheer (1984) have designed a microcomputer spread sheet simulation framework in which typical farms can be manipulated by changing one or more of the many parameters in the system (Fig. 3). Each activity of the farm is described on a "template" constructed on a microcomputer. These are used to develop a series of templates, e.g., farm land, forage system, forage storage, herd system, etc.,

48

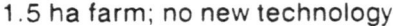

1.5 ha farm; no new technology

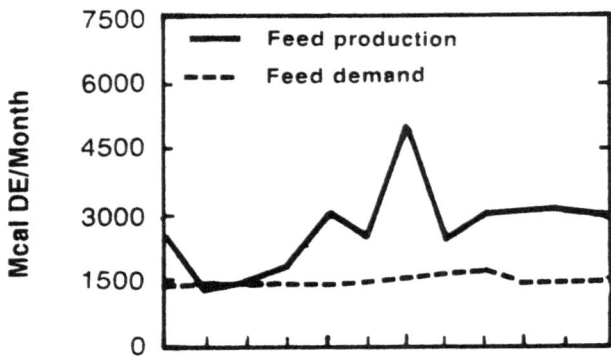

1.5 ha farm; feed and goat technology

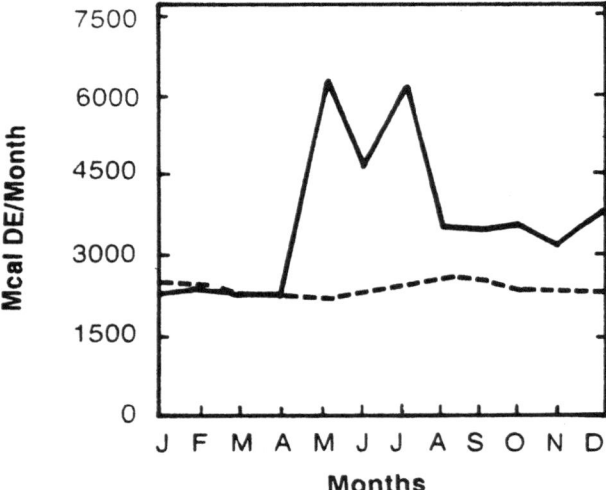

Months

Fig. 3. Annual feed balance in western Kenya using computer based spreadsheets (Hart and Knipscheer 1986).

which are used to build flow charts and finally diagrams of the system. It is a dynamic model that follows the system during the year.

They conclude, "feed availability is a major constraint for livestock production on these farms, but the design of appropriate technological alternatives to increase feed is complicated by the fact that most farms have multiple feed resources (cropped areas, fence rows, off-farm, etc.), each with varying relative importance during different seasons".

The framework is useful in understanding complex interrelationships and it has been used to test new technologies with a view to increasing the feed supply. Being able to simulate the new technology was a distinct contribution of the method. Similar diagrams can be constructed for other parts of the system and for other technological innovations.

Under the sustainability theme, a number of examples could be cited where livestock scientists have become involved, but two in particular fall under the socioeconomic and systems management constraint categories. The management of public land and common lands is currently being intensely investigated. The conflict between forestry departments, livestock herders, landless settlers, etc., has led to deforestation and other problems of land deterioration. Often the problems are "downstream", far away from the source. Because people are so closely tied to the problem, they must become a part of the solutions. Too often national governments have passed legislation that is not followed by local people or enforceable. Social scientists can and have contributed to understanding these issues.

Agroforestry has become popular and practitioners look at agroforestry in a systems context. One of the problems confronting farmers and scientists in Africa is converting slash and burn agriculture to more intensive land uses. The International Institute for Tropical Agriculture (IITA) and the International Livestock Centre for Africa (ILCA) have been successful in developing alley cropping in which crops are grown between rows of leguminous shrubs. One of the keys to this system has been its ability to maintain soil fertility under continuous cropping. With the high protein fodder provided by the shrubs, small ruminants are also important to the system's economic viability.

Conclusion

Because the production of sheep and goats is such an integral part of farming systems and can be one of the problems constraining rural development, there seem to be substantial opportunities to conduct research and development on small ruminants within the context of larger development programs. In search of rapid solutions, the development community tends to shift its priorities to current themes that look promising. In doing so, they threaten the continuous support that is needed if researchers are to make progress on complex development problems. A solution seems to be to look for research opportunities within these themes. There are numerous options for livestock scientists to make a contribution to improving livestock production.

References

FAO (Food and Agriculture Organization). Production Yearbooks, Various Issues. FAO, Rome, Italy.

Fitzhugh, H.A. 1987. Systems Approach to Small Ruminant Research and Development. Small Ruminants in the Middle East. FAO, Rome, Italy.

Fresco, Louise, Nygaard, D. and Tchamitchian, L. 1987. Farming Systems Research in Tunisia: A Review of the Goubellat Project. IDRC, Ottawa, Canada.

Hart, Robert and Knipscheer, Hendrick C. 1986. An Analytical Framework for the Design and Evaluation of Crop and Livestock Technology. Winrock International, Petit Jean Mountain, Arkansas, USA.

Hart, Robert, Onim, M., Russo, S., Matuva, M., Otieno, K. and Fitzhugh, H. 1984. An Analytical Framework for Feed Research on Mixed Farms in Western Kenya. Winrock International, Petit Jean Mountain, Arkansas, USA.

Johnson, W.C., van Eys, J.E. and Fitzhugh, H.A. 1986. Sheep and goats in tropical and subtropical agricultural systems. Journal of Animal Science 63 (5): 1587–1599.

Nordblom, T.L. and Thomson, E.F. 1987. A Whole-farm Model Based on Experimental Flocks and Crop Rotations in Northwest Syria. ICARDA-102 En. ICARDA, Aleppo, Syria. 78 p.

Schultz, T.W. 1964. Transforming Traditional Agriculture. Yale.

Scoville, O.J. and Sarhan, M. 1978. Objectives and constraints of ruminant livestock production. World Review of Animal Production 14 (1): 47.

Winrock International. 1978. The Role of Ruminants in Support of Man. Winrock International, Petit Jean Mountain, Arkansas, USA.

Winrock International. 1982. Livestock Program Priorities and Strategies (USAID). Winrock International, Petit Jean Mountain, Arkansas, USA.

World Bank. 1983. Sheep and Goats in Developing Countries. World Bank, Washington, D.C., USA.

E.F. Thomson and F.S. Thomson (eds), Increasing Small Ruminant Productivity in Semi-arid Areas
© 1988 ICARDA . ISBN 978-94-010-7086-7

Increasing Feed Resources for Small Ruminants in the Mediterranean Basin

P.S. Cocks and E.F. Thomson

Introduction

Livestock are an integral part of farming systems in the Mediterranean basin where crop production is limited by large seasonal variations in rainfall and temperature. These variations lead to a marked seasonality of feed supply which is a major constraint to livestock production. As it is generally agreed that a plentiful and balanced nutrient supply is the foundation of efficient livestock production, research at ICARDA during the past 10 years has focused on developing cereal-based crop rotations which include leguminous forage crops and pastures and using cereal straws. This paper outlines that research and presents some solutions. However, this focus does not imply that non-nutritional factors are less important. Indeed, the main aim of this workshop is to identify non-nutritional constraints that limit small ruminant productivity in Mediterranean areas. By turning our attention in the future to non-nutritional constraints, we imply that we have some understanding of nutritional constraints. The geographical area covered includes North African countries with a Mediterranean coast and West Asian countries with cool, wet winters and hot, dry summers. Areas with steppe vegetation will be briefly discussed, but generally the paper focuses on areas receiving above 250 mm rainfall. Much of the research also applies to southern Europe.

Farming systems in the Mediterranean basin

Farms are generally small, with over 95% being less than 50 ha and more than 70% less than 5 ha (Cooper et al. 1987). The main agricultural products are wheat, barley, and milk and meat from small ruminants and cattle. Grain legumes are also grown, mainly in high rainfall and irrigated areas where cattle are also found. In areas with less than 300 mm rainfall there are few alternatives to cereals and small ruminants are predominant. Their products are the main source of income and an important component of people's diets (Table 1; Thomson et al. 1986).

Crop rotations vary significantly. At 200 mm rainfall, cropping is risky and farmers attain good yields only when rainfall is above average. Crops are usually followed by one or more years of fallow. Towards 300 mm, cropping intensity increases and farmers traditionally use a cereal/fallow rotation but

Table 1. Contribution of commodities to human diets in West Asia and North Africa and the proportion of the value of total agricultural production from each commodity.

Commodity group	Protein contribution (%)	Calorie contribution (%)	Value (%)
Cereals [1]	58	59	25
Food legumes	4	2	3
Livestock [2]	17	5	31
Other food commodities [3]	21	34	41

Source: FAO (1987).

[1] Includes rice.

[2] Includes poultry.

[3] Includes roots, tubers, starchy foods, vegetables, fruits, oilseeds, and fish.

more recently have turned to continuous cereal. Above 300 mm, legumes and other crops enter the rotation.

There is a high degree of integration between livestock and cereal production. Indeed, below 300 mm, the huge areas sown to barley are failing to meet an ever-increasing demand for grain to feed livestock. In fact, it has been estimated that demand for barley will increase by more than 5% each year until the year 2000 (FAO 1986), an amount which cannot be met by increased productivity. Cereal straw and the grazing of weedy fallows contribute significantly to livestock production (Thomson 1987).

Livestock also graze native pastures, both the degraded shrub steppe below 200 mm and non-arable land within the cereal zone. The latter comprises about 30% of the surface area of, for example, western Syria. Within the cereal zone native pastures consist of Mediterranean annual grasses and legumes, typical of Mediterranean-type climates throughout the world (Rossiter 1966). Like the shrub steppe, annual pastures are severely degraded and the original perennial component has almost disappeared.

ICARDA has identified three ways in which livestock nutrition can be improved: replacing fallows in cereal/fallow rotations with pasture or forage legumes, improving productivity of native pasture, especially within the cereal zone, and increasing straw utilization by improving straw quality and using appropriate supplementary feeds.

Replacing fallows with pastures or forages

Two separate systems are being developed: replacing fallows with annually re-sown forage legumes or with self-regenerating pasture legumes. Both systems focus on legumes because of their beneficial effect in crop rotations, their independence of expensive nitrogenous fertilizer, and because they are excellent sources of dietary protein.

Table 2. Daily *ad-libitum* intake and daily liveweight changes of Awassi sheep offered fresh herbage (g dry matter) of barley, vetch, peas, and chickling, and dry matter digestibility of the forages.

	Barley	Vetch	Pea	Chickling
Daily intake (g)	1954	2411	506	2080
Liveweight change (g)	309	395	−210	383
Dry matter digestibilty (%)	69	77	64	76

Source: ICARDA (1986).

Breeding and selection of forage legumes are an important component of the research. At least three species of vetch (*Vicia sativa, V. narbonensis,* and *V. villosa* subsp. *dasycarpa*), two species of chickling (*Lathyrus ochrus* and *L. sativus*), and field peas (*Pisum sativum*) receive detailed attention. However, beyond stating that the principal objectives are to increase seed retention, select for cold tolerance, breed for disease resistance, and develop cultivars with high seed and straw yield, we will not discuss breeding further. Of more relevance is the way in which forage crops are used and their effect on farm profitability.

There are three methods of using forage crops: grazing to fatten lambs or for milk production, and harvesting as grain and straw. In all cases, feed value depends primarily on voluntary intake, which varies widely. For example, when penned sheep were fed the fresh immature herbage, hay (harvested at full flowering), and straw of barley, field peas, chickling, and common vetch, intake of field peas was very poor, such that at both the fresh herbage and hay stages sheep lost weight (Table 2). Subsequent grazing experiments have confirmed that sheep prefer weeds to the peas on offer (Thomson, unpublished).

Common vetch and chickling are easily the most palatable of the forage legumes, and on-farm experiments have shown that, together with the use of phosphate fertilizers, replacing fallows with either forage can more than double farm profitability. The aim of the on-farm research was to study the adoption of forage crops by resource-poor farmers, test the effect that forages have on the yield of subsequent barley crops, study the most appropriate way to use the crops, and measure the productivity and profitability of barley/forage rotations. The experiment was conducted on 18 farms near Breda, a small village south-east of Aleppo, where average rainfall is 280 mm. On each farm, adjacent areas separated by a 10m fallow strip were sown to vetch (V) and chickling (C) and 20 kg per ha of phosphorus was applied to half the area of each species. After each forage year a uniform, unfertilized barley crop was sown, and grain and straw yields were measured. The forages were either grazed by lactating ewes or lambs, or harvested for seed and straw.

Replacing fallow with unfertilized forages for grain and straw resulted in at least a 50% increase in net revenue (Table 3). Profitability was more than doubled when phosphorus was applied, particularly to chickling. Using the

54

Table 3. Net benefits from barley/fallow and barley/forage rotations. BF = barley/fallow; BV = barley/vetch; BC = barley/chickling; o = zero phosphorus; with p = phosphorus).

	BoFo	BoVo	BoVp	BoCo	BoCp
Gross revenue (SYP [1]/ha/2 years)					
Forage grain	0	1115	2156	2430	3349
Forage straw	0	785	1130	745	1027
Barley grain	1305	1213	1698	1449	1949
Barley straw	839	831	1091	906	1141
Average (SYP/ha/year)	1072	1972	3038	2765	3733
Direct costs (SYP/ha/2 years)					
Cultivations	200	400	400	400	400
Broadcasting	127	254	381	254	381
Seed (140 kg/ha)	231	756	756	756	756
Fertilizer	0	0	120	0	120
Hand harvesting [2]	300	600	900 [3]	600	900 [3]
Average (SYP/ha/year)	429	1005	1279	1005	1279
Net revenue (SYP/ha/year)	643	967	1760	1760	2455

Prices and costs in November 1986; forage grain 3.75 SYP/kg; barley grain 1.65 SYP/kg; all straws 0.80 SYP/kg; seed costs = grain prices; fertilizer 1.1 SYP/kg TSP; hand-harvest costs based on 20 SYP per labourer day and 15 labour days/ha.
[1] 1.00 USD = 10.00 SYP.
[2] Excludes cost of transport and threshing.
[3] Increased by 50% due to higher crop density.

forages for grazing, either to fatten lambs or to produce milk, resulted in even higher profits.

There is now ample evidence that replacing fallows with forage crops has only a slight, if any, adverse effect on cereal yields. In the above experiment barley yield after forage either exceeded that after fallow, in the case of chickling, or equalled it, in the case of vetch (Table 4). Work on Cyprus shows that barley yields after forage are significantly more than barley after barley (Papastylianou 1987; Papastylianou and Samios 1987), while in northern Syria barley after peas has equalled barley after fallow and considerably exceeded barley after barley (Keatinge et al. 1985). In this respect it is important to note that using legume/cereal mixtures for forage production will reduce subsequent cereal yields relative to pure legumes (Osman and Nersoyan 1986).

Replacing fallow with self-regenerating pastures is based on the ley farming system developed in southern Australia (Puckridge and French 1983; Chatter-

Table 4. Grain and straw yields (kg/ha) of barley after fallow, vetch (V). and chickling (C), with (p) and without phosphorus (o) (average of 3 years).

	Fallow	Vo	Vp	Co	Cp
Grain yield (n = 13)	791	735	1029	878	1181
Straw yield (n = 9)	1049	1039	1364	1133	1426

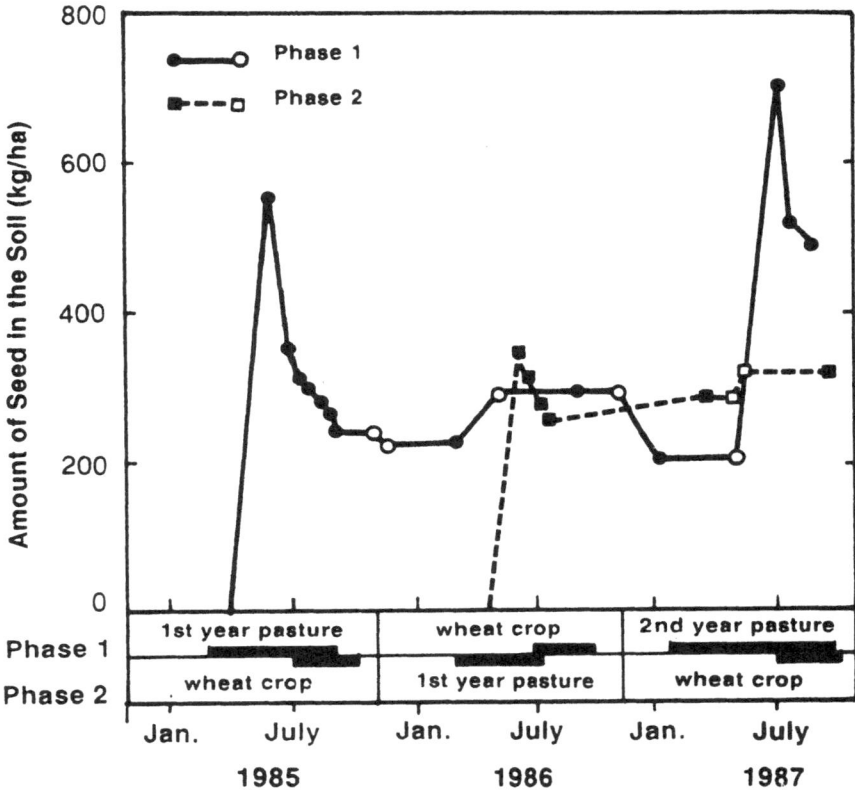

Fig. 1. Amount of medic seed in the soil of phase 1 (solid line) and phase 2 (broken line) of medic/wheat rotations in north-west Syria. The closed symbols are actual measurements and the open ones are estimates. The horizontal black bars below the figure are the periods of sheep grazing on medic pastures in the spring and early summer, and medic residues and wheat stubbles from July to September each year. Sheep alternate between phases 1 and 2 of the rotation.

ton and Chatterton 1984). In ley farming, fallows are replaced with self-regenerating annual legumes, usually annual medics (*Medicago* spp.) or subterranean clover (*Trifolium subterraneum*). While pasture productivity may be no more than in a forage-legume based system, costs are less because annual re-sowing is not necessary. Fig. 1, based on data obtained in northern Syria, shows the mechanism by which the system works: seeds produced in the first year remain dormant in the soil through the cropping phase and germinate in the next pasture phase.

Constraints to adoption of the system have been discussed by Cocks (1986) and Springborg (1986). It is clear that in West Asia a major constraint is lack of frost tolerance in the Australian medic cultivars (Cocks and Ehrman 1987). Lack of adapted rhizobia (Materon and Cocks 1987), inappropriate tillage machinery, poor grazing management, and lack of local seed production are also recognized constraints. It is also highly probable that a lack of sound data on profitability contributes to the limited success in introducing ley farming. Other sociological problems probably play a part, but resolution of the technical problems against a background of understanding local farming systems will eliminate these imponderables.

The major recent breakthrough has been recognizing the importance of using native legumes. The approach developed by ICARDA has been to survey the distribution of annual legumes within the target area and to choose from the most frequent those best able to survive. In this way, *M. rigidula* has been selected as adapted to ley farming in northern Syria (Abd El Moneim and Cocks 1986). It is likely that *M. rotata* will play a similar role in Jordan.

As with forage legume systems, on-farm research is the key to developing ley farming. Medic fields have been established at several villages north and south of Aleppo, and sheep productivity, effect on cereals, and returns from various farm enterprises are being monitored. The medics being sown are those selected by ICARDA, those occurring naturally at the villages concerned, and the Australian cultivars. In 1987 regenerating pastures yielded up to 7 t herbage per ha and carried a mean (over five farms) of 7.8 ewes per ha per year.

The experimental farms grew a variety of crops including lentils, barley, watermelons, and cumin in rotation with wheat. The yield of wheat after medic was compared to yield after whatever other crop was chosen by the farmers: after medic, wheat yielded 1.4 t per ha, significantly more than after the control crops – 1.1 t per ha.

It is still too early to conduct the kind of economic analysis shown in Table 3. However, costs and returns of other crops can be compared with returns from milk and meat produced on pasture. Assuming that pastures carried 7.8 ewes per ha per year, taking into account actual milk production and adding only half of the return from 0.8 lambs per ewe, the return from pastures was almost double the next most profitable crop (Table 5).

The impact of replacing fallows with either pasture or forage legumes is clearly enormous: throughout both the wheat and barley zones of Syria profitability could be increased by 50–200%. Perhaps one note of caution should be sounded. In some experiments wheat yields after medic have been substantially below wheat after fallow, especially when nitrogen fertilizer is

Table 5. Estimated profitability from alternative forms of land use (1986/87 prices).

Crop	Profit (SYP/ha)
Pasture [1]	6800
Lentils	2660
Watermelon	2600
Cumin	4000
Wheat	2010

[1] Pasture, lentils, watermelon, and cumin are grown in rotation with wheat.

used. This is probably due to poor weed control, which reinforces the need to consider all aspects of the farming system in such research.

Increasing productivity of native pasture

Within the cereal zone, communally grazed native pasture is usually available to sheep and access to it makes it possible to increase both the number of sheep farmers should own and farm profitability. In a study at ICARDA headquarters, Nordblom and Thomson (1987) considered that increasing herbage production by applying phosphorus to native pasture would increase profitability still more.

Apart from available soil water, there are three inter-connected factors limiting productivity from native pastures: excessive stocking rate, low plant numbers, and low soil fertility. Excessive grazing reduces seed production and

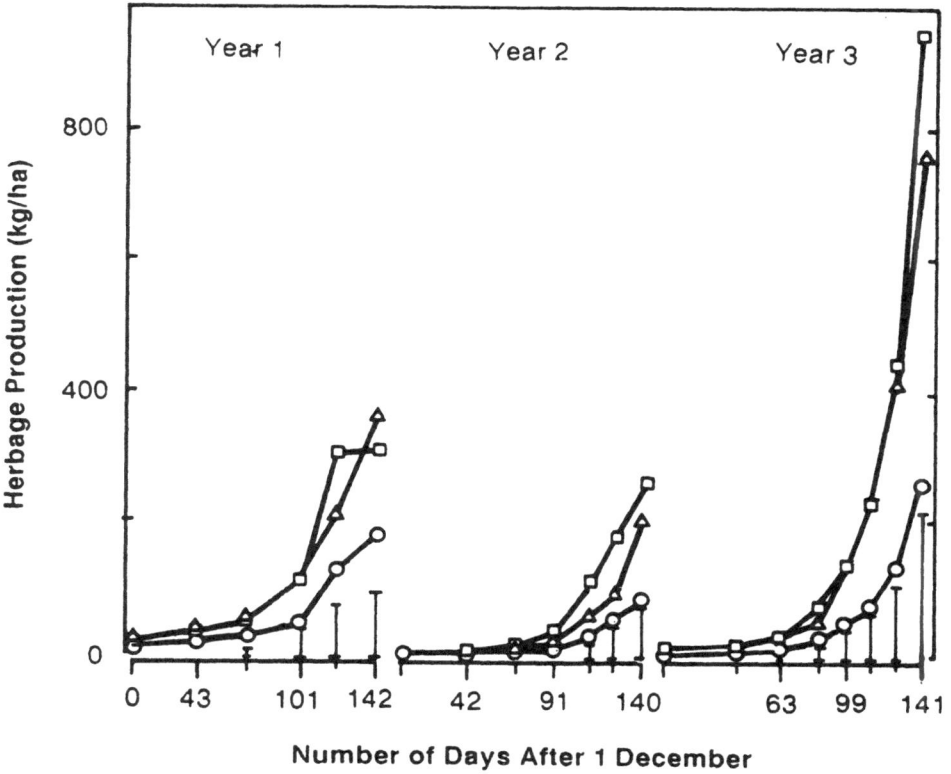

Fig. 2. Total herbage yield of legumes in grazed native pasture on marginal land at Tel Hadya in years 1, 2, and 3 at 0 (circles), 8 (triangles), and 25 (squares) kg of P_2O_5/ha. Bars represent LSD at $P < 0.01$.

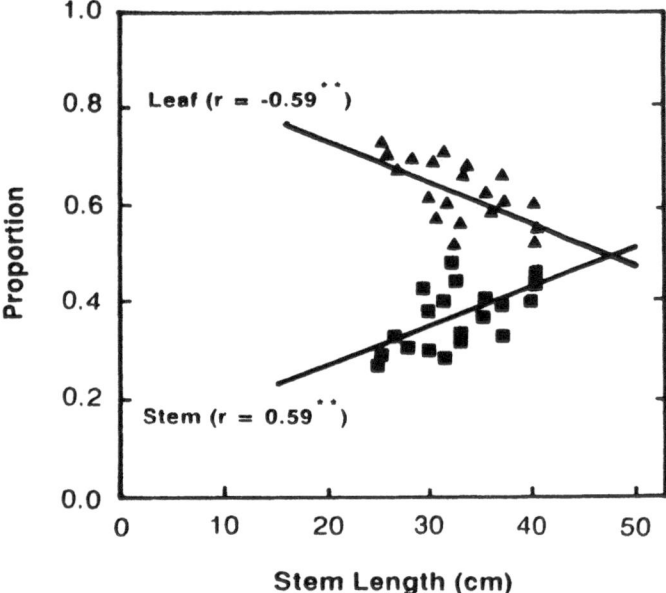

Fig. 3. Proportion of leaf and stem in barley straw of landraces at Breda, near Aleppo in north-west Syria.

hence plant number, low numbers of legumes restricts biological nitrogen fixation and hence soil fertility, and low soil fertility reduces plant growth and hence available pasture and production of seed.

In fact, native pasture is botanically extremely diverse and would seem to offer the possibility of improving productivity without expensive resowing programs. For example, at one 100 ha site, where the average yield of legume seed was 29 kg per ha, there were 43 different legume species. More widely, 97 different annual legumes have been collected from the cereal zone of Syria, almost exclusively from areas of native pasture.

A sensible approach to improving native pasture would therefore seem to be manipulation of either or both grazing management and soil fertility. Since the former has strong socio-economic implications, ICARDA has chosen the latter. While it is clear that improvement of soil fertility is a slow process, the results are clear (Fig. 2): in the third year herbage production of native pasture receiving only 8 kg per ha of phosphorus per year had increased by 70% in the presence of grazing animals. The experiment is typical of at least 25% of non-arable soils in Syria where available phosphorus is less than 10 ppm.

In drier areas (< 200 mm) the use of shrubs may be necessary. In these areas degradation of the native vegetation is more severe than in wetter areas, legumes are almost absent, and the original perennial vegetation has been lost. While improvement with shrubs is very expensive, preliminary analysis reveals that annual returns may be as high as 20% of capital invested (Cocks et al. 1986). Implementation would depend on improved grazing management but Draz (1978) believes that, by using techniques based on tribal land management and provided benefits could be demonstrated, farmers would be keen to improve management.

Clearly, improving native pasture continues to pose many problems, but recent research is suggesting that the rewards may be considerable.

Improving utilization of cereal straw and residues

In contrast to pastures and forages, straw is already an extremely important component of the diet of small ruminants, some 50 million tonnes of cereal straw being available for livestock in the Mediterranean basin. Until recently straw was from traditional varieties, indeed it remains so for barley in many countries. It is of surprisingly high quality as ewes are able to maintain liveweight on the local barley variety, Arabi Abiad, while losing weight on improved varieties (Table 6).

The high quality of Arabi Abiad is associated with late maturity, short stems, and a high proportion of leaf (Capper et al. 1986), factors which are inter-related (Fig. 3). As might be expected, they are also affected by environment, but the evidence suggests that genotypic differences remain consistent in different years and different environments. Agronomic treatment is believed to have relatively little effect, with nitrogen fertilization, time of sowing, seed rate, and grazing not affecting the nutritive value of barley straw significantly, although these conclusions need confirmation.

For wheat, the relationships seem similar, especially in that the traditional variety, Hourani, has better straw quality than the improved varieties, Sham 1 and Sham 2. It is noteworthy that Hourani was not able to maintain liveweight, in contrast to traditional barleys (ICARDA 1987).

Supplementation with small amounts of protein greatly increases the nutritive value of both wheat and barley straw. Limited supplementation with

Table 6. *Ad-libitum* intakes (g DM per $W^{0.75}$ per day) and liveweight changes (g per day) of Awassi sheep offered straw from seven improved and one traditional barley variety.

Variety	Intake	Liveweight change
Arar	34.8	−143
ER/Apam	39.0	−134
Rihane	40.3	−107
Beecher	38.9	−107
Badia	43.8	−80
Antares	45.2	−80
C63	50.9	−9
Arabi Abiad	51.1	+18
SEM	0.93	16.3

Source: Capper, Thomson and Rihawi (unpublished data).

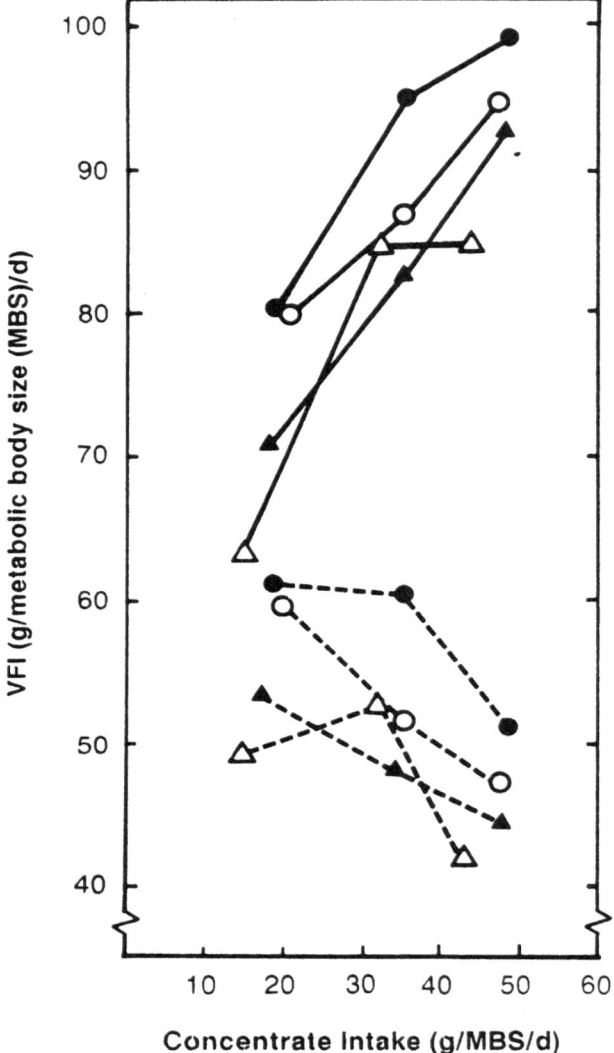

Fig. 4. Total voluntary feed intake (VFI) (solid lines) and VFI of straw (broken lines) of the barley varieties Abiad (closed circles), ER/Apam (open circles), Beecher (closed triangles), and C63 (open triangles) in ewes offered three levels of concentrate.

barley grain may increase voluntary intake of straw, but grain is far less effective than cottonseed cake, a locally available protein supplement. Considering the very low protein content of straw, this is not surprising and it has implications for the use of legume straws and residues which contain moderate amounts of protein. Perhaps grazing of cereal stubbles and medic residues on

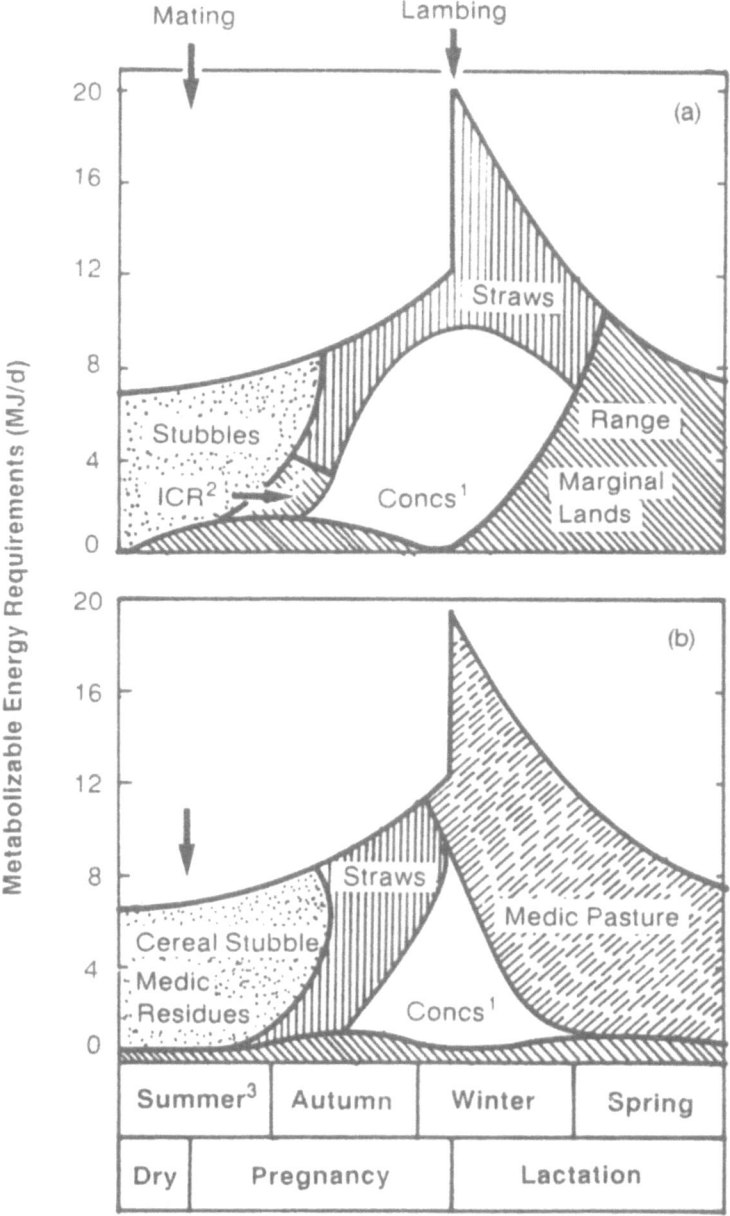

Fig. 5. Schematic presentation of the metabolizable energy requirements of sheep and the contribution of different feedstuffs during (a) traditional and (b) improved feeding cycles in north-west Syria. [1] Concs = feed grains (including forage legume grains) and industrial by-products (brans and oil-cakes); [2] ICR = irrigated crop residues; [3] starts 1 June.

Table 7. The effect of feeding ewes with barley straw and four levels of energy supplementation (four ewes per treatment).

	Low	Medium	High	Very high	SED
Straw intake (g per day)	911	1012	761	672	93.1
Concentrate intake (g per day)	649	889	1136	1310	183.6
Lamb gain[1] (g per day)	172	182	234	244	25.1
Milk yield[2] (kg)	37	39	46	48	–

[1] Weaned at 56 days.
[2] Total milk yield after weaning.

alternative days would increase the nutritive value of the former and extend utilization of the latter.

In addition to its effect on liveweight, supplementation of straw diets with barley grain also increases milk production and lamb growth rates (Table 7). Moreover, the effects of barley variety are also expressed even when moderate amounts of supplements are offered to ewes given *ad-libitum* access to straw (Fig. 4).

Matching feed resources and nutrient needs

In traditional systems herbage from native pasture and weedy fallows becomes available in winter and continues so until late spring. After harvest cereal and legume stubbles are grazed until, in late autumn, it becomes necessary to feed livestock with barley and conserved straw. Thomson (1987) has used survey information to show that barley grain and straw and native pasture provide 53 and 27%, respectively, of the annual metabolizable energy (ME) needs of lactating Awassi ewes. The remaining 20% comes from industrial by-products (such as cottonseed cake) and irrigated crop residues (Fig. 5a).

If the concepts discussed in this paper are implemented, the traditional feeding cycle will be substantially altered (Fig. 5b). Firstly, medic pasture will provide a high proportion of the ME needs of ewes and lambs during most of lactation. The energy and protein content of medics during winter and spring should be more than sufficient to allow ewes producing 1.5 kg of milk per day to cover their requirements. Secondly, a combination of cereal stubbles and dried medic pasture will provide the energy and protein needs of ewes before and after mating in summer. Ewes are able to gain liveweight on these residues, the amount varying from 20 to 50 g per day depending on stocking rate (Smith, personal communication). Such gains are essential if ewes are to achieve maximum lambing rates (Thomson and Bahhady, unpublished).

Thirdly, cereal and legume straws will provide most of the energy and protein needs during pregnancy, except during the last month when extra nutrients will be fed to cover increasing demands of the foetus, and to allow synthesis of body tissue reserves. In particular the straws of vetches and lentils

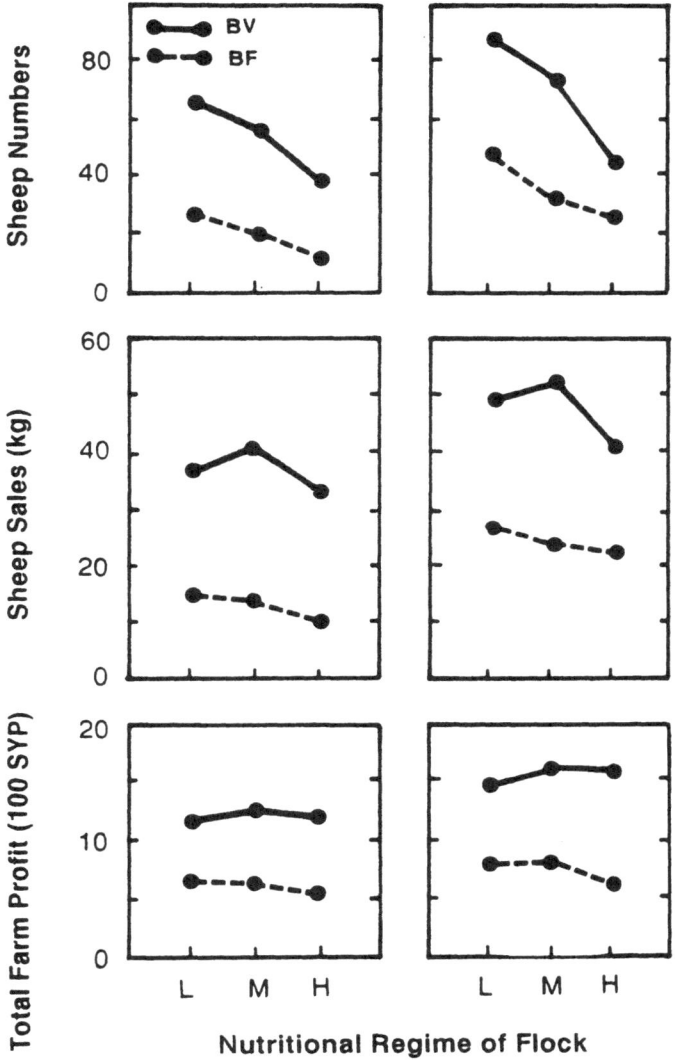

Fig. 6. Linear programming results showing sheep numbers and sales (milk, lambs, and cull ewes) and total farm profits (100 SYP/ha) of farms using barley/vetch (BV) and barley/fallow (BF) rotations and unimproved (left) and improved (right) native pasture. (100 USD = 9.75 SYP.)

are able to cover maintenance plus 250 g milk per day (ICARDA 1988), which is adequate to cover the nutrient needs of ewes during the first 4 months of pregnancy. Fourthly, the proposed feeding cycle will greatly reduce dependence on feed grains and industrial by-products. This is significant for two reasons. Feed grains, which are scarce in the region, can be used to fatten lambs, which is probably the most efficient way to use them, and there is a shortage of protein feeds which should be used to feed poultry. Grain harvested from legumes will also supply valuable protein.

Finally, the dependence on native pasture, especially in steppe areas with less than 200 mm rainfall will be minimized. If it becomes possible to increase stocking rates on high rainfall native pasture, even less pressure will be placed on the steppe. This will give governments more time to reverse the current process of degradation.

The possibility of more abundant feed makes it even more important to derive maximum benefit from these feeds. Nordblom and Thomson (1987) have shown that liberal feeding of lactating Awassi ewes is uneconomic, suggesting that farmers in Syria could increase flock profits by offering less feed, especially in winter (see Fig. 6). However, improving the genetic potential of Awassis through selection may be a more sensible alternative in the long run.

Conclusions

Research on pastures, forages, and livestock at ICARDA applies an agro-eco-logical approach, where farming systems are related to climate, especially rainfall. Attempts are also made to assess the economic significance of the newly developed farming practices and their effect on the sustainability of farming systems.

More information is needed on the agro-ecological boundaries of the various options described in this paper. For example, where is it best to use ley farming, what should be the boundary of the arid steppe, where should intensive annual cropping begin? We need to know more about how the various options are integrated, extend our work on ley farming to drier areas, facilitate and monitor adoption by farmers, respond to new problems, and establish a better economic base. Seed production of both pastures and forages needs to be encouraged. As well as an expanded plant breeding program, we need more information on the effect of new rotations on soil fertility and crop yields. In this context biological nitrogen fixation remains a high priority.

Nevertheless, the ICARDA work on meeting the nutritive needs of ever-increasing numbers of livestock is truly exciting. Our results indicate that in many areas livestock production and farm profitability could be doubled. By broadening the scope of our research to include some of the non-nutritional constraints we expect to further increase the usefulness of our existing results and create possibilities for even larger increases.

References

Abd El Moneim, A.M. and Cocks, P.S. 1986. Adaptation of *Medicago rigidula* to a cereal-pasture rotation in north-west Syria. Journal of Agricultural Science, Cambridge 107: 179–186.

Capper, B.S., Thomson, E.F., Rihawi, S., Termanini, A. and Macrea, R. 1986. The feeding value of straw from different genotypes of barley when given to Awassi sheep. Animal Production 42: 337–342.

Chatterton, B. and Chatterton, L. 1984. Alleviating land degradation and increasing cereal and livestock production in north Africa and the Middle East using annual *Medicago* pasture. Agriculture, Ecosystems, and Environment 11: 117–129.

Cocks, P.S. 1986. Integration of cereal-livestock production in the farming systems of north Syria. Pages 186–211 in Potentials of Forage Legumes in Farming Systems of Sub-Saharan Africa (Haque, I., Jutzi, S. and Neate, P.J.H., eds). ILCA, Addis Ababa, Ethiopia.

Cocks, P.S. and Ehrman, T.A.M. 1987. The geographic origin of frost tolerance in Syrian pasture legumes. Journal of Applied Ecology 24: 673–683.

Cocks, P.S., Thomson, E.F., Somel, K. and Abd El Moneim, A.M. 1986. Degradation and rehabilitation of agricultural land in north Syria. In Proceedings of a Conference on Degradation and Rehabilitation of Agricultural Land, March 1986, Canberra, Australia. In press.

Cooper, P.J.M., Gregory, P.J., Tully, D. and Harris, H.C. 1987. Improving water use efficiency of annual crops in the rainfed farming systems of west Asia and north Africa. Experimental Agriculture 23: 113–158.

Draz, O. 1978. Revival of the hema system of range reserves as a basis for the Syrian range development program. Pages 100–103 in Proceedings of the First International Rangeland Congress, 14–18 August 1978, Denver, Colorado (Hyder, D.N., ed.). Peerless Printing, Denver, Colorado, USA.

FAO (Food and Agriculture Organization). 1987. CGIAR Priorities and Future Strategies. FAO, Rome, Italy. 246 p.

ICARDA (International Center for Agricultural Research in the Dry Areas). 1986. Nutritive value of forages. Pages 318–320 in ICARDA Annual Report 1985. ICARDA, Aleppo, Syria.

ICARDA (International Center for Agricultural Research in the Dry Areas). 1987. Quality of wheat straw. Pages 178–185 in Pasture, Forage and Livestock Program Annual Report 1986. ICARDA 111 En. ICARDA, Aleppo, Syria.

ICARDA (International Center for Agricultural Research in the Dry Areas). 1988. Nutritive value of forage legume straws. Pages 87–89 in Pasture, Forage and Livestock Program Annual Report 1987. ICARDA, Aleppo, Syria.

Keatinge, J.D.H., Cooper, P.J.M. and Hughes, G. 1985. The potential of peas as a forage in the dryland cropping rotations of western Asia. Pages 185–191 in Proceedings of the 1984 Nottingham School of Agriculture, The Pea Crop – The Basis for Improvement. Butterworths, London, UK.

Materon, L.A. and Cocks, P.S. 1987. Biological nitrogen fixation by medic systems in western Asia. In Proceedings of a Symposium on Microbiology in Action, July 1986, University of Sydney, Australia. In press.

Nordblom. T.L. and Thomson, E.F. 1987. A Whole-Farm Model Based on Experimental Flocks and Crop Rotations in Northwest Syria. ICARDA-102 En. ICARDA, Aleppo, Syria. 87 p.

Osman, A.E. and Nersoyan, N. 1986. Effect of the proportion of species on the yield and quality of forage mixtures, and on the yield of barley in the following year. Experimental Agriculture 22: 345–351.

Papastylianou, I. 1987. Effect of preceding legume or cereal on barley grain and nitrogen yield. Journal of Agricultural Science, Cambridge 108: 623–626.

Papastylianou, I. and Samios, Th. 1987. Comparison of rotations in which barley for grain follows woollypod vetch or forage barley. Journal of Agricultural Science, Cambridge 108: 609–615.

Puckridge, D.W. and French, R.J. 1983. The annual legume pasture in cereal-ley farming systems of southern Australia: a review. Agriculture, Ecosystems, and Environment 9: 229–267.

Rossiter, R.C. 1966. Ecology of the Mediterranean annual-type pasture. Advances in Agronomy 18: 1–56.

Springborg, R. 1986. Impediments to the transfer of Australian dry land agricultural technology to the Middle East. Agriculture, Ecosystems, and Environment 17: 229–251.

Thomson, E.F. 1987. Feeding Systems and Sheep Husbandry in the Barley Belt of Syria. ICARDA-106 En. ICARDA, Aleppo, Syria. 20 p.

Thomson, E.F., Bahhady, F., Termanini, A. and Mokbel, M. 1986. Availability of home-produced wheat, milk products and meat to sheep-owning families at the cultivated margin of the NW Syrian steppe. Ecology of Food and Nutrition 19: 113–121.

E.F. Thomson and F.S. Thomson (eds), Increasing Small Ruminant Productivity in Semi-arid Areas
© 1988 ICARDA. ISBN 978-94-010-7086-7

A Comparison of Grazing and Browsing Ruminants in the Use of Feed Resources

P.J. Van Soest

Introduction

Differences in digestive ability and feeding behavior are among the various possible evolutionary adaptations by which herbivores obtain their dietary needs and maintain some control or assurance of feed supply. The differences are integrated to give the nutritional strategy of each species. The anatomy of the mouth parts (feeding apparatus) and the organization of the gastrointestinal tract impose behavioral strategies on herbivores that are optimal under the particular feeding conditions to which they are adapted.

The evolutionary adaptation of ruminants to a diet is commonly thought to have involved maximal extraction of energy from fibrous carbohydrates. This particular adaptation is in fact a characteristic of grazing bovids and may not apply to selective feeders and/or browsing types. Hofmann (1973) has divided herbivores into two categories: bulk and roughage eaters, including deer and small antelope, and intermediate feeders, including the goat and some of the more versatile antelope. Bulk and roughage eaters and the concentrate selectors are thought to have comparatively fixed strategies, the morphology of the mouth parts and digestive apparatus preventing more varied feeding behavior as seen in goats and other intermediate feeders. Hofmann's classification has been criticized as overly simplistic, and a two-dimensional system has been proposed (Demment and Van Soest 1983) that recognizes variable selectivity within both grazing and browsing strategies (Fig. 1).

Digestive physiology and feeding behavior

Various explanations have been suggested to account for differences between species in digestive physiology. These have included differences in buffering capacity and volatile fatty acid (VFA) absorption, rumen microbial population, efficiency of rumination, retention time, and faecal metabolic output. Selectivity must be included, a complex factor that involves the interaction between animal capability and the morphological differentiation of forage plants. Important subsidiary factors are the influence of environment upon forage morphology and compositional differentiation and the physicochemical nature of the food components.

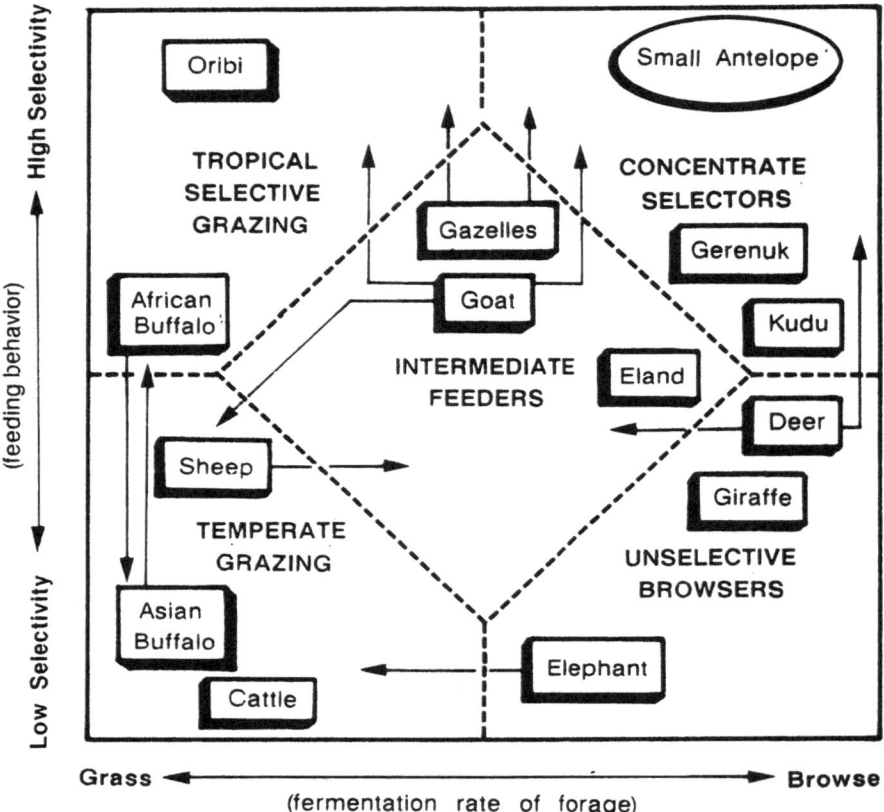

Fig. 1. An ordination of herbivore species based on diet. The axes are the degree of feeding selectivity and the amount of grass versus browse in the diet. The arrows indicate mobility of a species with respect to these axes.

The rates of digestion of forage components vary considerably. Generally, non-cell wall components like sugars, starch, and protein may be digested at rates which even animals with short retentions can digest. However, the digestion of cellulose, which is the fraction of forages most slowly digested, may set limits on the amount of energy extracted. One of the major limitations of digestion trials, which tend to be conducted at maintenance, is that when the same feeds are fed at a given production level, digestibility is often depressed because of the faster passage associated with high feed intake (Van Soest 1982).

A further weakness of conventional digestion trials is that they prevent selection, which is an important factor influencing results. They either allow very limited levels of feed refusal or do not measure them at all. This is a serious problem with many tropical forages or browses where there can be large differences in refusal levels and in the composition of what is and is not eaten. Selectivity may account for the purported difference in the ability of goats and cattle to digest fibre (Devendra 1978; El Hag 1976), since the more selective goat eats the less lignified tissue, and the more lignified refusal is not debited against the digestion balance.

Buffering and VFA absorption

Volatile fatty acids (VFA) are the major energy resource from anaerobic microbial fermentation in the digestive tracts of all animals. Whether or not the fermentation site is pregastric as in ruminants or postgastric as in most non-ruminants, the metabolic regulation is essentially the same. The VFA are absorbed across the gut wall in the free acid form, while sodium, bicarbonate, and urea flow in the reverse direction. Butyrate is extensively metabolized by the mucosa and is involved in its maintenance. The rate of absorption is directly proportional to the luminal concentrations. The net effect of this system is buffering of the produced acid via the pumping of hydrogen ions as free acids toward the blood side. The ions and the urea in the reverse flow plus the buffering substances in secreted saliva combine to provide regulation of rumen pH i.e., in the normal range of pH 6–7. If pH drops below 6 inhibition of digestion and fermentation occurs (Van Soest 1982).

Small antelope like dikdik and suni are reported to have higher VFA concentrations relative to sheep and cattle, reflecting a greater yield of VFA from fermentation of up to five-fold (Hoppe 1977). These high values reflect the high concentrate nature of their naturally selected diets. These species appear to have greater mucosal absorption surface, probably stimulated by VFA production (Hofmann 1973). Thus there is no evidence that inefficient VFA absorption will retard cellulolytic digestion, since for this to occur concentrations would need to accumulate to the point of either exceeding the buffering capacity with a drop in pH, or rise to inhibitory levels of osmotic pressure, neither of which appear to occur in small ruminants.

On the other hand, rumen acidosis is well known in cattle fed on high starch diets with all of the associated pathological problems including inhibition of cellulolytic digestion. It may be countered that these large grazers are being fed beyond their ecological and evolutionary dietary adaptation (Van Soest 1982). In the small concentrate-selector ruminants (Fig. 1) energy from cellulolytic fermentation is minor and the major function may be in part detoxification of tannins and alkaloids present in their food (Hofmann 1987).

Rumen microbial adaptation

Microbial adaptation is dependent upon substrate and therefore diet. The claim that a particular ruminant species can exclusively digest a certain plant depends on the rumen bacteria. For example, reindeer digest lichens with an efficiency of about 85% but *in vitro* digestion using fluid from a cow fed grass is only 15% (unpublished observations). Increasing the incubation time *in vitro* to 10–14 days allows microbial adaptation to occur and digestion increases. Rumen adaptation can be seen in Holstein heifers at the Alaska Agricultural Experimental Station which are commonly summer-pastured in the mountains near Palmer and eat a lot of lichen.

A similar situation exists with *Artimesia* (sage brush) which contains inhibitory terpenoid oils (Oh et al. 1968). Wapiti can digest *Artimesia* if exposed to the plant but find it unpalatable and so only eat it when other forage is limited. In contrast, although mimosine-degrading bacteria have been found in some Indonesian ruminants mimosine is not adaptable by the ordinary rumen organisms, suggesting that ruminal adaptation is not possible in this case and that specific inoculation is required to overcome the limitation.

Rumination, retention, and digestive capacity

All homeothermic animals require energy for maintenance which is a function of heat loss through body surfaces. The intraspecific relationship of this energy requirement to body mass is essentially a function of body weight to the power 0.75. On the other hand, the power relationship between fermentation contents or gastrointestinal capacities and body weight is 1.00–1.09 (Parra 1978; Demment and Van Soest 1983).

An equation can be derived from these two relationships (Van Soest 1982) showing that turnover i.e., retention time, is a function of body weight to the difference between the powers.

$$T = 31.4 \, DFGW^{0.25}$$

where T is rumen turnover time, D is digestibility, F is the ratio of wet rumen contents to body weight, G is rumen dry matter percent, and $W^{0.25}$ is the power of body weight. Because rumen turnover is related to body weight raised to the exponent 0.25, small ruminants need a shorter rumen turnover time (rumen contents replaced by new feed more often) than large ruminants to meet their maintenance energy requirements when eating diets of the same digestibility. This implies that the retention time in small animals is less than that in larger animals, and therefore they are generally less able to retain and use slowly fermented feeds. However, in posing this problem compensatory factors need consideration. These might include selective feeding to avoid slow digesting components, enlarged rumen capacity, or concentration of ingesta dry matter to avoid volume constraints.

Rate of passage and digestion balance measurements have been made at Cornell University on 46 species of mammals, including man. The various experiments have focused on the problem of animal size and digestive capacity (Van Soest et al. 1982).

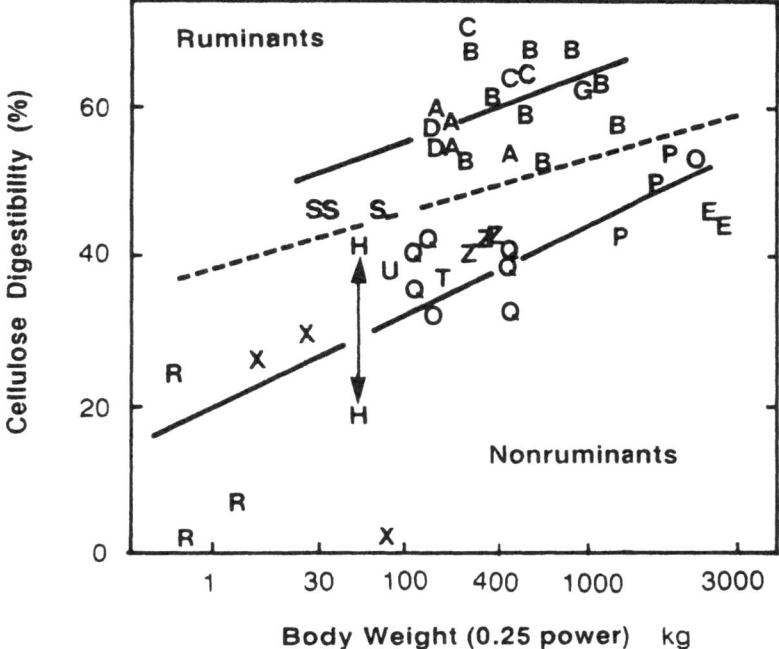

Fig. 2. Relationship between body weight and cellulose digestibility of various animal species fed grass-based diets. Range of values on high-fibre cereal diets observed in man (H) is designated by arrows. Regression equation for ruminants denoted by the upper solid line is $y = 42.0 + 4.0x$; $r = 0.56$; 21 degrees of freedom. Dashed line separates ruminants from nonruminants. Regression line for nonruminants (lower solid line) is $y = 14.5 + 5.4x$; $r = 0.74$; 24 degrees of freedom. H = man; X = beaver, panda, monkey; R = rodent; E = elephant; Q = horse, ass; A = antelope; T = tapir; C = camelid; Z = zebra; D = deer; P = rhinoceros; G = giraffe; O = hippopotamus; S = sheep, goat; Y = swine.

The capacity of both ruminant and non-ruminant mammalian herbivores to digest cellulose is related to body size (Fig. 2), with ruminants having a greater digestive capacity relative to size than non-ruminants. The capacity to digest cellulose is highly correlated with gastrointestinal retention time ($r^2 = 0.86$) and the same relationship appears to apply to both ruminants and non-ruminants. The comparison between mean retention time and body size is more varied (Fig. 3) but a strong association exists within the ruminant and non-ruminant subclasses.

The principal differences between ruminants and non-ruminants are that ruminants specialize in utilizing cellulosic carbohydrates and have sacrificed maximal intake for optimal extraction of the energy in cellulose. They retain food residues longer than non-ruminants of an equivalent size and rumen fermentation involves selective retention of fibre and comparatively fast passage of liquid. Restricted intake is the price of longer retention of slow digesting fibre, due to the volume devoted to fermentation and the time

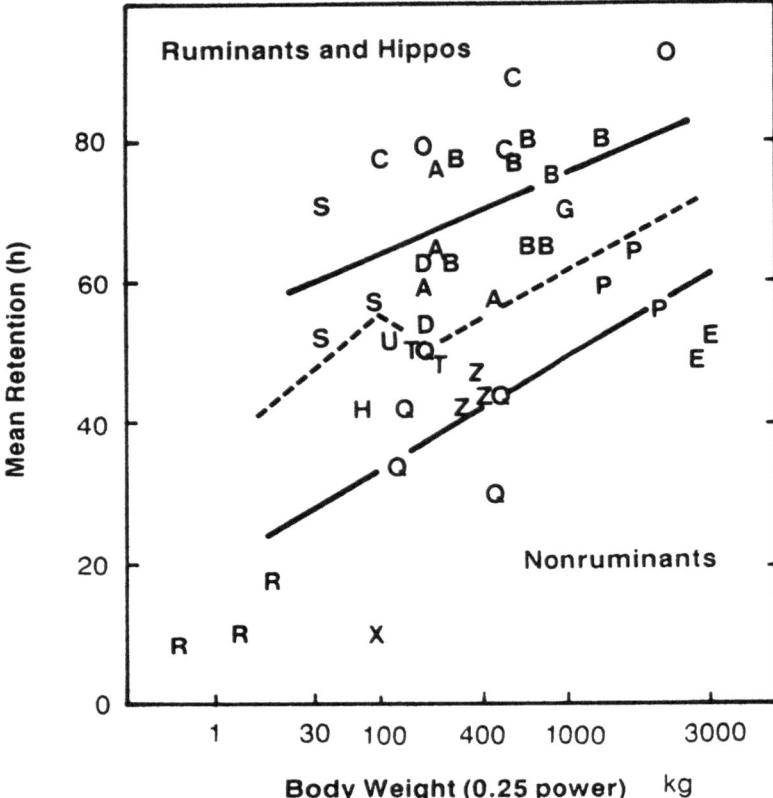

Fig. 3. Relationship between mean retention of fibre residues in the gastrointestinal tract and body weight. Upper solid line represents regression for ruminants, y = 49.6 + 0.49x; r = 0.45; 19 degrees of freedom. Dashed line separates nonruminants and hippos (pregastric fermentors). Lower solid line represents regression for nonruminants (excluding hippos), y = 13.4 + 6.4x; r = 0.68; 19 degrees of freedom. Letters as in Fig. 2.

required to process the ingesta. This presents a special problem for small ruminants that require more food energy per kg of body weight. Adaptations to overcome this limitation may include a larger omasal orifice (Hofmann 1987), larger rumen volume, and selective feeding.

Rumen bacteria that digest poor quality forages are limited by their substrate and are unable to increase the rate of digestion beyond the physicochemical limit reached after nutrient requirements are satisfied. There is no convincing evidence that small ruminants have more efficient bacteria and indeed some studies show that small ruminants have limited cellulolytic capacity (Hofmann 1973; Van Soest 1982).

There is no evidence that rumination or fine grinding increase digestion rates (Sequeira 1982). In fact, comminution increases transit and reduces

Table 1. Comparison of fibre particle size in the rumen and faeces of ruminants.

Type of animal	Body weight (kg)	Rumen particle size (microns)	Faecal particle size (microns)
Large heifers	550	2290	830
Small heifers	243	1670	640
Sheep	30	1290	460
Goats	29	1470	460

Source: Uden and Van Soest (1982).

rumen load and retention time, and so is associated with lower digestibility and greater faecal loss of potentially digestible matter.

Rumination capacity is also related to body size with an interspecific power of 0.95 (Van Soest 1982; Welch 1983). Small ruminants must chew to a smaller particle size (Uden and Van Soest 1982) and these particles must pass through a smaller orifice than in large ruminants (Table 1).

Shkolnik et al. (1987) have made interesting observations on the Bedouin goats in the Sinai. The rumen becomes a water-storage organ associated with slower liquid passage and rumen washout. Thus these goats are able to achieve longer rumen retention under conditions of limiting water and so increase the extent of digestion. This advantage disappears if the animals have access to unlimited water.

Faecal metabolic output

Faecal metabolic output is the faecal matter of non-dietary origin and constitutes the difference between apparent and true digestibility (Van Soest 1982). It is largely composed of the indigestible remnants of rumen microorganisms (Mason 1979) with the endogenous component being only about 15% of the total (Van Soest 1982). The amount of microbial matter in faeces is thus a reflection of the amount of gut fermentation. Ruminant species with a greater capacity for cellulolytic digestion tend to have larger metabolic losses so faecal metabolic loss is greater in cattle than in sheep and goats (Table 2).

The biological factors determining metabolic losses are influenced by retention. Small species, which have a larger energy requirement per unit of

Table 2. Values of true digestibility and metabolic losses of neutral-detergent solubles.

Animal species	True digestibility (slope)	Metabolic fraction (% of intake)	Source
Cattle	98	15.2	Van Soest 1982
Sheep	98	11.0	Van Soest 1982
Sheep	83	10.7	Parra 1978
Goats	100	9.9	McCammon-Feldman 1980

body size than large species, cannot retain digesta for as long or digest as much as larger grazing species. Therefore, smaller species derive less energy for maintenance from fermentation. This implies that smaller species digest more dietary matter post ruminally i.e., it escapes or by-passes the rumen, and this contributes to their lower metabolic losses.

Variation in metabolic losses accounts for some of the differences in digestive capacity between species. Those species with smaller metabolic losses will exhibit greater apparent digestibility with goats ranked over sheep and cattle (Huston et al. 1986), which is the opposite of what is expected from retentive capacities. Thus, reduced metabolic losses compensate for higher digestive losses of potentially digestible fibre.

The slower digesting fractions are those which will be selectively lost in faeces. These tend to be cellulose and the cellulosic carbohydrates peculiar to monocots, mature grasses in particular. Furthermore, since plant quality declines with age, so goats will be less able than cattle to digest fibre at lower potential digestibilities, but more able at higher digestibilities where the quantity of fibre is better. While there is an inadequate range of data for goats, this difference can be seen by comparing sheep and cattle. Mertens and Ely (1983) found that at digestibilities above 66%, sheep digested forages with higher digestion coefficients than cattle. Below 66% digestibility, they were increasingly inferior to cattle as digestibility decreased. The slope of the regression of cattle digestibilities upon sheep digestibilities was only 0.88, significantly less than unity. Thus it can be expected that on more digestible feeds goats will perform much better than grazing ruminants. This is consistent with their observed ability to select for quality.

Selection and morphology of forages

The inability of small ruminants to digest slow-fermenting dietary fractions is compensated for by their ability to selectively browse. Their prehensile lips and other aspects of mouth morphology are also important in selective feeding behavior. Another factor is the morphology of the forage plant itself and the differentiation of plants into fractions of diverse nutritional quality has been important in the evolution of selective feeders.

Reported digestibilities imply that tropical forages contain about 15 total digestible nutrient units less than temperate forages (McDowell 1972). This results from differences in climate and management. It may be difficult to harvest tropical forages at their optimum nutritive value because of rapidly changing quality and adverse conditions at harvest. However, the reported maximum and minimum digestibilities of forage grasses from extreme immaturity to full maturity show a definite pattern related to latitude and temperature during growth (Van Soest 1982).

Forages grown in cool or dry environments are more stressed than those grown in tropical environments (Van Soest et al. 1978). They use several strategies to survive in these conditions. One is to invest in energy reserves and reduce conversion of photosynthetic materials into structural substances such as lignin or cellulose which are unrecyclable sinks (Deinum et al. 1968). This produces a more nutritious plant, and is seen in adventitious plants that are grazed or browsed and require resources for regeneration. Adventitious plant species include most of those exploited in animal feeding and are included mostly in the Graminae and the Leguminosae. Other plants produce toxic substances when they are stressed, thereby protecting themselves against grazing, and some of these substances may be recyclable. A third category includes plants which reduce their growth rate to produce non-recyclable protective substances. These plants are not browsed or grazed, have an extremely low nutritive value, and are usually quite toxic.

The digestibility of forages grown at high temperatures is reduced because of increased structural cell well components. This is caused by increased metabolic activity at high temperatures, including greater activity of enzymes associated with lignin biosynthesis, and more rapid conversion of photosynthetic products into structural components such as lignin (Deinum et al. 1968). This reduces the pool size of nitrate, protein, soluble carbohydrates, and other metabolites in the cell. In tropical forages the pool size of the soluble carbohydrates is further reduced by respiration during the long dark periods.

Lack of water causes plants to adjust their photosynthetic resources. Therefore, desert plants may be highly nutritious but may produce tannins, terpenoids, or alkaloids as a means of defence against grazing or browsing. The early annual growth of browses is of much higher nutritional value than the older woody parts. Thus selective feeding behavior would be of an advantage where such feed is available.

In warm environments there is often a wide range in quality between different parts of a plant (Table 3). The difference in digestibility of leaves and leaf sheaths and stems is promoted by growth temperature. The leaves and stems of temperate grasses often have similar quality, and thus do not offer the

Table 3. Effect of temperature of growth upon digestibility [1] of leaf blade and of leaf sheath plus stems in *Brachiaria ruziensis* and *Setaria sphecelata*.

	Temperature (°C)		
	20–23 [2]	23–29	27–31
Brachiaria			
Leaf blade	76	72	67
Leaf sheath and stem	72	60	53
Setaria			
Leaf blade	74	68	67
Leaf sheath and stem	65	52	51

Source: Deinum and Dirven (1975; 1976).

[1] Original values in the publication were given as true digestibility and are converted to apparent values by subtraction of the metabolic constant 12.9.

[2] Range of night-day temperatures, respectively.

same possibilities for selective feeding as the tropical grasses. Some tropical grasses may show greater ranges in quality than those shown in Table 3. Unpublished analyses of Puerto Rican grasses at Cornell show that at 60 days of growth the digestibility of young leaves of Pangola grass was 60–70%, while in old leaves it was 53–62%. Digestibility of upper stems ranged from 46 to 56% and of lower stems from 41 to 45%. A similar analysis on Napier grass showed that young emerging leaves had a digestibility of 75–80% and that of lower stems was as low as 28%. The quality of tropical grasses also tends to vary with soil type. Poor soils may yield forages of higher digestibility because these plants are energy stressed and cannot produce so much lignin.

Shrubs and other browses

There is a large difference in nutritive value between the vegetative and woody parts of perennial shrubs, which may be browsed for their leaf or annual growth. Leaves of leguminous shrubs are high in protein and very low in true lignin and fibre because they have little structural function unlike grass leaves and sheaths. They tend to contain inhibitors such as tannins and alkaloids, which require less energy to produce than lignin.

The ability of ruminants to tolerate tannins is not completely understood. It may be that resistant species have enlarged salivary glands and salivate extensively so that mucins bind the tannin and make the protein available for digestion. This may imply evolutionary adaptation in browsing species (Hofmann 1987). Alternatively, there may be adaptation of the rumen microbes so that cell protein synthesis increases in order to bind tannins. This mechanism would increase the need for recycled urea and non-protein nitrogen sources (Horvath 1981).

Selection

Selective feeding allows animals of small digestive capacity to coexist with larger forms, provided that the available diet is sufficiently varied to allow selection. Thus, the diet of deer and cattle appears to be the same on high quality ryegrass pastures in New Zealand, but in North America deer eat browse almost exclusively and are crop pests.

Small ruminants probably receive only part of their energy from rumen fermentation, with more of the potentially digestible nutrients escaping the rumen than in larger grazing species (Hoppe 1977; Van Soest 1982). Hofmann (1987) postulates that small ruminants may temporarily open the omasal orifice to allow woody material to be expelled from the rumen, so relieving the load on rumination. He also suggests that small ruminants are non ruminant-like due to the quantities of digested feed that by-pass or escape the rumen to be directly digested in the abomasum and small intestine. In small ruminants, a smaller proportion of maintenance energy comes from VFA than in larger grazing species (Hoppe 1977), even though the former tend to have faster rates of fermentation and VFA production. The faster fermentation is a reflection of the higher nutritional quality of their selected diets.

Goats exhibit a considerable versatility in feeding behavior and are adaptable to a wide range of conditions, provided there is a supply of quality forage or browse. In tropical regions they exploit the better quality fractions of forages and this may allow them to perform better than cattle on the same diet. For example, when goats are fed Napier grass, refusals are about 30–60%.

Sheep that graze more and are less selective than goats could not be forced to consume all of an average Guinea grass hay. When forced to consume all the feed, severe underfeeding resulted (Tessema 1972). By comparison, cattle could be easily made to consume all of the same hay. This selective behavior is characteristic of all small ruminants and has been observed in dwarf sheep in Nigeria (Olubajo et al. 1974) and in goats in Western Kenya (Sands 1983).

Therefore, goats and other small ruminants are specialists and do not truly utilize cellulosic matter. Overgrazing and unavailability of high quality selective material will severely stress goats forced to eat highly lignified matter. However, goats maintain weight better than cattle during dry periods as they eat many browses and tropical legumes, selectively choosing leaves and parts of higher quality which cattle are unable to do (McCammon-Feldman et al. 1981).

Discussion

Sheep and goats are near the minimum limiting body size for efficient digestion of cellulosic carbohydrates (Demment and Van Soest 1983). These two species have the largest average gastrointestinal capacities (as percent of body weight). There is also a considerable variation in feeding both within and between the species. The smaller types may have compensated by investing more in dietary selection and reduced metabolic requirements for maintenance. This strategy presumes the existence of quality selectable forage browse that such small ruminants could exploit. Such environments would include desert and tropical regions. Temperate and cold-temperate adapted species may need to be larger in order to reduce surface heat losses and these animals exist in environments where nutritional uniformity of herbage offers less advantage for the selection mechanism.

The question also arises over the feasibility of animal selection for digestibility and food intake. These two seemingly desirable traits are probably inversely related. Most production studies (Van Soest 1982) have shown that feed intake is far more often the limiting factor in animal production and response than is digestibility.

Measurement of feed intake and passage characteristics of animals would be a very interesting exercise, since preliminary information on dairy cattle suggests large between-animal variation in situations where equal amounts of a standard diet are offered (Mertens, personal communication). However, such trials are expensive and require careful control of the standard diet so as to avoid confusion with dietary variation. Also, when a uniform standard diet is offered in a proper intake study the ability to select is abolished by the experimental management. There are no experimental models or procedures for measuring the ability to select, but this would theoretically become a relevant characteristic to study in sheep and goats.

References

Deinum, B. and Dirven, J.G.R. 1975. Climate, nitrogen and grass. 6. Comparison of yield and chemical composition of some temperate and tropical grass species grown at different temperatures. Netherlands Journal of Agricultural Science 23: 69–82.

Deinum, B. and Dirven, J.G.R. 1976. Climate, nitrogen and grass. 7. Comparison of production of *Brachiaria ruziensis* and *Setaria sphecelata* grown at different temperatures. Netherlands Journal of Agricultural Science 24: 67–78.

Deinum, B., Van Es, A.J.H. and Van Soest, P.J. 1968. Climate, nitrogen and grass. 2. The influence of light intensity, temperature and nitrogen on *in vivo* digestibility of grass and the prediction of these effects from some chemical procedures. Netherlands Journal of Agricultural Science 16: 217–233.

Demment, M.W. and Van Soest, P.J. 1983. Body size, digestive capacity and feeding strategies of herbivores. Winrock International Livestock Research and Training Center, Petit Jean Mountain, Morrilton, AR, USA.

Devendra, C. 1978. The digestive efficiency of goats. World Review of Animal Production 14: 9–22.

El Hag, G.A. 1976. A comparative study between desert goat and sheep efficiency of feed utilization. World Review of Animal Production 13: 43–48.

Hofmann, R.R. 1973. The Ruminant Stomach: Stomach Structure and Feeding Habits of East African Game Ruminants. East Africa Literature Bureau, Nairobi, Kenya.

Hofmann, R.R. 1987. Morphophysiological evolutionary adaptations of the ruminant digestive system. Pages 1–26 in Aspects of Digestive Physiology in Ruminants (Dobson, A., ed.). Cornell University Press, New York, USA.

Hoppe, P.P. 1977. Rumen fermentation and body weight in African ruminants. Pages 141–150 in Proceedings of the 13th International Congress of Game Biologists (Peterle, T.J., ed.). The Wildlife Society, Washington, D.C., USA.

Horvath, P.J. 1981. The nutritional and ecological significance of Acer-tannins and related polyphenols. MS thesis. Cornell University, Ithaca, New York, USA.

Huston, J.E., Rector, B.S., Ellis, W.C. and Allen, M.L. 1986. Dynamics of digestion in cattle, sheep, goats and deer. Journal of Animal Science 62: 208–215.

Mason, V.C. 1979. The quantitative importance of bacterial residues in the non-dietary faecal nitrogen of sheep. Zeitschrift fuer Tierphysiologie, Tierernaehrung und Futtermittelkunde 41: 131–139.

McCammon-Feldman, B. 1980. A critical analysis of tropical savanna forage consumption and utilization by goats. PhD thesis. University of Illinois, Urbana, USA.

McCammon-Feldman, B., Van Soest, P.J., Horvath, P. and McDowell, R.E. 1981. Feeding Strategy of the Goat. Cornell International Agricultural Mimeograph 88. Division of International Agriculture, Cornell University, Ithaca, New York, USA.

McDowell, R.E. 1972. Improvement of Livestock Production in Warm Climates. W.H. Freeman Co., San Francisco, USA.

Mertens, D.R. and Ely, L.O. 1983. Relationship of rate and extent of digestion to forage utilization–a dynamic model evaluation. Journal of Animal Science 54: 895.

Oh, H.K., Jones, M.B. and Longhurst, W.M. 1968. Comparison of rumen microbial inhibition resulting from various essential oils isolated from relatively unpalatable plant species. Applied Microbiology 16: 39–44.

Olubajo, F.O., Van Soest, P.J. and Oyenuga, V.A. 1974. Comparison and digestibility of four tropical grasses grown in Nigeria. Journal of Animal Science 38: 149–153.

Parra, R. 1978. Comparison of foregut and hindgut fermentation in herbivores. Pages 205–229 in The Ecology of Arboreal Folivores (Montgomery, G., ed.). Symposium of the National Zoological Park, 29–31 May 1975. Smithsonian Institute Press, Washington, D.C., USA.

Sands, M.S. 1983. Role of livestock on smallholder farms in Western Kenya: prospects for a dual purpose goat. PhD thesis. Cornell University, Ithaca, New York, USA.

Sequeira, C.A. 1982. Effect of grinding on the in vitro digestibility of forages. MS thesis. Cornell University, Ithaca, New York, USA.

Shkolnik, A., Brosh, A. and Choshniak, I. 1987. Goats and the desert ecosystems. Pages 115–119 in Proceedings of the Fourth International Conference on Goats, 8–13 March 1987, Brasilia, Brazil.

Tessema, S. 1972. Nutritional value of some tropical grass species compared to some temperate grass species. PhD thesis. Cornell University, Ithaca, New York, USA.

Uden, P. and Van Soest, P.J. 1982. The determination of digesta particle size in some herbivores. Animal Feed Science and Technology 7: 35.

Van Soest, P.J. 1982. Nutritional Ecology of the Ruminant. O & B Books, Corvallis, USA. 374 p.

Van Soest, P.J., Jeraci, J.L., Foose, T. Wrick, K. and Ehle, F. 1982. Comparative fermentation of fibre in man and other animals. Pages 75–79 in Proceedings of the Dietary Fibre in Human and Animal Nutrition Symposium (Wallace, G. and Bell, L., eds). 23–28 May 1982, Massey University. Royal Society of New Zealand, Palmerton North, New Zealand.

Van Soest, P.J., Mertens, D.R. and Deinum, B. 1978. Preharvest factors influencing quality of conserved forages. Journal of Animal Science 47: 712.

Welch, J.G. 1983. Rumination, particle size and passage from the rumen. Journal of Animal Science 54: 885.

E.F. Thomson and F.S. Thomson (eds), Increasing Small Ruminant Productivity in Semi-arid Areas
© *1988 ICARDA . ISBN 978-94-010-7086-7*

Improving Livestock Production from Straw-Based Diets

H.B. Perdok, R.A. Leng, S.H. Bird, G. Habib and M. Van Houtert

Introduction

Straw alone is a poor quality feed. It is deficient in the soluble nitrogen and minerals needed to support an active and efficient rumen microbial ecosystem and therefore a high feed intake and digestibility. It contains little or none of the nutrients which escape rumen degradation and lacks nutrients that augment the products of fermentative digestion. It is also low in lipid and, although it has a high content of potentially fermentable carbohydrate, it has a low actual digestibility due to the close association of the carbohydrates with lignin. In addition, depending on soil and growing conditions, straw is also deficient in the nutrients required by the microbes that digest straw e.g., Co and S, and in the minerals essential to the well-being of the animal e.g., P, Na, Mg, Cu, and Zn.

The digestibility of cereal crop residues can vary widely depending on variety, growth characteristics as affected by water and fertilizer availability during growth and plant diseases, and method of harvesting (Nicholson 1984). For example, in Indonesia, rice is harvested as the grain is required. The straw is often fed to livestock immediately, so it contains some green leaf and therefore has a higher digestibility and protein content than the average straw. In parts of China, the wheat crop is pulled from the ground and often includes lower stems and roots which are of low digestibility.

Improving the nutritional value of straw

Methods for improving the nutritional value of straw can be divided into two broad categories which are often complementary and additive. The first category includes those methods that increase actual digestibility in the rumen, for example supplementation and physical or chemical treatment. The other category includes supplementation or manipulation to balance the nutrients absorbed more closely to those required for production.

Increasing digestibility

Straw has a potential digestibility of 80% (Jackson 1977) but the actual digestibility rarely exceeds 55%. There is therefore scope for increasing the straw is governed by its residence time and its rate of digestion in the rumen. In turn, the latter can be affected by pretreating the straw and the rate and extent of colonisation by fungi and bacteria.

Increasing digestibility by manipulating the crop

Fractionation of the cereal plant

Fractionation of cereal crop residues into portions with high and low digestibility is rational when the straw is to be used for more than one purpose i.e., as feed or fuel. In general, the digestibility of the upper parts of the plants is 5–10 units higher than that of the lower stems and roots, and simple physical fractionation methods can be applied after harvest. Alternatively, the crop can be fractionated by selective feeding. Goats and sheep will select the leaves and upper stems and so increase their total feed intake, provided they are given sufficient feed to be able to readily select (Table 1) (Zemmelink 1986; Owen and Wahed 1986).

Treatment with alkali or acid

Chemical treatment of straw with alkali or acid improves digestibility. Treatment causes swelling of the vascular bundles, solubilisation of hemicellulose,

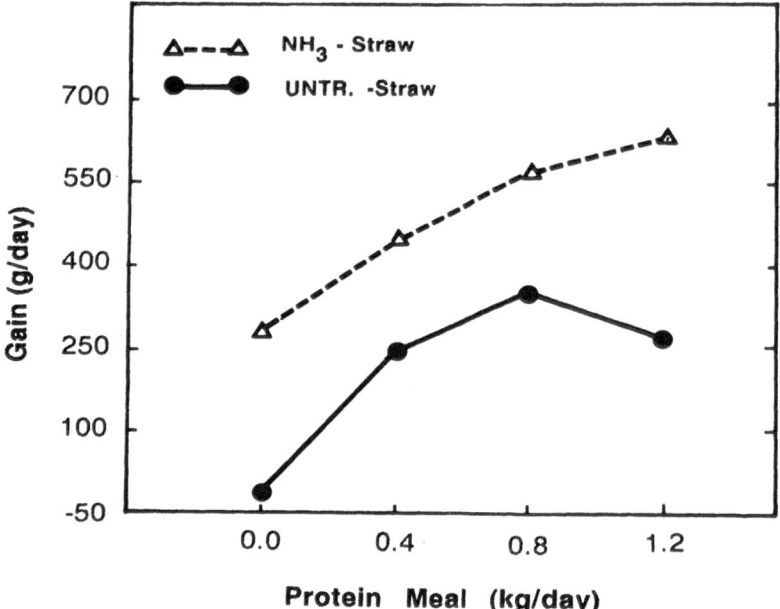

Fig. 1. Growth rate of young cattle on a basal diet of ammoniated rice straw or untreated rice straw supplemented with various levels of a bypass protein meal (Perdok and Leng 1987).

Table 1. Intake of straw dry matter by goats offered straw at 120 or 150%. Intake when no selection is allowed is 100% (18 goats/group).

Feed	Straw allowance as % of intake	
	120	150
Straw intake (kg DM/100 kg lwt)	1.4	1.8

Source: Owen and Wahed (1986).

separation of the highly lignified materials, and some hydrolysis of the lignocellulose bonds. This increases the accessibility of cell wall components to rumen microbes and usually increases digestibility from approximately 45 to 55%. Rigorous hydrolysis with strong acids and alkalis can result in a digestibility of 80% (Dryden and Leng 1986).

Treating straw with gaseous-, aqueous-, or urea-ammonia is currently the most practical and potentially economic means of increasing digestibility. The increase in productivity that can be achieved by feeding treated straw is shown in Fig. 1.

Balancing the rumen with essential nutrients for microbes

The effect of a deficiency in any nutrient that limits microbial growth is a net decrease in the efficiency of utilization of the energy (ATP) made available in fermentation for microbial cell synthesis. The overall effect is a decreased pool size of microbes and, in some cases, single species with specific or high requirements for the deficient nutrients may be eliminated. For example, fungi disappear from the rumen of sheep on low sulphur diets (Akin et al. 1983).

Rumen ammonia concentrations must be above 150 mg N/l to optimise straw intake (Fig. 2) (Perdok and Leng unpublished; Boniface et al. 1986). At these levels, optimum intake of straw is supported although digestibility, as measured by the nylon bag technique, is apparently constant when rumen ammonia levels exceed approximately 50–100 mg N/l (Perdok and Leng unpublished; Boniface et al. 1986). The apparently lower ammonia requirement for optimum digestibility than for maximising intake may be an artefact of the nylon bag technique. It is probable that at low levels of rumen ammonia, the *in sacco* technique overestimates organic matter digestibilities, as would arise if small particles are lost from the bag during washing. At higher ammonia levels, when most small particles in the nylon bags have been largely digested, the *in sacco* digestibility is closer to true digestibility. This is clearly shown when cotton wool, which is not broken down into small particles, is used as the substrate (Krebs and Leng 1984; Perdok and Leng unpublished; Fig. 2).

There is considerable controversy as to whether or not other nitrogenous compounds, such as amino acids, peptides, or branched chain and higher volatile fatty acids (VFAs), are essential nutrients affecting efficiency of microbial growth in the rumen.

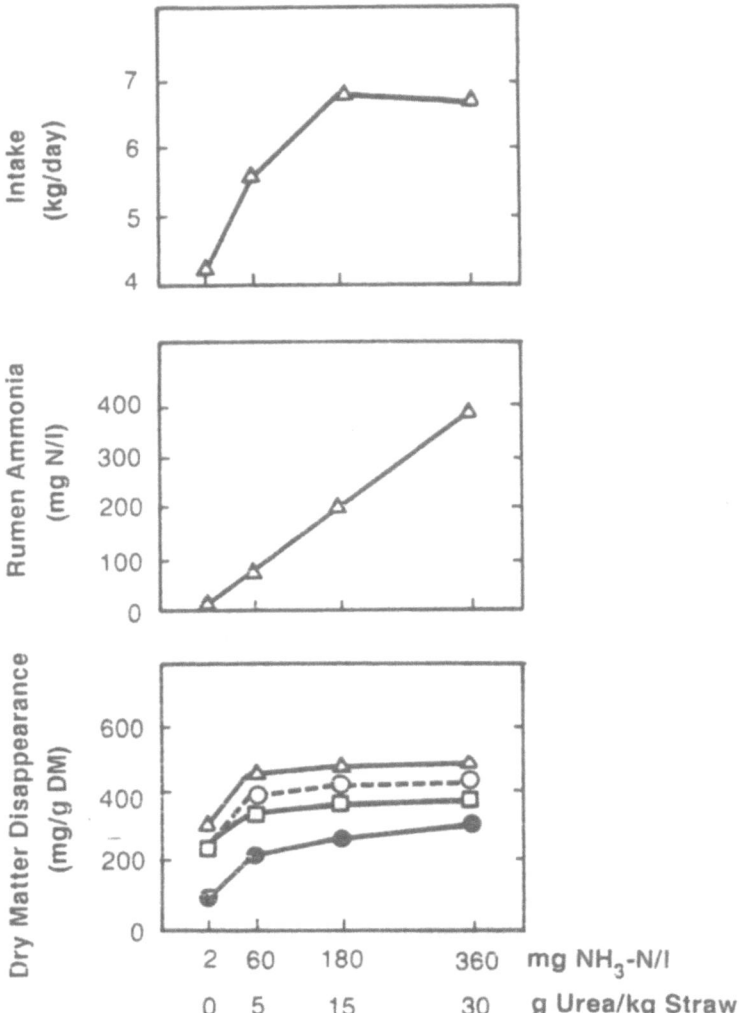

Fig. 2. The effects of urea infused into the rumen on rumen ammonia concentrations, straw intake, and dry matter digestibility in cattle fed rice straw plus minerals (Perdok and Leng, unpublished). Dry matter digestibility at 24 h of NH_3-treated straw (triangles), urea ensiled (open circles), untreated (squares), and cotton wool (closed circles).

Manipulating the size of the colonising microbial pool

Supplementing a basal straw diet of low digestibility with a small quantity of a readily and highly digestible forage increases straw digestibility (Juul-Nielsen 1981; Silva and Ørskov 1985). Data illustrating this are shown in Table 2. The

Table 2. The effects of supplementing with high digestibility fibre at 10% of a wheat straw-based diet on the DM disappearance of straw, ammoniated straw, or cotton wool from nylon bags in the rumen. Sheep were fed diets of straw or ammoniated straw with supplements to ensure adequate minerals and ammonia in the rumen.

Material in nylon bag	Supplement	DM disappearance (%) from nylon bag at		
		12h	24h	48h
Basal diet untreated straw				
Untreated	nil	17	27	35
straw	+ lucerne	20	32	42
Ammoniated	nil	26	41	58
straw	+ lucerne	32	41	62
Cotton wool	nil	25	48	81
	+ lucerne	31	54	91
Basal diet ammoniated straw				
Untreated	nil	13	23	32
straw	+ lucerne	16	28	37
Ammoniated	nil	28	41	55
straw	+ lucerne	30	47	58
Cotton wool	nil	27	40	63
	+ lucerne	31	47	85

Source: Romulo, B., Bird, S.H. and Leng, R.A., unpublished.

highly digestible forage may increase the number of free bacteria in the rumen fluid that can colonise straw particles, or it may stimulate the growth of rumen fungi. Even a small fungal biomass growing on the high quality forage could produce a massive number of zoospores to infect the major forage component of the diet. Stimulated fungal growth on the forage may result in more rapid development of fragile straw particles (Akin et al. 1983), easier rumination, more rapid comminution of feed particles, increased fermentation, and faster outflow from the rumen of the less digestible components. Whatever the effect, small farmers in developing countries have recognised the benefits of supplementing straw with a more digestible forage and traditionally give a handful of green forage to straw-fed ruminants.

Manipulating the balance of organisms in the rumen

Effects on productivity of the unfaunated rumen

Studies at the University of New England over the past 10 years have clearly shown that the absence of protozoa in the rumen i.e., the unfaunated state, has increased wool growth of sheep on both green and dry pasture (Table 3) and in those given treated or untreated straws with various supplements (Table 4; Fig. 3). The increases in productivity have all been related to increases in the bacterial and fungal biomasses in the rumen and to higher straw digestibility (Table 4).

Table 3. Wool growth rate and body weight gain of faunated (+ P) and defaunated (− P) sheep grazing native pasture.

Sheep type and year		No. of animals	Study period (weeks)	Bodyweight gain (g/d)		Wool growth (g/d)	
				+ P	− P	+ P	− P
Ewes	1982	32	23	− 48	− 48	3.6 [a1]	4.4 [b]
	1983	39	23	67	73	6.6 [a]	7.0 [b]
	1984	37	52	8	0	7.5	7.5
Weaner lambs	1983	49	16	85 [a]	98 [b]	7.2	7.6

Source: Bird and Leng (1985).
[1] Means in the same row with a different superscript differ significantly (P < 0.05).

Table 4. Disappearance of dry matter from nylon bags incubated in the rumen of faunated (+ P) and defaunated (− P) sheep given untreated or ammoniated wheat straw.

Basal diet	Material in nylon bag	DM disappearance (%) at			
		6 h		24 h	
		+ P	− P	+ P	− P
Wheat straw	Wheat straw	18 [a1]	23 [b]	37	40
NH_3-wheat straw [2]	NH_3-wheat straw	15 [a]	20 [b]	50 [a]	55 [b]
	Cotton wool	4	6	63 [a]	72 [b]
Wheat straw [2]	Wheat straw	5	6	32 [a]	37 [b]
	Cotton wool	12	12	74 [a]	88 [b]

[1] Means in the same row and same incubation time with a different superscript differ significantly (P < 0.05).
[2] *Source*: Romulo et al. (1986).

Greater wool growth in unfaunated sheep than in control sheep (Bird and Leng 1985; Habib and Leng unpublished) indicates increased sulphur amino acid absorption from the small intestine. This is difficult to explain in the straw-based diets without a concomitant increase in digestibility and/or feed intake. With these diets, protozoal numbers are usually very low and probably form only a small proportion of the total microbial biomass. It is difficult to associate defaunation (i.e., the removal of protozoa by detergents) with a large increase in microbial protein availability to sheep on such diets (Veira et al. 1983). Recent feeding trials from our laboratories have shown that defaunated lambs on wheat straw diets consumed more straw and had greater bodyweight gains and wool growth than faunated lambs (Figs 3 and 4).

The development of methods to create and preserve the unfaunated state in sheep and cattle on straw-based diets together with supplementation could contribute to improving production of animals on such diets.

Modifying rumen organisms

The advent of recombinant DNA technology has created the possibility of improving the ability of the rumen microbes to digest fibrous feeds. In

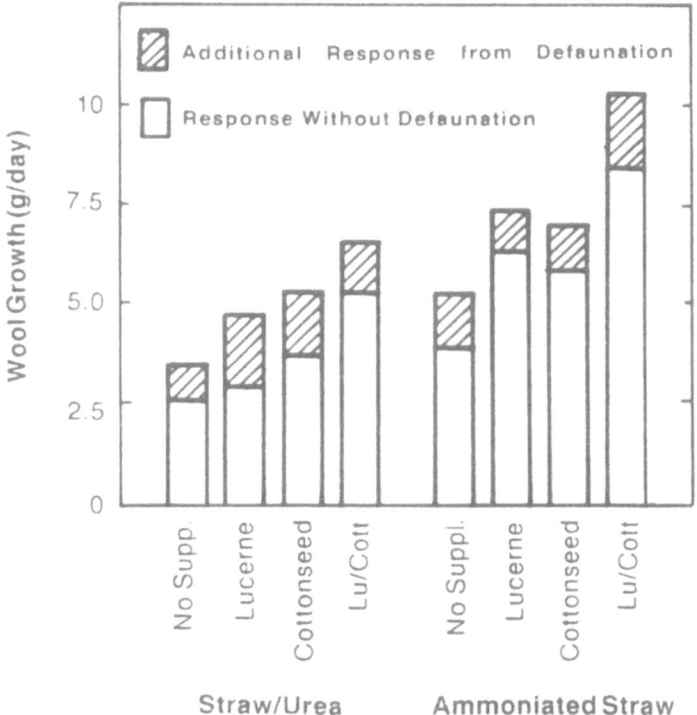

Fig. 3. The effects of straw treatment, supplementation, and defaunation on wool growth of sheep fed straw-based diets (Bird, Romulo, and Leng, unpublished).

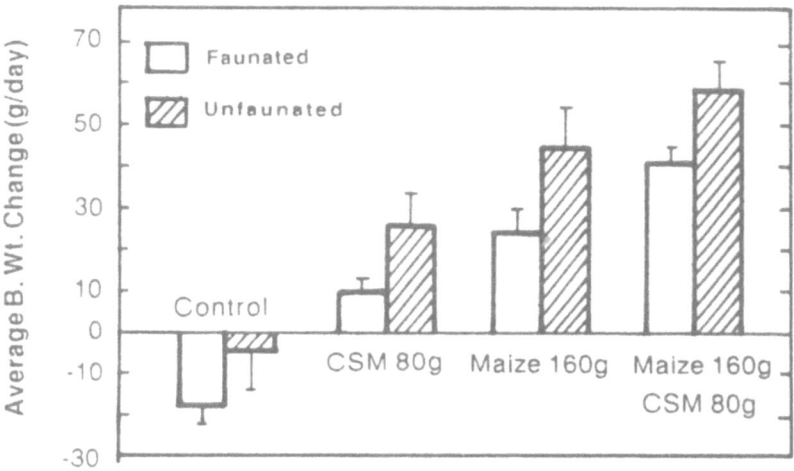

Fig. 4. The effects of supplementation of straw-based diets with maize and/or bypass protein (cottonseed meal, CSM) in faunated and unfaunated lambs (Habib and Leng, unpublished). Vertical bars show standard errors of mean.

addition, there is the potential for improving the composition of nutrients absorbed from the rumen to provide a better balance of nutrients to meet productive needs. A number of strategies have been suggested. The overall cellulolytic activity of the microbial pool could be improved or cellulolytic activity could be developed in microbes previously demonstrating only xylanolytic activity, thereby increasing the efficiency of a single organism faced with mixed substrates. Organisms growing on xylan will run out of substrate before those growing on cellulose so the latter will only be able to colonise cellulose at some later time after feeding. The protein content and amino acid balance of microbes and the efficiency of substrate utilisation could also be improved. This would make them more efficient users of ATP. Rumen organisms could be developed with the capability to detoxify some plant toxins and solubilise lignins, thus increasing the range of feeds and supplements suitable for ruminants.

Accelerating fibre degradation by increased cellulolytic activity of the microbial pool in the rumen is an attractive objective, especially if the antibacterial properties of lignin can be moderated by solubilisation. The objective is to increase the rate and extent of fibre breakdown in the rumen, thus increasing both nutrient extraction and the amount of straw consumed. When developed, the techniques will only be beneficial when there are no deficiencies of nutrients that are essential for microbial growth in the rumen. This means that in an intensive feeding or field situation, nutrient limitations for the rumen microbes must be identified and corrected if research modifying rumen microbes is to be successfully applied.

Achieving a balance of absorbed nutrients compatible with requirements

Ruminants use an array of nutrients which include acetate, propionate, butyrate, dietary and microbial amino acids, and long-chain fatty acids (LCFAs). The efficiency of feed utilisation depends on the balance of nutrients available, which in turn depends on the efficiency of rumen microbial growth, the pattern of VFA production, and the extent to which dietary nutrients escape the rumen and are digested in the lower intestine.

The requirements for nutrients depend on the physiological state of the animal. Thus, the amounts of amino acids, glucose, LCFAs, and oxidisable substrates needed to meet the nutrient requirements for work, maintenance, and synthesis of tissues and milk are obviously variable. The nutrient requirements are shown in Table 5. Glucose and amino acids are undoubtedly essential and the availability of either one could be a primary constraint to production. Providing a bypass protein meal as a supplement is a practical means of improving the balance of glucogenic or aminogenic substrates to ruminants on straw-based diets (Leng and Brumby 1986).

The effects of supplying bypass protein as a supplement to cattle on ammoniated or untreated straw diets are shown in Fig. 1. The overall effect in

Table 5. The critical nutrients limiting production in different physiological states. These nutrients must be supplied and absorbed in sufficient quantities and ratios for the particular function. When the balances of absorbed nutrients are optimised, both feed intake and feed efficiency are increased.

Physiological function	Limiting nutrients
Growth (lean)	Amino acids
Growth (fattening)	Glucose, LCFAs, amino acids
Puberty	Glucose, amino acids
Conception	Glucose, amino acids
Pregnancy	Glucose, amino acids
Lactation	Glucose, amino acids, LCFAs
Work	Glucose, LCFAs
Wool growth	Amino acids

Source: Preston and Leng (1986).
LCFAs = Long-chain fatty acids.

this trial was increased efficiency of feed utilisation rather than increased straw intake. An increase in basal diet intake often occurs when bypass protein is used to supplement straw-based diets and, in general, increases in feed intake stimulate productivity (Leng et al. 1977; Preston and Leng 1984). This means that balancing the nutrients closer to production requirements reduces the amount of metabolic heat generated by ruminants on straw-based diets and so minimises the wasteful expenditure of nutrients.

Fibrous crop residues are low in fats (Theander and Aman 1984) and considerable quantities of glucose must be oxidised to promote fat synthesis from acetate. Recent studies (Van Houtert and Leng 1986) have demonstrated that fats are efficiently utilised when protein and fat are supplemented simultaneously (Fig. 5).

Tissue growth requires less glucose, LCFAs, and amino acids than foetal growth in late pregnancy or milk production. It is therefore not surprising that

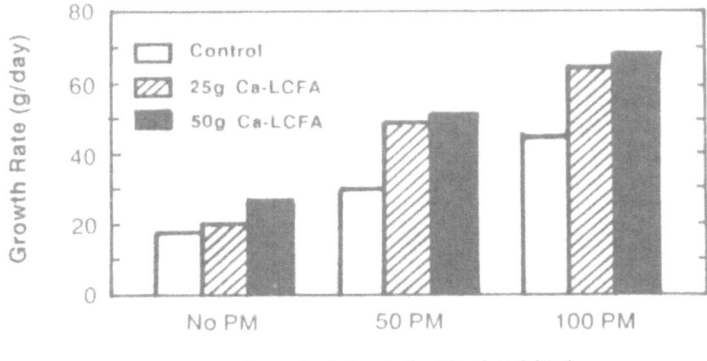

Fig. 5. The effects of feeding unreactive forms of long-chain fatty acids (Ca-soaps) and bypass protein on growth of lambs given ammoniated rice straw.

during pregnancy and lactation animals show a greater response to a balanced nutrient supply and improved intake.

The fact that tissue and foetal growth, and milk and wool production respond to balanced nutrition on straw-based diets appears now to be irrefutable (Leng and Brumby 1986; Leng et al. 1987; Preston and Leng 1986). What is only casually apparent is that ovulation, conception, and male fertility are also influenced by the nutrient balance during the mating season (Preston and Leng 1986).

Conclusions

Straw cannot be regarded as a poor quality forage since with correct supplementation, moderate levels of production can be achieved. It is better therefore, to refer to straw as an unbalanced forage, as this emphasises the primary constraint to production of animals consuming straw-based diets. The growth rates of cattle and sheep given treated straw that is supplemented with a variety of specific nutrients may approach that which would be achieved on so-called high quality pasture.

There are a number of manipulations that can be used to improve straw utilisation by ruminants. These could be very important in those Third World countries where straw forms a major proportion of the diet of ruminants for part or all of the year, provided that simple means of application can be found.

References

Akin, D., Gordon, G.L.R. and Hogan, J.P. 1983. Rumen bacterial and fungal degradation of *Digitaria pentzii* grown with or without sulphur. Applied and Environmental Microbiology 46: 738–748.

Bird, S.H. and Leng, R.A. 1985. Productivity responses to eliminating protozoa from the rumen liquor of sheep. Pages 109–117 in Biotechnology and Recombinant DNA Technology in the Animal Production Industries–Reviews in Rural Science 6 (Leng, R.A., Barker, J.S.F., Adams, D.B. and Hutchinson, K.J., eds). University of New England Publishing Unit, Armidale, Australia.

Boniface, A.N., Murray, R.M. and Hogan, J.P. 1986. Optimum level of ammonia in the rumen liquor of cattle fed tropical pasture hay. Proceedings of the Australian Society of Animal Production 16: 151–154.

Dryden, G. McL. and Leng, R.A. 1986. Treatment of barley straw with ammonia and sulphur dioxide gases under laboratory conditions. Animal Feed Science and Technology 14: 41–54.

Jackson, M.G. 1977. The alkali treatment of straw. Animal Feed Science and Technology 2: 105–130.

Juul-Nielsen, J. 1981. Nutritional principles and productive capacity of the Danish straw-mix system for ruminants. Pages 287–299 in Maximum Livestock Production from Minimum Land (Jackson, M.G., Dolberg, F., Haque, M. and Saadullah, M., eds). Bangladesh Agricultural University, Mymensingh, Bangladesh.

Krebs, G. and Leng, R.A. 1984. The effect of supplementation with molasses/urea blocks on ruminal digestion. Proceedings of the Australian Society of Animal Production 15: 704.

Leng, R.A. and Brumby, P. 1986. Cattle production in the tropics. Pages 884–887 in Proceedings of the 13th International Congress of Nutrition, Brighton (Taylor, T.G. and Jenkins, N.K., eds). John Libbey, London, UK.

Leng, R.A., Nolan, J.V. and Kempton, T.J. 1977. Non-protein nitrogen and bypass proteins in ruminant diets. Pages 1–21 in Australian Meat Research Council Review No. 33 (November).

Leng, R.A., Perdok, H.B. and Kunju, G.P.J. 1987. Supplementing fibrous feeds to increase ruminant production. Pages 70–73 in Proceedings of the Fourth Asian-Australian Animal Production Congress, 1–6 Feb 1987. New Zealand Society of Animal Production, Hamilton, New Zealand.

Nicholson, J.W.G. 1984. Digestibility, nutritive value and feed intake. Pages 340–372 in Rice Straw and Other Fibrous By-Products as Feed (Sundstol, F. and Owen, E., eds). Elsevier Press, Amsterdam, The Netherlands.

Owen, E. and Wahed, R.A. 1986. The effects of amount offered on selection and intake of barley straw by goats. Pages 312–315 in Rice Straw and Related Feeds in Ruminant Rations (Ibrahim, M.N.M. and Schiere, J.B., eds). Agricultural University, Wageningen, The Netherlands.

Perdok, H.B. and Leng, R.A. 1988. Effect of supplementation with protein meal on the growth of cattle given a basal diet of untreated or ammoniated rice-straw. Accepted by Animal Feed Science and Technology.

Preston, T.R. and Leng, R.A. 1984. Supplementation of diets based on fibrous residues and by-products. Pages 373–413 in Straw and Other Fibrous By-Products as Feed (Sundstol, F. and Owen, E., eds). Elsevier Press, Amsterdam, The Netherlands.

Preston, T.R. and Leng, R.A. 1987. Ruminant Production with Available Feed Resources in the Tropics and Sub-Tropics. Penambul Books, Armidale, Australia.

Romulo, B.H., Bird, S.H. and Leng, R.A. 1986. The effects of defaunation on digestibility and rumen fungi counts in sheep fed high-fibre diets. Proceedings of the Australian Society of Animal Production 16: 327–330.

Silva, A.T. and Ørskov, E.R. 1985. Effect of unmolassed sugar beet pulp on the rate of straw degradation in the rumens of sheep given barley straw. Proceedings of the Nutrition Society 44: 50A.

Theander, O. and Aman, P. 1984. Anatomical and chemical characteristics. Pages 45–78 in Straw and Other Fibrous By-Products as Feed (Sundstol, F. and Owen, E., eds). Elsevier Press, Amsterdam, The Netherlands.

Van Houtert, M. and Leng, R.A. 1986. Strategic supplements to increase the efficiency of utilisation of rice straw by ruminants. Pages 282–284 in Rice Straw and Related Feeds in Ruminant Rations (Ibrahim, M.N.M. and Schiere, J.B., eds). Agricultural University, Wageningen, The Netherlands.

Veira, D.M. 1986. The role of ciliate protozoa in nutrition of the ruminant. Journal of Animal Science 63: 1547–1560.

Veira, D.M., Ivan, M. and Jui, P.Y. 1983. Rumen ciliate protozoa: effects on digestion in the stomach of sheep. Journal of Dairy Science 66: 1015–1022.

Zemmelink, G. 1986. Evaluation and utilisation of tropical forages. Pages 285–298 in Rice Straw and Related Feeds in Ruminant Rations (Ibrahim, M.N.M. and Schiere, J.B., eds). Agricultural University, Wageningen, The Netherlands.

Part II

Breeding

E.F. Thomson and F.S. Thomson (eds), Increasing Small Ruminant Productivity in Semi-arid Areas
© 1988 ICARDA . ISBN 978-94-010-7086-7

Breeding Strategies for Small Ruminants in Arid and Semi-Arid Areas

G.E. Bradford and Y.M. Berger

Introduction

Sheep and goats that have evolved in arid or semi-arid environments are usually well adapted to their environment. The productivity of these animals is low compared to performance of these species in more favorable environments, but their ability to survive and reproduce in bad years as well as good is remarkable. Because of this, sheep and goats help ensure the survival of people in dry areas in years of drought and provide extra income in years of normal rainfall.

With increasing human population in many areas where sheep and goats are important, an urgent goal is to increase the offtake of small ruminant products i.e., meat, fiber, milk, and skins, without degrading the grazing resource.

Flamant et al. (1979) point out that in environments where adaptation is critical, natural selection favors the development of animals with a balance among reproduction, growth rate, and maintenance requirements. Crossing locally adapted breeds with breeds selected for higher performance can upset this balance, leading to a loss of adaptation which may impact unfavorably on the lives of many people. Even selection for performance within the adapted breeds may result in a loss of adaptation, though less so than from crossing with exotic breeds. The possibility of changing the genetic potential of animals highly adapted to a particular environment is therefore limited unless environmental constraints are reduced. A critical question is whether or not it is feasible to alter environmental constraints sufficiently to permit genetic improvement, while maintaining essential adaptability.

Environmental constraints

High temperatures

Many studies have shown that high temperatures have a negative effect on reproductive performance and lamb survival (MacFarlane 1964; Terrill 1968; Aboul-Naga and Afifi 1980). Adapted animals generally have a lower respiration rate and rectal temperature under heat stress (Hopkins et al. 1979) and these two traits may be good means of identifying adapted animals with better reproductive performance for a given environment. With extensive management, there is no known way of artificially reducing the ambient temperature. However, with more intensive management and smaller flocks, providing shade during the hot hours of the day might help to improve conception rate and reduce prenatal and neonatal lamb and kid mortality.

Feed scarcity

In arid and semi-arid climates, years of drought are interspersed with years of normal rainfall, making forage availability very unpredictable. Improving feed resources in dry regions is often difficult or not economically feasible, and at best the improvement possible is usually only moderate. Most sheep and goats in arid and semi-arid climates will continue to be primarily dependent on natural forage, which fluctuates in quantity and quality between seasons as well as years. In such environments, productivity cannot be greatly improved. However, in areas of higher and more predictable rainfall where agricultural by-products may be available and forage production possible, the constraint of feed scarcity can be partially reduced or completely eliminated.

Therefore, breeding programs for at least two different systems of production should be considered. The first is the very extensive system, where specialized adaptation to the environment is essential for survival. Because of the difficulties of reducing constraints, significant improvement of genetic potential may be limited to traits not closely associated with fitness, such as fleece quality, or positively associated with fitness, such as some reduction in size of the fat tail. The second system is that seen in areas of mixed livestock and crop production where environmental constraints can be considerably reduced and therefore genetic improvement is more feasible.

For any system, major changes in genetic potential will usually have a limited impact on overall productivity unless feeding and management practices are also improved. Similarly, improvements in feeding and management with animals of low genetic potential for reproduction and growth will produce only a limited response, unless the animals were severely underfed or diseased. Thus, a genetic improvement program should always be accompanied by a management and feeding improvement program.

Methods of genetic improvement

Genetic improvement can be effected by selecting within local populations, utilizing the different breeds of the region in crosses, or importing improved breeds to cross with or replace the local breeds.

Selection

Improving a breed by selection is slow and requires consistent, long-term effort. It is the most important approach in the long run, but requires continuity of personnel and funding, which are often lacking. International aid programs frequently have a short (2–5 years) planning horizon and funding period, which is quite inadequate to implement successful selection programs. Galal (1987) reports that, in Egypt, although considerable effort has been put into estimating phenotypic and genetic parameters of local breeds, no serious attempt has been made to use this information in a selection program because of the long-term planning required and the high cost involved.

Crossing among breeds of the region

This approach can be very effective, if appropriate breeds are available, and improvement is more rapid than with selection. Costs of proper evaluation are substantial but less than those for importing exotic stocks and the chances of failure, biologically or in terms of acceptance by local farmers and markets, are usually lower than when exotics are used.

An example of this approach comes from Morocco, where sheep are extremely important. One of the local breeds is the D'man, a small breed of high prolificacy (ovulation rate 2.85) and productivity. Generally located in oases south of the High Atlas and raised in small confined flocks of less than five ewes, the D'man reaches puberty at an early age (219 days) and shows estrus cyclicity throughout the year (Lahlou-Kassi and Marie 1985). When crossed with the Sardi breed, of much lower prolificacy but larger and with better carcass quality, the F_1 ewes are intermediate between the parental breeds for litter size, age at puberty, and year round breeding. However, in two out of three parity season groups, the productivity, in terms of weight of lambs at weaning per ewe present at breeding, was higher for the F_1 crossbred ewes than for either parent breed (Table 1).

In this project Sardi, D'man, and crossbred ewes are raised in a semi-intensive system with one lambing approximately every 8 months. The animals graze every day for about 8 h on fallow land, wheat stubble, and under olive trees. Supplementation is given to ewes only at certain times, such as mating or early lactation, or when feed resources are inadequate. There was no problem of adaptation to this system of production in the D'man or in the F_1 crossbred ewes.

The relatively poor performance of the Sardi in season II (Table 1) is attributed to the seasonal breeding pattern of this breed as not all ewes were cycling in May and June. This also appeared to be the case for F_1 ewes at second parity, but not at third.

In season II, mating was directly after weaning, with many of the F_1 ewes having raised twins, and this may have affected the performance of second

Table 1. Fertility, litter size, and weight of lambs produced by two Moroccan breeds and their F_1 cross in two seasons.

Breed Parity	Season I [1]				Season II [2]					
	D'man	Sardi		DxS F_1	D'man		Sardi		DxS F_1	
	>3	2	>3	2	2	>3	2	>3	2	3
No. ewes	43	19	136	42	20	46	26	135	64	42
Mating weight (kg)	28.2	37.2	45.3	34.3	27.6	28.8	37.8	44.6	33.8	34.1
Fertility	95.3	94.7	94.9	97.6	90.0	89.1	65.3	61.5	68.8	95.2
Litter size	2.49	1.06	1.26	1.76	2.11	2.07	1.12	1.17	1.45	1.95
Lamb mortality at 0–60 d (%)	20.6	0.0	2.5	5.6	7.9	11.8	5.3	5.2	10.9	14.1
Lambs weaned /ewe present (kg)	1.88	1.00	1.17	1.62	1.75	1.63	0.69	0.68	0.89	1.59
Weight at 60 d /ewe present (kg)	18.2	15.5	18.6	20.2	19.9	17.6	10.7	11.8	11.6	20.6

Source: Berger et al. (1985).

[1] Mated Oct/Nov.

[2] Mated May/June.

parity ewes in season II. The results emphasize the very large effect of variation in fertility on meat production and the advantage of breeds which do not have seasonal anestrus.

Importation of exotic breeds

Exotic breeds, usually of European origin, should be imported only after thorough evaluation of local breeds and of evidence from comparisons between local breeds and exotics from countries with similar climate and production systems. The generally poor adaptability of exotic breeds to an environment different from their own is the major disadvantage in using these breeds. Casu et al. (1981) imported Berrichon du Cher and Ile de France into Sardinia for a terminal sire crossing system and found that the mortality of rams was 28–60% under extensive management on private farms. Fertility of pure bred ewes was only 70–80%. They concluded it would be impossible to establish a terminal sire crossing system using rams of these two imported breeds because of the difficulties of producing enough males for a crossing program.

Taneja (1974) reported very low fertility and poor lamb and adult survival rates for Rambouillet sheep introduced into an arid zone in India. Also, F_1 Rambouillet × Chokla ewes were less fertile than pure Chokla ewes, although survival of F_1 lambs was better than that of either parent breed. Adult survival was good in the F_1, but poor in 3/4 Rambouillet ewes. In goats, Garcia and

Gall (1981) reported significantly higher mortality in 3/4 Alpine or Nubian, 1/4 Native goats than in F_1 Alpine or Nubian × Native in a semi-arid tropical environment in Venezuela. Kidding interval was also higher in 3/4 than in 1/2 exotic breed females. These results are typical of many experiments, showing a decrease in adaptability i.e., poor reproduction and viability, as the proportion of imported breed inheritance increases.

Bradford et al. (1987) suggested a number of indicators for lack of adaptability of exotic or exotic × local crossbred stock, including fertility from a 2-month mating season of less than 80% or more than 10% below that of adapted local stocks and lamb or kid mortality from birth to weaning exceeding 20% of all young born. A frequent contributor to high mortality is multiple births; in an environment in which mortality of singles, twins, and triplets is 12, 25, and 60%, respectively, stocks with a significant (> 10%) incidence of triplets are not adapted. Other indicators include lambing or kidding intervals greater than 12 months, growth rates or milk yields of introduced breeds less than 50% of those typical of these breeds in their home environment, and annual mortality of animals aged 1–6 years exceeding 5%.

The first step in planning a breeding program is to define the breeding objectives (James 1982). In industrialized economies, the objective is generally to increase profit, if economic parameters are fairly stable, or productivity, defined as amount of product produced per breeding animal in a specified period, per hectare, or per unit of feed input. In arid environments, well-being of the livestock owners and their families may depend more on the numbers of animals surviving in poor feed years than on amount of product sold in normal years. In this situation, there will be much more emphasis on adaptability than in industrialized production systems, where the environment may be adjusted to achieve high productivity.

Meat and milk are probably the two most important products from small ruminants in arid lands, although wool and skins may also be important.

Increasing meat production

Meat production may be improved by increasing fertility, frequency of parturition, prolificacy, lamb or kid survival, growth rate, milk production, or some combination of two or more of these.

Fertility

Good fertility is essential for good productivity while poor fertility is a clear indicator of lack of adaptability. However, fertility is not often included as a selection criterion in breeding programs as it is always subject to natural selection and has a low heritability. To achieve high genetic potential for fertility, a breed or cross should be used which has high fertility in the particular environment. In subsequent selection, breeding males from poor fertility parents should be avoided e.g., from females that produce offspring only in alternate years.

Systematic culling of unproductive animals may be the most important management practice to increase the number of lambs born in a flock. According to the Range Management Improvement Project in Morocco (Range Management Improvement Project 1986), about 25% of adult ewes surveyed in the project are estimated to be incapable of raising offspring because of sterility, disease, old age, and/or congenital defects. A high proportion of barren ewes was also observed in a flock of Blackheaded Persian sheep in Colombia (Pastrana et al. 1983), and this is believed to be widespread in unculled flocks. Where the primary goal of maintaining animals is to have an animal to sell when cash is needed and price is similar for animals of different productive capacity, this may not be a serious problem. Where the goal is to increase productivity of the flock, culling is potentially a very effective first step.

Frequency of parturition / breeding season

In favorable environments, small ruminant producers can use the short gestation of their animals to achieve mean parturition intervals of 7–9 months. thus potentially increasing annual production of young per breeding female very substantially. In arid environments where there are several months with little or no rain, it is critical that reproduction is timed so that lactation and early growth of the young coincide with the period of best forage growth. This dictates once-a-year reproduction, and selection for more frequent parturitions is not a goal. However, it is important that the stocks used have a natural breeding season which permits reproduction in the optimum season. Many European breeds have restricted breeding seasons and they and their crosses do not reproduce well or at all at the optimum season in Mediterranean or other arid climates. This is one of the most important considerations in deciding whether to import or work only with local stocks.

Prolificacy

Number of young born per parturition is often the variable with greatest influence on meat production from small ruminants. Prolificacy is also closely related to adaptability. Where feed is often scarce, optimum prolificacy will usually be single births. Twins may have poor survival during the neonatal period and low weaning weights because the dam cannot produce enough milk. If the extra nutrients required for gestating and particularly for nursing twins are not available, the dam will become thin and more susceptible to disease, parasites, or predators. Fertility the following year and even ability to survive drouth may be jeopardized by multiple births. In this situation, neither introduction of prolific breed inheritance nor selection for multiple births is advised.

Where deficiencies in the nutrients of natural forages can be compensated for by using crop residues, cultivated forages, or by-products in an economically feasible way, twinning may be advantageous. The critical times are the 2–3 week period prior to mating, the last month of gestation, and the first few weeks of lactation. Timing the reproductive cycle so that lambing occurs early in the best feed season may mean that supplements are needed for only a short period each year. An increase in weight of 50– 60% in young weaned per dam from twins compared to singles can be expected. This estimate comes from data on sheep at the Hopland Field Station in California with a Mediterranean climate. It is obtained by assuming that ewes with a single lamb have 88% lamb survival, a 35 kg lamb at 4 months, and 30.8 kg lamb weaned per ewe, and that ewes with twins have 82% lamb survival, 30 kg lambs at 4 months, and 49.2 kg lamb per ewe.

Actual values will vary with mature size of the breed, weaning age, etc. and production will be increased more in very good environments. However, these improvements are indicative of the potential in a fairly harsh environment where supplemental feed is provided for only 4–8 weeks per year.

Prolificacy in excess of twins is never desirable in sheep or goats dependent on grazing in arid lands. Thus the goal is to increase the mean litter size born from 1.0–1.2 to 1.5–1.8. A mean above 1.8 usually involves a significant incidence of triplets and is therefore often undesirable.

An increase in prolificacy may be achieved by selection or crossing with a prolific breed, the latter being much quicker in achieving the goal. Litter size appears to be transmitted additively in crosses of several prolific breeds e.g., the Finnish Landrace (Land et al. 1974; Dickerson 1977), Romanov (Ricordeau et al. 1976), and D'man (Table 1) with breeds of low prolificacy. Aboul-Naga (1985) reviewed the results of several crossbreeding experiments with prolific breeds (Finnish Landrace, Romanov, Chios, and D'man) conducted in North Africa and the Middle East, all of which show this was an effective means of increasing prolificacy. Most, if not all of these experiments were conducted under better feed conditions than would be available to the majority of sheep in these regions (e.g., Eyal et al. 1984), and the reports deal with number of lambs born rather than number weaned. Thus, the net effect of such crossing on increasing productivity under field conditions has not yet been adequately tested, although the potential for increase clearly exists.

If the F_1 (50% prolific breed) has litters which are too large, as is frequently the case, a lower percentage such as 25% or 38% may be used. Also, adaptability is usually better with the lower percent prolific breed inheritance. All prolific breeds have developed in environments where extra feed and care could be provided so they are not well adapted to extensive range conditions. It may be possible to use them to increase prolificacy, but because of their lack of adaptation to harsh environments it is usually desirable to use the minimum proportion of their inheritance which will produce the desired level of prolificacy. Also, quantity and quality of wool, size, and conformation may be superior in the adapted local breed, making it important to stay as close to that type of animal as possible.

Selection for multiple births in sheep has been shown in several studies to increase litter size by 1–2% per year and occasionally more (Bradford 1985). Screening a large population to create a nucleus flock, with continued infusion of superior females from the larger (base) population, should accelerate this rate. However, an increase in mean litter size from say 1.1 to 1.6, is likely to require 15–20 years or more with the best selection schemes. Thus selection will be the method of choice only when no suitable prolific breed is available for crossing or where fleece or adaptability of the local breed relative to those of any available prolific breed dictate use of the pure local breed.

Use of major genes such as the Booroola gene (Bindon 1984) is not generally indicated as a means of increasing twinning rate under extensive conditions because of the magnitude of increase and the increase in variability in litter size (e.g., Beetson and Lewer 1985). With a major gene, it is not possible to set the mean prolificacy level at a range of intermediate values in the same way as with quantitative variation from a prolific breed.

Survival

Poor survival, like low fertility, is an effective indicator of lack of adaptability. The low survival of pure exotic or high percentage exotic breed crosses in many experiments (Aboul-Naga 1978; Aboul-Naga and Afifi 1980; Casu et al. 1981; Zervas et al. 1975) provides some of the most compelling evidence against importation of breeds from other environments. Lamb survival rate has a low heritability and so will respond slowly to genetic selection. Also, rate of response will decrease as survival increases toward 100%. In a well structured selection program, stud rams should be selected from dams which have raised a high percentage of their lambs and although more emphasis on selection for survival may not be warranted, several steps can be taken to improve survival. The first is to set mean prolificacy at a level appropriate to the feeding and management system feasible. Secondly, the mating season should be controlled and scheduled so that parturitions occur at a time favorable for survival based on weather and feed availability. Thirdly, improvements in feeding and management before and at parturition, e.g., supplemental feeding, shelter, and fostering, can substantially increase survival rates.

Growth rate

Given that prolificacy and viability are at or near optimum, the next most important variable affecting meat production is growth rate of the offspring.

This is determined by nutrition, mature size potential, and the inherent shape of the growth curve. Nutrition after birth, for both dam and young, should be the best which is economically feasible. Mature size potential and inherent shape of the growth curve are both moderately heritable genetic traits.

A primary goal of many importations of exotic breeds is to increase growth rate. Comparing gains of 300–500 g per day in European or North American sire breeds of sheep with 50–100 g per day in local sheep suggests that importation of the former for crossbreeding will effect improvement. Often, the F_1 lambs do grow faster than local purebred animals but the crossbred will only be more productive if the extra growth is not offset by lower fertility of the crossbred mating (Aboul-Naga 1978) or lower viability of the crossbred offspring. This means it is essential to measure production per breeding female, not just average weight of the progeny weaned. If weight of F_1 (exotic breed male × local breed female) progeny weaned is improved, but F_1 daughters are not suitable because of poor adaptability, a limited breeding season, low fleece quality, or other traits, then the high growth exotic breed must be used only as a terminal sire in a repeat crossbreeding system. This requires good control of the breeding program and the cost of the males used as terminal sires must not be too high (Casu et al. 1981). Thus biological, organizational, and economic factors must be considered in deciding whether or not to recommend introduction of a breed with high growth rate.

Selection for improved growth rate within local breeds should result in faster growing, larger animals. Two relatively long-term experiments involving single trait selection for weaning weight have been carried out (Pattle 1965a; 1965b; Lasslo et al. 1985a; 1985b). Substantial response in growth rate was obtained in both cases. In the experiment reported by Pattle, which used Merino sheep not previously intensely selected for weaning weight, there was little if any correlated change in overall reproductive rate. In the experiment by Lasslo et al. using Targhees, a larger breed of sheep, fertility and lamb viability decreased in the weight-selected lines in each of two environments. The decrease offset or more than offset the increase in individual lamb weight so production per ewe was not improved, although mature ewe weight and thus feed requirement per ewe increased substantially. This decrease in fitness may not be a problem for many generations in stocks previously unselected for growth rate, but it would seem best to select for high reproductive fitness as well as growth rate, and not for growth rate (size) alone.

There is between-breed variation in shape of the growth curve with some breeds reaching mature size earlier than others. In principle, this is desirable in meat animals as it means a shorter period of maintenance to a given percentage of mature weight. However, most early maturing breeds, e.g., Dorset and Finnish Landrace sheep, have evolved in very favorable environments. Such breeds and those selected for rapid growth are expected to have higher maintenance requirements. In contrast, breeds evolved in and adapted to harsh environments tend to grow slowly and to have low maintenance requirements. Selection for growth rate to weaning or older will eventually have an adverse effect on adaptability; selection for an early maturing pattern of growth might accentuate this problem and, based on current knowledge, is not recommended for arid environment breeds.

Milk production

Dairy production in general requires a higher level of feeding, in terms of both quantity and quality, than meat or fiber production. Nevertheless, milk production from both sheep and goats in arid and semi-arid regions is often important; it does of course tend to occur in the better seasons and feed areas of such regions.

Increasing genetic potential for milk production is desirable for either dairy production or increased weaning weights of offspring for meat production. The constraint is that a milk production potential which is too high for the feed resources of a particular area will result in a loss of condition of the breeding female. This in turn can increase susceptibility to disease and decrease fertility and fecundity in the next reproduction period. Thus for milk, as for prolificacy and growth, it is essential to match genetic potential to environment and management.

The difference in milk yield potential between breeds selected for dairy production and those not so selected is usually larger than the differences in meat production ability between selected and unselected meat breeds. There may be important differences in behavior related to milking between "dairy" and "non-dairy" stocks. Also, the labor required for milking makes it desirable to have a certain minimum production level. These factors suggest that development of dairy from non-dairy stocks should involve crossing with breeds with high milk potential. However, this need not mean importing breeds of European origin. In both sheep and goats, there are breeds with high milk production potential which have been selected in and are adapted to the East Mediterranean/West Asia region. These include Chios sheep, dairy strains of Awassi sheep, and Damascus and Black Bedouin goats.

Results of an 8-year comparison in Greece of the Chios breed and the Friesian, a European dairy sheep breed, reported by Zervas et al. (1975) and Kalaissakis et al. (1977) illustrate the advantages of using a breed adapted to the region (Table 2).

Mean milk production of Awassi ewes was nearly tripled from 131 to 356 kg in milk recorded flocks in Palestine between 1937/38 and 1964/65 (Epstein 1985). The effect of selection and of improved feeding and management cannot be separated but both undoubtely contributed. The figures indicate the great potential for improvement in milk production. The review of milk production values for different breeds of goats by Garcia and Gall (1981) indicated that Damascus goats were the highest producing breed of goats of non-European origin. The Black Bedouin goat has exceptionally good milk production for its size and yet appears to have low dietary energy require-

Table 2. Reproductive performance and milk production of Chios and Friesian sheep and their crossbreds, in Greece [1].

| | Breed or cross | | | | |
	Chios (C)	CXF F$_1$	3/4F	7/8F	Friesian (F)
Fertility	81	91	83	78	70
Litter size	1.72	1.75	1.51	1.40	1.55
Lamb mortality (%)					
0–24 h	4.5	5.5	10.7	6.0	6.6
1–56 d	1.2	3.2	3.3	4.6	8.4
Lambs weaned/					
ewe mated	1.14	–[2]	–	–	0.94
Longevity					
Years	–	4.8	2.8	2.3	–
Lambings	–	3.9	1.9	1.3	–
Milk yield (kg) [3]	161	184	152	147	148
Lactation (d)	172				153

[1] From Zervas et al. (1975) and Kalassaikis et al. (1977).
[2] No estimate.
[3] Following a 56-day suckling period.

ments for maintenance. The breed also has remarkable physiological adaptation to water deprivation, enabling it to maintain good lactation performance while drinking at only 2–4 day intervals in a hot desert environment (Shkolnich et al. 1980). Where improved milk production is a goal in arid and semi-arid areas, use of or crossing with such breeds is likely to produce much better results than introducing breeds which have evolved in cool, wet climates.

Wool

Quantity and quality of wool can probably be changed more rapidly and with fewer adverse effects on adaptability than most other production traits. This is because wool requires less dietary energy than lactation, gestation, or growth. Wool quantity and quality traits are also relatively easy to measure, can be evaluated in both sexes prior to maturity, and are fairly heritable. There are large differences between improved and unimproved wool breeds in amount and efficiency of wool production, suggesting that crossing with improved breeds would be useful. However, most improved wool breeds are either fine-wooled (Merino and derivatives) or not adapted to arid areas (e.g., Romney). Because wool in arid countries is frequently used for carpets and hand-made products which require relatively coarse wool, the wool of exotic breeds or their crosses often does not meet local market demands. Phillips (1949) points out that in the Southwestern United States, crossbreeding of the local Navajo sheep, which are highly adapted to the arid environment, with the Corriedale breed not only did not increase the number of lambs weaned per ewe but also considerably reduced the quality of the carpets produced by the

Navajo Indians because the wool was too fine for hand weaving. This factor, and the fact that wool tends to be more important the drier the area because of the lack of forage to support milk or a high level of meat production, strongly suggests that wool production by sheep in arid lands should be improved by selection within local breeds.

Taneja (1974) has suggested that selection against medullation is an effective means of improving wool quality in native breeds. There appears to be very large variation, within breeds and flocks, in incidence of kemp and in fiber diameter in indigenous breeds of sheep in North Africa and West Asia. Assuming kemp is always undesirable and that there is an optimum fiber diameter for particular markets, a selection program based on visual scoring of fleeces for these two traits should result in rapid improvement in fleece quality. Objective measurements available will increase accuracy, but selection programs need not depend on equipment, especially in situations where phenotypic variation is large. The advantages of on-the-spot selection and the feasibility of scoring large numbers of animals at low cost are important factors in favor of visual scoring. Proper training in scoring is important and readily possible.

Fat tail

Many sheep breeds in arid areas of Asia and Africa have fat tails, and such sheep have existed in Southwest Asia since very early times (Epstein 1985). These fat tails are often assumed to be important as an energy reserve during drought and hence are essential to adaptability to an arid environment. However, in some arid areas e.g., Morocco and parts of the Sahel, there are large numbers of apparently well adapted sheep without fat tails. Also, there are apparently no fat-tailed goats. Juma et al. (1971) reported that body temperature was lower for docked than for undocked fat-tailed rams while the review by Shelton et al. (1987) indicates that although fat-tailed sheep were less affected by high temperature stress than Rambouillets, this did not appear to be directly related to the fat tail. There does not seem to be objective evidence that possession of a fat tail itself improves adaptability, and the maintenance of populations with large fat tails may reflect tradition and breeder preference for a certain appearance.

For those areas where fat-tailed sheep are the only or preferred type, an important question is whether productivity can be improved by changing the size of the tail. Very large tails impair fertility (Obst et al. 1980; Shelton et al. 1987) and as percent lean in the whole carcass is inversely related to size of the tail, selection for smaller fat tails may be advantageous. Crossing between fat-tail and non fat-tail breeds will of course reduce tail size and this may be one advantage of crossing with exotic breeds.

Conclusion

Genetic improvement programs for small ruminants in arid and semi-arid environments should be based on locally adapted breeds. Adaptability, as indicated by viability, fertility, and regularity of reproduction, is usually lower for exotic, improved breeds and often for the crossbreds produced by mating these to local breeds. The possibilities for genetic improvement increase as the level of feeding and management increase; a breeding strategy based on these factors and the traits to be considered is shown in Table 3.

Improvements in productivity of 20–50% are feasible by improving genetic potential (Bradford et al. 1987; Shelton et al. 1987). Return on investment in breeding programs is often very favorable, but substantial time is required to achieve goals. A sound breed or crossbreeding evaluation with small ruminants will require 6–10 years and a similar period will often be required to establish a significant response to selection, although effective screening of a large population can establish a significant and visible difference between a nucleus flock and the base population in one generation. The great advantages of selection are that the effects are cumulative over time and relatively permanent. Selection within local stocks has the added advantages of utilizing animals familiar to producers and producing products known and accepted in local markets.

The conclusion that importation of exotic breeds may not be the best means of effecting genetic improvement in difficult environments is not new (Phillips 1949). We still believe this to be generally true, based on physiological aspects of adaptability and disease susceptibility. Unfortunately, this has very frequently been overlooked during the past 4 decades, and while there have been a few successes, there have been many more failures from importa-

Table 3. Breeding strategies according to level of feeding and management.

Environment	Selection within local stocks only						Crossbreeding [1] based on	
	cull on fleece defects and barenness	select on recorded performance					improved local breed	exotic breed
		fleece wt	growth	milk	twin-ning			
least favorable	*							
	*	*						
	*	*	*					
	*	*	*	*				
	*	*	*	*	*			
most	*	*	*	*	*	*		
favorable	*	*	*	*	*	*		[2]

[1] Usually most useful for improving milk production and prolificacy.

[2] Only after critical comparison of the exotic breed and its crosses with local animals, under feeding and management conditions feasible for producers in that environment.

tions. We recommend that importation of improved breeds should be undertaken only after very carefully evaluating the performance of local breeds under the nutritional and management conditions which would be provided for the imported animals and their crosses. Also, imported breeds should be released only after they or their crosses have been shown to be superior in lifetime performance to local animals under feasible management conditions.

References

Aboul-Naga, A.M. 1978. Using Suffolk sheep for improving lamb production from subtropical Egyptian sheep. 1. Reproductive performance. Journal of Agricultural Science 90: 125–130.

Aboul-Naga, A.M. and Afifi, E.A. 1980. Crossing subtropical Egyptian sheep with Hampshire to improve their lamb production. Journal of Agricultural Science 95: 365–370.

Aboul-Naga, A.M. 1985. Crossbreeding for fecundity in subtropical sheep. Pages 55–62 in Genetics of Reproduction in Sheep (Land, R.B. and Robinson, D.W., eds). Butterworths, London, UK.

Beetson, B.R. and Lewer, R.P. 1985. Productivity of Booroola cross ewes in Western Australia. Pages 391–398 in Genetics of Reproduction in Sheep (Land, R.B. and Robinson, D.W., eds). Butterworths, London, UK.

Berger, Y.M., Lahlou-Kassi, A., Boujenane, I. and Bradford, G.E. 1985–86. Annual reports SR-CRSP.

Bindon, B.M. 1984. Reproductive biology of the Booroola Merino sheep. Australian Journal of Biological Science 37: 163–189.

Bradford, G.E. 1985. Selection for litter size. Pages 3–17 in Genetics of Reproduction in Sheep (Land, R.B. and Robinson, D.W., eds). Butterworths, London, UK.

Bradford, G.E., Subandriyo and Iniguez, L.C. 1987. Breeding strategies for small ruminants in integrated crop-livestock production systems. Pages 318–331 in Proceedings of a workshop on Small Ruminant Production Systems in South and South East Asia (Devendra, C., ed.), Bogor, Indonesia, 6–10 October 1986. IDRC Proceedings Series 256 E. IDRC, Ottawa, Canada.

Casu, S., Sanna, A., Cappai, P. and Ruda, G. 1981. Problemes lies a l'introduction et l'utilisation de beliers de race a viande pour le croisement industriel en Sardaigne. In Le Croisement Industriel Ovin en Mediterranee. Options Mediterraneenne. CIHEAM.

Dickerson, G.E. 1977. Crossbreeding evaluation of Finn sheep and some US breeds for market lamb production. North Central Regional Publication No. 246. University of Nebraska, Lincoln, USA.

Eyal, E., Goot, H., Kali, J., Amir, D., Rosenberg, Miriam, Schindler, H., Davidson, M., Tamarin, Ruth, Foote, W.C., Mattews, D.H. and Hogue, D.E. 1984. The promotion of prolific strains of sheep by nutritional and managerial means. Agricultural Research Organization, Institute of Animal Science, The Volcani Center, Bet Dagan.

Epstein, H. 1985. The Awassi Sheep with Special Reference to the Improved Dairy Type. FAO Animal Production and Health Paper No. 57. FAO, Rome, Italy.

Flamant, J.C., Bibe, B., Gibon, Annick and Vu Tien Khang, Jacqueline. 1979. Approche pour une amelioration genetique des races locales ovines. Notion de rusticite. Journees Recherches Ovine et Caprine (5e). INRA-ITOVIC.

Galal, E.S.E. 1987. Sheep and goat production and research in Egypt. Pages 117–156 in Small Ruminants in the Near East. FAO Animal Production and Health Paper No. 54. Vol. 1. FAO, Rome, Italy.

Garcia, O. and Gall, C. 1981. Goats in the dry tropics. Pages 515–556 in Goat Production (Gall, C., ed.). Academic Press, New York, USA.

Hopkins, P.S., Pratt, M.S. and Knights, G.I. 1979. The impact of environmental factors on sheep breeding in the semi-arid tropics. Pages 131–134 in Sheep Breeding (Tomes, G.J., Robertson, D.E. and Lightfoot, R.J., eds, revised by Haresign, W.). Butterworths, London, UK.

James, J.W. 1982. Economic aspects of developing breeding objectives: general considerations. Pages 107–118 in Future Developments in the Genetic Improvement of Animals (Barker, J.S., Hammond, K. and McLintoch, A.E., eds). Academic Press, Sydney, Australia.

Juma, K.H., Gharib, F.H. and Eliya, J. 1971. A note on studies on heat tolerance in Awassi sheep. Animal Production 13: 369–370.

Kalaissakis, P., Papadimitious, P., Flamant, J.C., Boyazoglu, J.G. and Zervas, N. 1977. Comparaison des races ovines Chios et Frisone avec leur croisements en Grece continentale. II. Production laitiere. Annales de Genetique et de Selection Animale 7 (3): 181–201.

Lahlou-Kassi, A. and Marie, M. 1985. Sexual and ovarian function of the D'man ewe. Pages 245–260 in Genetics of Reproduction in Sheep (Land, R.B. and Robinson, D.W., eds). Butterworths, London, UK.

Land, R.B., Russell, W.S. and Donald, H.P. 1974. The litter size and fertility of Finnish Landrace and Tasmanian Merino sheep and their reciprocal crosses. Animal Production 18: 265–271.

Lasslo, L.L., Bradford, G.E., Torell, D.T. and Kennedy, B.W. 1985a. Selection for weaning weight in Targhee sheep in two environments. I. Direct response. Journal of Animal Science 61: 376–386.

Lasslo, L.L., Bradford, G.E., Torell, D.T. and Kennedy, B.W. 1985b. Selection for weaning weight in Targhee sheep in two environments. II. Correlated effects. Journal of Animal Science 61: 387–397.

McFarlane, M.V. 1964. Terrestrial animals in dry heat, ungulates. Pages 509–539 in Handbook of Physiology of Environment (Oill, B.R., ed.). American Physiology Society, Washington D.C., USA.

Obst, J.M., Boyes, T. and Chaniago, T.D. 1980. Reproduction performance of Indonesian sheep and goats. Proceedings of the Australian Society of Animal Production 13: 321–324.

Pastrana, R., Camacho, R. and Bradford, G.E. 1983. African sheep in Colombia. Pages 79–84 in Hair Sheep of Western Africa and the Americas (Fitzhugh, H.A. and Bradford, G.E., eds). Westview Press, Boulder, Colorado, USA.

Pattie, W.A. 1965a. Selection for weaning weight in Merino sheep. I. Direct response to selection. Australian Journal of Experimental Agriculture and Animal Husbandry 5: 353–360.

Pattie, W.A. 1965b. Selection for weaning weight in Merino sheep. II. Correlated responses in other production characteristics. Australian Journal of Experimental Agriculture and Animal Husbandry 5: 361–368.

Phillips, R.W. 1949. Breeding livestock adapted to unfavourable environments. FAO Agricultural Studies No. 1. FAO, Rome, Italy.

Range Management Improvement Project. 1986. Final report of activities, findings and conclusions. USAID-MARA, Rabat, Morocco. 291 p.

Ricordeau, G., Razungles, I., Eychenne, F. and Tchamitchian, L. 1976. Performance de reproduction des brebis Berrichonnes du Cher, Romanov et croisees. Annales de Genetique et de Selection Animale 8: 25–35.

Shelton, M., Lewis, R., Willingham, T., Smith, G.C. and Savell, J.W. 1987. Investigations relating to fat-tail sheep. SR-CRSP Technical Report No. 91. TAMU Experimental Station, San Angelo, USA.

Shkolnick, A., Maltz, E. and Gordin, S. 1980. Desert conditions and goat milk production. Journal of Dairy Science 63: 1749–1754.

Taneja, G.C. 1974. Problems and perspectives in breeding for sheep improvement in arid environment. Pages 801–813 in Proceedings of the First World Congress on Genetics Applied to Livestock Production, October 1974, Madrid, Spain, Volume 1.

Terrill, C.M. 1968. Adaptation of sheep and goats. Pages 246–276 in Adaptation of Domestic Animals (Hafez, E.S., ed.). Lee and Febiger, Philadelphia, USA.

Zervas, N., Boyazoglu, J.G., Kalaissakis, P., Papadimitious, P. and Flamant, J.C. 1975. Comparaison des races ovines Chios et Frisone avec leur croisements en Grece continentale. I. Viabilite et reproduction. Annales de Genetique et de Selection Animale 7 (3): 277–291.

E.F. Thomson and F.S. Thomson (eds), Increasing Small Ruminant Productivity in Semi-arid Areas
© *1988 ICARDA . ISBN 978-94-010-7086-7*

A Strategy for the Exploitation of Sheep Genotypes for Improved Flock Performance

J.B. Owen

Introduction

There are two main methods for the genetic improvement of sheep in North Africa and West Asia. One is within-breed improvement of the native, mainly fat-tailed sheep while the other is the importation of genotypes from other areas to replace or be incorporated into the existing genotypes.

The main advantage of a breeding system based on within-breed improvement of native sheep is that the foundation sheep are already well adapted to the local environment by being resistant to parasites, heat tolerant, and having a buffering capacity–the fat tail–against widely fluctuating feed supplies. Unless the effects of the obvious environmental constraints such as parasites, climate, and irregular feed supply are considerably reduced, the main avenue of genetic improvement is likely to be within-breed selection. But when the environmental constraints are removed, some of the possible disadvantages of the native genotypes can become apparent, such as lower inherent prolificacy and poor carcass quality.

The use of foreign genotypes can be a short cut for genetic improvement, but the environmental constraints must be removed otherwise these unadapted genotypes are likely to perform worse than the existing native types. When imported stock are indicated, existing native types are seldom completely replaced; gradual introduction and judicious fusing of the two stocks is likely to be the best strategy.

The central issue is genotype-environment interactions. Although there is little formally documented evidence for such interactions in sheep (e.g., Woolaston 1985; Jankowski et al. 1983; Saoud and Hohenboken 1984), their existence is obvious to all practical sheep men operating in difficult environments e.g., semi-arid range or mountain areas. The underlying component traits contributing to genotype-environment interactions and giving rise to adaptation are numerous and interact in a complex way so the outcome of genotype changes and introductions are unpredictable. This emphasizes the need for carefully planned breeding schemes that minimize negative results whilst leaving sufficient possibilities for exciting new combinations.

Objectives and selection criteria

Traditionally, the main products from sheep in North Africa and West Asia are milk, meat, wool, and skins. Many of the traditional sheep systems are

Table 1. Trends in human and sheep populations in some countries of North Africa and West Asia.

Country	Human population (economically active)			No. of sheep (×1000)		
s	total (×1000)		% in agriculture			
	1975	1985	1975	1985	1979–81	1985
Afghanistan	4569	4971	63.6	58.4	18667	20000
Algeria	3455	4834	39.2	24.3	13111	18000
Egypt	10037	12837	48.8	42.5	1590	2500
Ethiopia	15912	19182	82.4	76.8	23250	23500
Iran	9493	13023	39.9	32.9	33833	34500
Iraq	2890	4259	37.1	23.5	9408	8500
Jordan	634	799	19.0	5.8	978	990
Lebanon	771	769	17.0	12.2	137	135
Libya	628	904	23.5	14.1	5046	5500
Morocco	4656	6676	51.5	39.7	14180	12000
Pakistan	17639	21385	64.8	51.7	24180	25037
Saudi Arabia	2042	3405	56.3	40.5	2904	3800
Somalia	1516	1999	77.5	73.5	10100	9700
Sudan	5328	6991	74.1	67.9	17628	19000
Syria	1850	2596	41.1	24.7	9311	13665
Tunisia	1608	2224	38.1	31.6	4651	5220
Turkey	17639	21385	64.8	51.7	46199	40391
Yemen AR	1336	1676	72.5	64.5	1688	1850
Yemen PDR	427	558	46.0	36.4	892	940

Source: FAO (1986).

unspecialized and all these products are produced to varying extents. It is likely that this pattern will continue in future although it is possible that there will be a tendency towards mainly meat with wool as a by-product or milk production with young lamb as a by-product. Specialist wool producing sheep are perhaps less likely to become important in a region dominated by family flock owners. In all cases, the object is to achieve efficient production of a high quality product.

In setting selection objectives, a balanced judgement must be made of the present situation coupled with perceived trends for the future since it takes several years to produce operating phenotypes. Table 1 shows some human and sheep population trends for North Africa and West Asia. These suggest an increasing tendency towards higher labour costs, greater urbanisation, and the possible need for sheep that can utilize semi-arid ranges in certain seasons and respond positively to supplementary feeding. Sheep production may shift towards a semi-intensive system, making the maximum use of the valuable range resources at the appropriate times of the year. In terms of inputs, judicious supplementary feeding of concentrates could be important, although it may be far wiser to rely on natural resistance to parasites rather than using full anti-parasitic drug control.

Selection criteria

To be effective, general objectives must be translated into specific selection criteria that can be operated by the breeder.

Adaptation

There is usually little argument about the importance of adaptation as an objective but it is harder to include it as a specific selection criterion. In many circumstances, it is best to ignore adaptation as a selection entity and assume that selection within a given environment for other production traits will automatically safeguard important genetic aspects of adaptation. In other circumstances, it is possible to devise specific tests for adaptation such as to climate (Slee 1984) or parasite resistance (Gray 1987). Several other specific indirect selection criteria have been advocated, including biochemical parameters of the blood (Haley et al. 1987). Some of the specific components of adaptation may be controlled by a single gene with a major effect although most appear to be polygenically controlled.

Milk yield

The interaction of natural suckling with artificial milking in many sheep systems makes milking ability a difficult trait to reduce to a specific measurable criterion. Fortunately, recent work on Awassi ewes in Syria (Hossamo et al. 1985; I. Fadel, personal communication 1987) indicates that simplified recording, where the milk yield of all ewes in a flock is measured during one 24 h period, can give an accurate ranking of the trait for the season. Milk quantity and quality are assessed and the method promises to be an important tool for the future and particularly useful for screening large numbers of ewes in adapted commercial flocks.

Milk is important for processing and as the main source of food for the young suckling lamb. Where the ewes are not hand milked, lamb weaning weight, suitably corrected for some of the main non-genetic effects, is likely to be an important selection criterion. Weights recorded on a single visit to the flock have been shown to be an efficient means of measuring this trait and of ranking lambs and ewes.

Prolificacy

Prolificacy is assessed by making individual observations of litter size and is defined as the total number of lambs born at a lambing. The trait is very important and assessment of the optimum level of prolificacy for the conditions and system of production is a major determinant of productive and economic efficiency in sheep systems (Nitter 1987). Optimum ewe prolificacy varies from unity in the harshest range environment to as high as 2.5 under intensive feeding and management systems (Owen et al. 1986).

Litter size is an easily measured trait under supervised lambing. Its component trait, ovulation rate, is reasonably easy to measure using endoscopy and is a more highly heritable trait than litter size (Hanrahan 1987). The number of lambs weaned per ewe mated, known as weaning rate, is directly relevant to the flock owner. But because of its higher component of environmental variance, it is better where possible to isolate barrenness, defined as the failure to achieve or maintain pregnancy, and lamb viability as separate components for selection purposes.

The discovery of a major gene effect influencing ovulation rate and prolificacy in sheep has been a major step towards quickly manipulating prolificacy in sheep. Published evidence is now available for the existence of such a gene in the Booroola Merino (Australia), Cambridge (United Kingdom), Icelandic (Iceland), D'man (Morocco), and Javanese (Indonesia) sheep (Piper et al. 1985; Hanrahan and Owen 1985; Jonmundsson and Adalsteinsson 1985; Lahlou-Kassi and Marie 1985; Bradford et al. 1986). The best documented occurrence is in the Booroola and indicates that the gene increases the basal mean ovulation rate by about 1.5 ova and that its effect on ovulation rate is not dominant. Because of the association of ovulation rate with embryo mortality, the effect on litter size is less than 1.5 and appears to be dominant with little increase in litter size between the heterozygous (one copy) and the homozygous (two copies) state. The gene seems to have a similar effect in the other breeds noted and it is possible that the arrangement of the DNA bases is identical. Although there is no published evidence of a gene of this kind in some sheep breeds that have been intensively investigated e.g., Finn sheep, it may be that such a gene is widespread in many sheep populations but at a very low gene frequency. It appears that certain breeding schemes, where there is intensive selection for prolificacy, tend to concentrate the gene to a frequency where its presence is more easily recognised.

Table 2 shows some of the evidence for the presence of the major prolificacy gene in the Cambridge sheep. This breed has been developed from a wide genetic base over a period of 25 years, with intense selection for prolificacy. The table shows that ewes in this flock can be categorised into

Table 2. Results of cluster analysis of ovulation rate (OR) values (1983 and 1984).

Criterion (sum of OR 1983 and 1984)	Genotype	No. of ewes	Mean ovulation rate	CV	Repeat- ability
7	+ +	37	2.6	0.29	0.17
8–12	C +	15	4.7	0.20	0.12
13	CC	9	8.0	0.19	0.22

Source: Owen and Hanrahan (1987).

three groups, uniform within group, showing the basal level of ovulation (group + +) and the effect of one copy (group C +) and two copies of the gene (group CC).

Meat production traits

Prolificacy and milk production are important components of an efficient sheep meat production system, as are growth potential and carcass characteristics. The latter two traits are associated with the mature size of the breed, and the weight and stage of development at which sheep are slaughtered are major non-genetic factors in determining the weight and composition of the final carcass. The optimum mature size for a sheep breed is a complex trait since body size not only influences meat production but is also associated with many other traits, not least those that form the complex of adaptation. Carcass quality in relation to the needs of particular markets is often difficult to describe as an objective in simple terms; it is even more difficult to translate these objectives into practicable and measurable selection traits. Work such as that of El-Karim et al. (1987) has attempted to set out appropriate sample joint techniques for the simple assessment of carcass composition in the Sudan Desert sheep.

A major technique in the improvement of growth and carcass traits in sheep is the use of *in vivo* measurements to enable the use of sire performance testing. These performance tests could be carried out under intensive feeding from birth to post weaning (Owen et al. 1978) or under field conditions. Tissue scanning techniques have been developed that should enable much better assessment of carcass attributes without killing the ram (Simm 1987).

Wool production

Where wool production is a major objective, many useful techniques are available to improve quantity and quality. These methods, based largely on measuring yearling fleece attributes, such as weight and wool fibre diameter, can be highly effective because of the relatively high heritability of these traits. However, it is important to ensure that other associated traits involved in adaptation and reproductive characters are not detrimentally affected.

Interrelationship of traits in selection programmes

Many selected traits are genetically associated with other traits. For example, prolificacy may be associated with many other important traits e.g., milk yield and precocity (Table 3). More information is required on these aspects in the sheep of North Africa and West Asia.

Table 3. Genetic and phenotypic correlations between prolificacy (total lambs born per ewe lambing) and some important traits.

	Genetic		Phenotypic
	r	S.E.	r
No. born alive	0.85	0.038	0.75
No. alive at 2 days	0.96	0.035	0.59
No. alive at 50 days	0.32	0.249	0.27
Mortality			
at birth	0.85	0.878	0.24
birth to 2 days	ne [1]	ne	0.27
birth to 50 days	0.85	0.158	0.59
2–50 days	0.81	0.198	0.48
Mating weight	0.40	0.240	0.05
Date of first oestrus	0.59	0.196	0.08
Mean lamb weight			
at birth	−1.0	ne	−0.68
at 50 days	0.16	0.363	−0.33

Source: Owen et al. (1986).

[1] ne = no estimate.

Genotypes available for a sheep improvement strategy

Aboul-Ela and Aboul-Naga (1987) have described some of the native sheep breeds found in the semi-arid areas of North Africa and West Asia (Table 4). These breeds are fat-tailed and well adapted to their environment but, because of husbandry constraints, the genetic basis and phenotypic manifestation of prolificacy have been kept at a low level and precocity and lambing frequency are poorly developed. However, native breeds should normally form the basis of any improvement programme and the importation of other stock should be evaluated objectively and only accomplished when sufficient positive information is available. The native breeds are likely to possess the required traits for adaptation and many of the dam characters required for improved dairy traits and suckling ability, which are the required genetic base for efficient lamb meat production.

Apart from wool production traits, there seem to be two main possibilities for imported stock; modifying carcass quality and increasing prolificacy.

Carcass quality

The use of a sire-line breed to produce crossbred lambs from native breed ewes appears to present few technical problems if the lambs are intensively fed in a feed-lot type system. Since most of the dams are fat-tailed, artificial insemination would be necessary for successful mating. A wide choice of sire-line breeds would be available, such as the Suffolk and Texel. However, some market research would be needed to find out whether the consumer in

Table 4. Reproductive performance of subtropical fat-tailed sheep breeds.

Breed	Country	Age at first lambing (month)	Lambing interval	Litter size		Reference
				Year-ling	Adult ewes	
Non-prolific breeds						
Ossimi	Egypt	15–22	–[1]	–	1.17	
Rahmani	Egypt	15–22	–	–	1.21	Aboul-Naga and
Barki	Egypt	18–25	–	–	1.07	Aboul-Ela (1986)
Tim Hadit	Morocco	21–23	10–12	–	1.02–1.07	
Serdi	Morocco	20–23	10–12	–	1.00–1.07	Lahlou-Kassi and
Beni-Guil	Morocco	21–23	10–12	–	1.04	Marie (1985)
Beni-Hsen	Morocco	21–23	10–12	–	1.04–1.20	
Nejdi	Saudi Arabia	13–18	–	–	1.10–1.38	
Nejdi	Kuwait	22	–	–	1.1	
Harri	Saudi Arabia	17–18	–	–	1.06	
Kurdi	Iraq	24	–	–	1.04	
Hamadani	Iraq	–	–	–	1.10	Ghanem (1980)
Awassi	Syria	24	12	–	1.05	
Barbary	Libya	–	–	–	1.00–1.10	
Barbary	Tunisia	24	–	–	1.20	
Barbary	Algeria	14–15	–	–	1.00	
White Karaman	Turkey	–	–	–	1.05	
Red Karaman	Turkey	–	–	–	1.00–1.05	
Daglie	Turkey	–	–	–	1.00–1.02	
Kellakui	Iran	–	–	–	1.11	
Bakhtiari	Iran	–	–	–	1.20	
Kizili	Iran	–	–	–	1.25	
Baluchi	Iran	–	–	–	1.16	
Karkul	Iran	–	7–8	–	1.16	
Bibrik	Pakistan	–	–	–	1.00–1.05	Sefidbakht et al. (1977) Osman (1985)
Prolific breeds						
Chios	Greece	> 13	6–12	–	2.3	Mason (1980)
Chios	Cyprus	–	–	–	1.69	Constantinou (1985)
D'man	Morocco	12–14	6–8	1.67–2.00	1.98–2.67	Lahlou-Kassi and
D'man	Morocco	11–17	6–8	–	1.85–2.40	Marie (1985)
Javanese	Indonesia	6–12	6–9	–	1.6	Mason (1980)
Horro	Ethiopia	–	–	–	1.6	Galal et al. (1986)
Hu-Yang	China	13–16	6–8	–	> 2.0	Mason (1980)

[1] No estimate

the region prefers the traditional lean carcass with its fat tail, or a more meaty crossbred lamb with less fat in the tail and omental region but more subcutaneous and intramuscular fat.

Prolificacy

It is possible that the development of sheep production systems using seasonal range and supplementary feeding, and with intensive lambing husbandry or even more intensively yarded systems, will create a demand for sheep of higher prolificacy. A system that might be especially suitable may involve differential management for ewes suckling twins and those with singles. Under such a system, single suckling ewes might follow a more traditional pattern with more extended periods of range grazing whilst the ewes suckling twins would be given more concentrate and high quality forage for longer periods.

Whilst within-breed selection for prolificacy would eventually produce results, many might wish more immediate results. This could be done by initial crossbreeding with a specialized imported genotype and then stabilizing by interbreeding into a true-breeding, self-replacing population. An alternative would be to base commercial production on a first or second cross female as is common in many temperate countries.

The strategy adopted determines the choice of genotype, particularly whether or not a genotype carrying a major gene would be advisable. If the strategy is to develop a stabilized new breed, then it would be advantageous to use an imported genotype whose prolificacy had a multigenic base since the final breed would tend to have a less variable litter size. On the other hand, if a system based on first cross females were adopted, rams from an imported dam line breed which were homozygous for the prolificacy gene would yield first cross females which were highly prolific (carrying one copy of the gene) and would have a low variance about the mean litter size (CV about 34%, see Owen 1987b).

Several promising genotypes from subtropical, semi-arid environments are possible candidates in providing prolificacy, coupled in many cases with earlier sexual maturity and the ability to breed more frequently. These include the Chios (Greece), D'man (Morocco), Javanese (Indonesia), Horro (Ethiopia), and Hu-Yang (China). The advantage of using these breeds in a breeding programme would be their greater adaptation to the environment.

Other alternatives for specialized meat production systems would be breeds from temperate areas like the Cambridge. This breed could be used either to transfer the prolificacy gene to breeds like the Awassi, grading back to the pure Awassi over several generations, or a Cambridge × Awassi ewe might be used. Many exciting possibilities are now practicable in this field particularly with the impending international commercial availability of stored semen and embryos. It is important that well designed trials are conducted that can give reasonable assurance that the genotypes used and the breeding plan adopted are suitable for commercial exploitation.

Breeding methods to improve commercial flocks

The transfer of planned breeding schemes into operation at flock owner level is crucial and recent developments indicate several useful methods of achieving this.

Screening commercial flocks

There is mounting evidence that the start of many successful improvement programmes is the screening of a wide range of commercial flocks for superior females. This intense selection for desired traits in a small group of females at the extreme of the commercial flock range has sometimes resulted in a substantial initial genetic improvement, often beyond expectation from the perceived genetic parameters for the population in question. Such unexpected results may be due to major gene effects at the extreme or could be another manifestation of disruptive selection as described by Belyaev and Trut (1986). The more flocks that are included in the initial screening process the better, particularly if they span a broad range of practising flock owners. Such screening does not depend on complicated recording procedures and it is possible to screen flocks efficiently in one visit for the best genotypes in terms of milk yield and suckling ability as judged by lamb weight.

Nucleus flock schemes

The rationale of screening is to set up nucleus flocks which can be used to concentrate improvement efforts and provide a ready source of rams. Good genetic material can be lost by random 'drift' in the early stages of the establishment of a nucleus and a sufficient number of males is required to maintain effective population size. A minimum of 10–12 sires per generation is suggested.

Group-breeding cooperation

A suitable vehicle for achieving the requirements for screening and nucleus maintenance in many cases has been group breeding (Owen 1985; 1987a). A group of 10–15 breeders act cooperatively and screen their own flocks to form the nucleus. They then maintain the nucleus partly by self replacement and partly by contributing ewes from their own flocks on a regular basis, thus forming an 'open' nucleus. The members of the group breeding schemes are directly rewarded by having selected rams from the nucleus flock for their own use. They may also benefit in many indirect ways from acting as a cooperative group, the benefits being partly genetic and partly operational and promotional.

Conclusions

In North Africa and West Asia there appear to be many possibilities for adopting important new initiatives in sheep breeding. Some will follow lines similar to those described in this paper although there will be modifications and differences appropriate to the differences of tradition and circumstances that are such a strong feature of sheep husbandry all over the world. Priorities for the semi-arid regions appear to be to study and characterise the genetic wealth of adapted genotypes, to screen them for the most efficient ewes and to explore their use in balanced semi-intensive systems making judicious use of range forage. Foreign genotypes need careful evaluation to assess what role, if any, they can play in complementing native genotypes.

References

Aboul-Naga, A.M, and Aboul-Ela, M.B. 1986. Performance of subtropical Egyptian sheep breeds, European breeds and their crosses. 1. Egyptian sheep breeds. World Review of Animal Production.

Aboul-Ela, M.B. and Aboul-Naga, A.M. 1987. Improving fecundity in subtropical fat-tailed sheep. Pages 163–171 in New Techniques in Sheep Production (Marai, I.F.M. and Owen, J.B., eds). Butterworths, London, UK.

Belyaev, D.K. and Trut, L.N. 1986. A new view on the old problem of genetical – evolutionary mechanisms of domestication. Paper presented at the 37th Annual Meeting of the European Association for Animal Production, Sept 1986, Hungary.

Bradford, G.E., Quirke, J.F., Sitorus, P., Inounee, I., Tiesnamurti, B., Bell, F.L., Fletcher, I.C. and Torell, D.T. 1986. Reproduction in Javanese sheep: evidence for a gene with a large effect on ovulation rate and litter size. Journal of Animal Science 63: 418–431.

Constantinou, A. 1985. Ruminant livestock genetic resources in Cyprus. Pages 1–8 in Animal Genetic Resources Information No. 4, FAO/UNEP Publication. FAO, Rome, Italy.

El-Karim, A.I.A., Owen, J.B. and Whitaker, C.J. 1987. Measurement of slaughter weight, side weight, carcass joints and their association with carcass composition of two types of Sudan Desert sheep. Journal of Agricultural Science: 109. In press.

FAO (Food and Agriculture Organization). 1986. FAO Production Yearbook 1985. Volume 39. FAO, Rome, Italy.

Galal, E.S.E., Gojjam, Y., Tiyu, U. and Woldgabriel, K. 1986. Horro sheep: development, reproductive efficiency and productivity in Ethiopia. International Goat and Sheep Research.

Ghanem, Y.S. 1980. (Arabian Sheep Breeds.) Publication of the Arab Organization for Education, Culture and Sciences. In Arabic.

Gray, G.D. 1987. Genetic resistance to haemonchosis in sheep. Parasitology Today 3: 253–255.

Haley, C.S., Cameron, N.D., Slee, J. and Land, R.B. 1987. Indirect selection. Pages 113–124 in New Techniques in Sheep Production (Marai, I.M.F. and Owen, J.B., eds). Butterworths, London, UK.

Hanrahan, J.P. 1987. Genetic variation in ovulation rate in sheep. Pages 37–48 in New Techniques in Sheep Production (Marai, I.M.F. and Owen, J.B., eds). Butterworths, London, UK.

Hanrahan, J.P. and Owen, J.B. 1985. Variation and repeatability of ovulation rate in Cambridge ewes. Animal Production 40: 529.

Hossamo, H.E., Owen, J.B. and Farid, M.F.A. 1985. The genetic improvement of Syrian Awassi sheep with special reference to milk production. Journal of Agricultural Science, Cambridge 105: 327–337.

Jankowski, S., Davidowicz, E. and Roguska, E. 1983. Examples of sex-environment and genotype-environment interactions in lamb growth. Pages 584–585 in Proceedings of the 34th Annual Meeting of the European Association for Animal Production, 3–6 Oct 1983, Madrid, Spain. Volume 2. Summaries. Study Commissions. Cattle, Sheep, Goats, Pigs, Horses.

Jonmundsson, J.V. and Adalsteinsson, S. 1985. Single genes for fecundity in Icelandic sheep. Pages 159–168 in Genetics of Reproduction in Sheep (Land, R.B. and Robinson, D.W., eds). Butterworths, London, UK.

Lahlou-Kassi, A. and Marie, M. 1985. Sexual and ovarian function of the D'man ewe. Pages 245–260 in Genetics of Reproduction in Sheep (Land, R.B. and Robinson D.W., eds). Butterworths, London, UK.

Mason, I.L. 1980. Prolific tropical sheep. FAO Animal Production and Health Paper No. 17. FAO, Rome, Italy.

Nitter, G. 1987. Economic response to increasing genetic potential for reproductive performance. Pages 271–280 in New Techniques in Sheep Production (Marai, I.M.F. and Owen, J.B., eds). Butterworths, London, UK.

Osman, A.H. 1985. Near East: sheep breeding and improvement. World Animal Review 54: 2–15.

Owen, J.B. 1985. The development and role of new sheep breeds to suit different conditions. Paper presented at the conference on Animal Production in Arid Zones, Sept 1985, Damascus, Syria.

Owen, J.B. 1987a. Group breeding schemes and simplified recording in sheep improvement. Pages 157–162 in New Techniques in Sheep Production (Marai, I.M.F. and Owen, J.B., eds). Butterworths, London, UK.

Owen, J.B. 1987b. Breeding for fecundity. Paper presented at the British Veterinary Association Congress, Warwick, Sept 1987.

Owen, J.B., Brook, L.E., Read, J.L., Steane, D.E. and Hill, W.G. 1978. An evaluation of performance testing of rams using artificial rearing. Animal Production 27: 247–259.

Owen, J.B., Crees, S.R.E., Williams, J.C. and Davies, D.A.R. 1986. Prolificacy and 50 day lamb weight of ewes in the Cambridge sheep breed. Animal Production 42: 355–363.

Owen, J.B. and Hanrahan, J.P. 1987. The development of the Cambridge breed in relation to a major gene for ovulation rate. Paper presented at the European Association for Animal Production, Sept 1986, Budapest, Hungary.

Piper, L.R., Bindon, B.M. and Davies, G.H. 1985. The single gene inheritance of the high litter size of the Booroola Merino. Pages 115–126 in Genetics of Reproduction in Sheep (Land, R.B. and Robinson, D.W., eds). Butterworths, London, UK.

Saoud, N.B. and Hohenboken, W.D. 1984. Genetic, environmental and interaction effects on lifetime production efficiency of crossbred ewes. Journal of Animal Science 59: 594–606.

Sefidbakht, N., Mostafari, M.S. and Farid, A. 1977. Effect of season of lambing on postpartum ovulation, conception and follicular development of four fat-tailed Iranian breeds of sheep. Journal of Animal Science, Cambridge 45: 305–310.

Simm, G. 1987. Carcass evaluation in sheep breeding programmes. Pages 125–144 in New Techniques in Sheep Production (Marai, I.F.M. and Owen, J.B., eds). Butterworths, London, UK.

Slee, J. 1984. Improving lamb survival. Animal Breeding Research Organisation. Pages 11–16 in AFRC Annual Report 1984. Her Majesty's Stationery Office, London, UK.

Woolaston, R.R. 1985. Genotype-environment interactions with sheep. In Proceedings of the Fifth Conference, Australian Association of Animal Breeding and Genetics, University of New South Wales, Sydney, New South Wales, 26–28 Aug 1985, Australia.

E.F. Thomson and F.S. Thomson (eds), Increasing Small Ruminant Productivity in Semi-arid Areas
© 1988 ICARDA. ISBN 978-94-010-7086-7

Sheep and Goats: Their Relative Potential for Milk and Meat Production in Semi-Arid Environments

J. Steinbach

Environmental setting and animal resources

Small ruminants originate from the semi-arid regions that are the focal point of this workshop. Here, sheep and goats have supplied man with food, fibre, and funds for the past 10000 years. The semi-arid and arid regions are characterized by protracted periods of soil water deficit, highly variable precipitation, temperature extremes, poor quality and inadequate forage, and frequently saline drinking water. In addition, small ruminant husbandry has always been governed by low-input strategies. In such a climatically and topographically diverse region, sheep and goat ecotypes have evolved in response to natural and artificial selection and they differ greatly in their physiological and morphological characteristics. Both sheep and goats have developed specific adaptations to forage and water shortages and although both species have certain specific differences their ecological niches and evolutionary developments overlap.

Frequently, sheep and goats are kept in the same flock, and in Arabic both species are called "ghanam". The coexistence of sheep and goats is particularly striking in extremely marginal environments and in nomadic flocks. Where good and poor locations occur side by side, sheep and goats may be kept separately, with sheep in more favourable areas such as the Medjerda Valley in Tunisia or the Barley Belt in Syria and goats in areas where sheep may find it difficult to survive such as on dense shrub vegetation of the Mediterranean marquis or on mountainous, rugged terrain. Also, goats convert high quality forage into milk protein more efficiently than sheep and so may be favoured in densely populated, irrigated systems and oases.

Consequently, there is a wide variety of sheep and goat ecotypes in arid and semi-arid regions. Mason (1969) has identified 22 goat (30% of the world total) and 46 sheep breeds (14% of the world total) indigenous to North Africa and West Asia. The term breed implies man-made, artificial selection pressure, which has largely been absent in most areas or in small ruminant populations in semi-arid or arid regions. Therefore, distinctive sheep and goat populations should be referred to as ecotypes, which have developed under environmental pressure over thousands of years. Accordingly, differences within may be greater than between the two species. This makes the discussion of the relative production potential of sheep and goats rather difficult, and evidence can be cited for higher biological and economic productivity for either sheep or goats depending on the interaction between genotype and environment. Moreover, there is little precise knowledge on the production potential of most sheep and goat populations. Of the 22 goat and 46 sheep types listed by Mason (1969), very few have been tested for their genetic merit; examples are Awassi, D'man, Omani, or Barbarine sheep and Damascus, Bedouin, or Tunisian Race locale goats. For most indigenous breeds only general descriptions are available. A precise knowledge of the characteristics of existing small ruminant populations is, however, necessary if sheep and goat production are to be improved with genetic methods. So far, with the exception of a few Mediterranean countries, systematic research and development in the genetic improvement of indigenous populations of small ruminants are non-existent, except perhaps for the occasional importation of exotic, high-yielding breeds for indiscriminate cross-breeding.

Genotype evaluation, and where sensible the conservation of genetic material, must precede planned and systematic genetic improvement of local sheep and goat populations.

Evaluation of genetic resources

The ultimate aim of comparative genotype evaluation is to identify genetic resources that should be conserved for improving present productivity within their region of origin or elsewhere, or for preserving genetic material for future use. To be useful, procedures for evaluating genotypes must be standardized to permit comparison between laboratories. The environmental setting in which evaluation takes place must be clearly defined since productivity is the result of the genotype, the environment, the production system, and their subcomponents.

So far, very little evaluation has been made of small ruminants in the semi-arid and arid regions of West Asia. While some traits have been measured in certain populations, comparable results have not been obtained due to a lack of standardized procedures. More recently, the FAO European Research Network on Sheep and Goats has been drawing up a list of descriptors of goat populations (Steinbach 1987a) and this has been successfully applied to sheep and in a survey that included North Africa and West Asia.

Criteria for evaluating populations

Flock owners must balance inputs such as labour, land, and capital against outputs in kind or cash. Thus, a concept on evaluation must include parameters of productivity, disease susceptibility, physiological adaptability to relevant stress factors, and economic criteria. It is important to distinguish between biological and economic productivity since in comparative trials increases in productivity may be obtained only with such an increase in maintenance costs that a larger profit margin is obtained in the lower yielding population. The production efficiency of the flock is derived from individual performance records of a number of different traits that can be combined in productivity indices such as those proposed by ILCA and others (Steinbach 1987a; Peacock 1987). Also, it is important that genotype comparisons or evaluations are carried on long enough for realistic estimates to be made of lifetime production (Turner 1982) of the parent and, where applicable, of the crossbred offspring. Finally, the estimation of genetic parameters is an important prerequisite for decisions relating to breeding policies. The descriptors of small ruminant genotypes can then be categorized into phenotypic characteristics, disease susceptibility, physiologically important adaptive traits, genetic parameters, and economic input and output criteria.

Phenotypic characteristics

The important phenotypic parameters are those that are directly related to production traits i.e., growth, reproduction, lactation, and fibre and skin characteristics. Important morphological criteria are mature size, coat characteristics, and udder conformation, while linear measurements e.g., the length of the body, ears, or horns, are not important for production. Sexual dimorphism may be important since small females require less feed for maintenance while large males may increase the growth potential of male offspring used for fattening. In addition, differences in growth rates can be observed absolutely and relative to mature weight. Hair coat descriptors include fibre quality, the number and ratio of primary and secondary follicles, and coat colour, all of which may affect the processing value of the fibre. Seasonal and sex differences are important for some of these characteristics (CSIRO 1982).

Udder conformation may determine milkability of dairy goats and the risk of injury in range goats so descriptions of the size and attachment of the udder are useful.

A high rate of reproductive efficiency is the most important prerequisite for the production of meat, milk, skins, and breeding stock and it has a considerable influence on the cost of production. Reproductive efficiency in the doe is characterized by the individual and compound parameters shown in Table 1.

These parameters should be measured and can be combined into an index of biological productivity. This expresses the annual weaning performance per unit metabolic doe weight and permits the comparison of reproductive efficiency in populations which differ in mature size. In addition, factors must be established to correct for differences in lactation numbers since a population with a high percentage of first kidding does will be penalized in a comparative trial, as may be the case in crossbreeding programmes. A correction for sex and litter size may also be necessary. When evaluating populations, it is useful not only to measure the production parameters and their

Table 1. Parameters characterizing reproductive efficiency in does.

Duration of the breeding season
Age and weight at puberty (1st oestrous)
Occurrence of oestrous a) after parturition
                               b) during suckling
Age at 50, 67, and 75% mature weight
Age and weight at first service
Age and weight at first, second, and third kiddings/lambings
Duration of first and second kidding/lambing interval
Weight changes during first, second, and third pregnancy
Duration of lactation/suckling
Weight changes during first, second, and third lactation
Litter size and litter weight (first, second, and third kidding/lambing)
Preweaning kid and litter weight gain (standardized to 100 days)
Preweaning mortality (percentage and causes)
Biological productivity: weaning weight per metabolic doe weight per year

variability but also to determine their specific contribution to the production index using sensitivity analyses. For example, Peacock (1987) reported that in Maasai flocks of sheep and goats, conception and mortality rates were more important than litter size or weaning weight. However, the ranking of traits may differ from population to population due to inheritance or environmental conditions.

In the male, the important criteria are age and weight at complete sexual maturity, seasonality of libido, ejaculate characteristics, testis size, storability of the spermatozoa, and the number of services per conception.

The meat production potential of the individual animal can be estimated from growth intensity, feed intake (where intensive fattening is envisaged), and carcass quality of weaned male kids and lambs. Details of the measurements are given in Table 2.

Different feeding intensities e.g., supplementation of the pasture with 0, 25, 50, and 75 g concentrate/kg metabolic liveweight would be desirable. For

Table 2. Measures of meat production potential.

Measure	Time of recording
Growth capacity	Mature weight
Growth intensity	Average daily gain at 3–6 or 9–12 months old or at 20, 40, or 60% of mature weight
Feed efficiency	At 3–6 or 9–12 months old or at 20, 40, or 60% of mature weight
Carcass quality to include slaughter weight, carcass weight, weights of skin, head, feet, GIT, and valuable cuts, and carcass composition (water, fat, protein, ash)	At 6, 9, or 12 months old or 20, 40, or 60% of mature weight

instance, a 10% (38–42%) increase in dressing rate was observed in Tunisia and this increase was smaller in the local breed than in the crosses between the Race locale and the European dairy breeds.

Milk yield and composition are important for milk, cheese, and butter production and for suckling kids. Genotypes differ in milk yield but estimates are also affected by the method of determination. The difference in milkability may account for considerable genotypic variation so several methods should be used when comparing meat, dual purpose, and dairy breeds for milk production potential.

Different periods and methods can be used to estimate milk yield: kidding to weaning (100 days) using suckling and hand milking (with and without oxytocin treatment) or postweaning milk yield using hand milking (with and without oxytocin treatment), until the milk yield becomes less than 200 ml/day. Testing the milk weekly for 4 h periods in the morning and at night has been found adequate. Chemical analyses should determine at least the fat, lactose, protein, and mineral contents but tests for specific constituents may be required in special circumstances.

Methods to determine the production value of the textile products have hardly been investigated, with the exception of cashmere and mohair, and knowledge of genotypic variations in the technological qualities of goat skin or fine undercoat wool is rather limited. Consequently, evaluation programmes should include quality testing of leather yield per animal in relation to age and liveweight, skin quality including thickness, softness, and tensile strength, pelt quality (e.g., Zhongwei goat), hair and wool yield per annum, and hair and wool quality including fineness, fibre length, colour, etc.

Disease susceptibility and mortality

Genotypes vary in their rusticity and ability to resist and overcome diseases. Diseases increase the cost of production, reduce productive performance, or increase mortality.

These responses, all of which reduce economic productivity, are naturally related to management and climatic and nutritional stresses. Adaptability to suboptimal environmental conditions interacts with disease risk so it is necessary to record the occurrence of important diseases in different age groups (kids, young stock, mature animals) and mortality rates in different age and sex groups to measure the suitability of a population for a marginal environment.

Physiologically important traits

Physiological characteristics differ among populations and several are related to goat management and to the performance traits already discussed. The most important of these characteristics are the following:

1. Biometeorological adaptations.

   a) Radiation balance.
   b) Physiological responses to increasing ambient temperatures.

2. Nutritional adaptations.
   a) Rate of metabolism and maintenance requirements.
   b) Feed intake, diet selectivity, and utilization of vegetation.
   c) Digestibility of fibre and other nutrients.
   d) Feed conversion efficiency.
   e) Response to fluctuations in feed supply (compensatory growth).
   f) Salt tolerance (feed and water).

For example, black goats gain twice as much heat from radiation as white goats (Finch et al. 1980), a disadvantage during the day but a possible advantage for cold nights which are typical for arid climates.

Nutritional adaptations are likely and also vary among populations. To date, genetic differences in the efficiency of diet utilization have been tested in inter-species rather than intra-species comparisons (Van Soest 1981). Using salt tolerance in goats as an example, indigenous goats lost absolutely and relatively less weight during watering with sea water and their weight losses levelled off earlier than in non-adapted European dairy goats.

Genetic parameters of populations

Decisions necessary for genetic improvement programmes require an adequate knowledge of the additive and non-additive genetic parameters of the populations involved. Moreover, genotype by environment interactions may be important. The relative magnitude of these values determines whether selection or crossbreeding is the appropriate improvement strategy.

Important additive genetic parameters are heritability, repeatability, and genetic correlations. They are not always easily estimated, due to confounding factors which arise when records from one single station are used, particularly as heritability values are thought to vary among populations. However, breeding values can only be computed and selection practiced if these values are known. Additive genetic parameters should be estimated under fairly standardized conditions and economically feasible management.

While inbreeding depressions in small populations have traditionally been over-estimated, heterotic effects may be very important and vary among environments and populations. Cunningham (1981) suggested that heterosis is more pronounced in marginal than in optimal environments, but this has never been tested. More work is needed to elucidate the mechanisms involved in the heterosis of farm animals managed under conditions of nutritional and environmental stress.

Economic evaluation

As livestock improvement aims to improve rural incomes, any evaluation programme must balance the gross income against the costs of production and marketing. Gross income is determined by the production of offspring (weaning performance × market price), liveweight gain and the value of slaughtered animals, milk yield and sales value, fibre production and market value, and possibly other products and their value e.g., manure. The costs of production and marketing include the replacement of stock and mating costs, concentrate and other feed costs, veterinary treatment, housing and fences, interest on invested capital, and marketing expenses. Whether or not labour costs should be included depends on the type and size of the enterprise. In a smallholder production system the inclusion of labour costs is questionable if alternative employment opportunities are scarce. Herding costs can be considerable in large flocks.

Systems of evaluation

Genotypes can be evaluated on experimental stations and in commercial or village flocks. Research flocks have the advantage of the standardized conditions and many precise records can be collected, albeit from a restricted number of animals. The disadvantages are the high cost per animal unit and a certain degree of artificiality that cannot be avoided.

In village flocks fewer and less accurate records can be collected from many animals under variable, usually more representative conditions. Larger commercial flocks are not very common in goat production, with the exception of Angora flocks, but data collection is more precise than in smallholder flocks and cheaper than in experimental flocks.

A prerequisite to genotype evaluation in rural flocks is the development of an adequate infrastructure and acceptable testing procedures. This can be achieved by combining extension with evaluation. Ideally, an extension worker should visit each flock once a month to identify and weigh the animals, record births, deaths, and sales, measure milk yield (where appropriate), and report the results of the last visit to the flock owner along with suggestions for improved management. Field data can be recorded on appropriate forms or using a data logger for subsequent computer analysis.

The number of animals necessary for evaluation and manageable for one extension worker depends on flock size, the distance between flocks, and the cooperation of flock owners but a field technician can handle 50–100 flocks or 1000–3000 animals on a regular basis. In many instances, sheep should be included in the evaluation procedures, since both small ruminant species are frequently kept on the same farm and compete for the same resources.

In private flocks a number of problems may arise that are less critical on research stations. For example, animals may be sold or slaughtered, records are often inaccurate, irrational changes in management may be made, or the flock owner may lose interest and become less cooperative. These problems can be minimized by convincingly demonstrating to the flock owner the economic benefit of the exercise and by developing an atmosphere of mutual confidence between the researcher and the flock owner. Frequent visits, avoiding unreasonable work loads and flock disturbance, and providing advice on improved management procedures will help.

The relative advantage of station or village flock evaluation will largely depend upon local conditions. Each has its own problems and merits and a combination of the two systems might help to balance the information and demonstrate the yield gap i.e., the difference between productivity values obtainable on- and off-station, which would be a measure of non-genetic improvement potential.

A specific case of genotype evaluation that has aroused interest in recent years is the screening of populations for major genes occurring at low gene frequencies. Examples are the Booroola gene which was detected in Australian Merinos (Davis et al. 1982) and the gene controlling the expression of alpha-S_1-casein in caprine milk (Boulanger et al. 1984). Timon (1987) has suggested that screening national flocks for similar major genes may be extremely rewarding if exceptional animals are about three standard deviations above the mean. Such animals may increase genetic progress. Booroola Merino sires were reported to increase ovulation rate by 64% on average in Rambouillet ewes (Willingham et al. 1986). However, in marginal environments increased ovulation rates may not be acceptable due to a lack of feed and high mortality rates.

Surveys: collection and dissemination of information

Genotype evaluation is only useful if standardized information is recorded, analyzed, collated, and disseminated. The FAO has started to publish an information bulletin of Animal Genetic Resources. Since very little standardized information has been published, an attempt was made to collect whatever information was available on sheep and goats in the Mediterranean basin and Africa (Steinbach 1987b). The survey was conducted by mail and revealed a great scarcity of the required data. In total, 25 institutions (17%) returned 69 questionnaires (65% sheep, 35% goat), of which less than half contained sufficient information to calculate productivity values. The results indicate little difference between sheep and goats when biological productivity is expressed in relation to mature metabolic dam weight (Fig. 1) and only Eastern Mediterranean goats fall significantly below the average of 1.5 kg. Due to the poor return of acceptable information, the results can only be considered preliminary but they illustrate what a survey could achieve when precise experimental records from village and station populations become available. With more and better information it should be possible to demon-

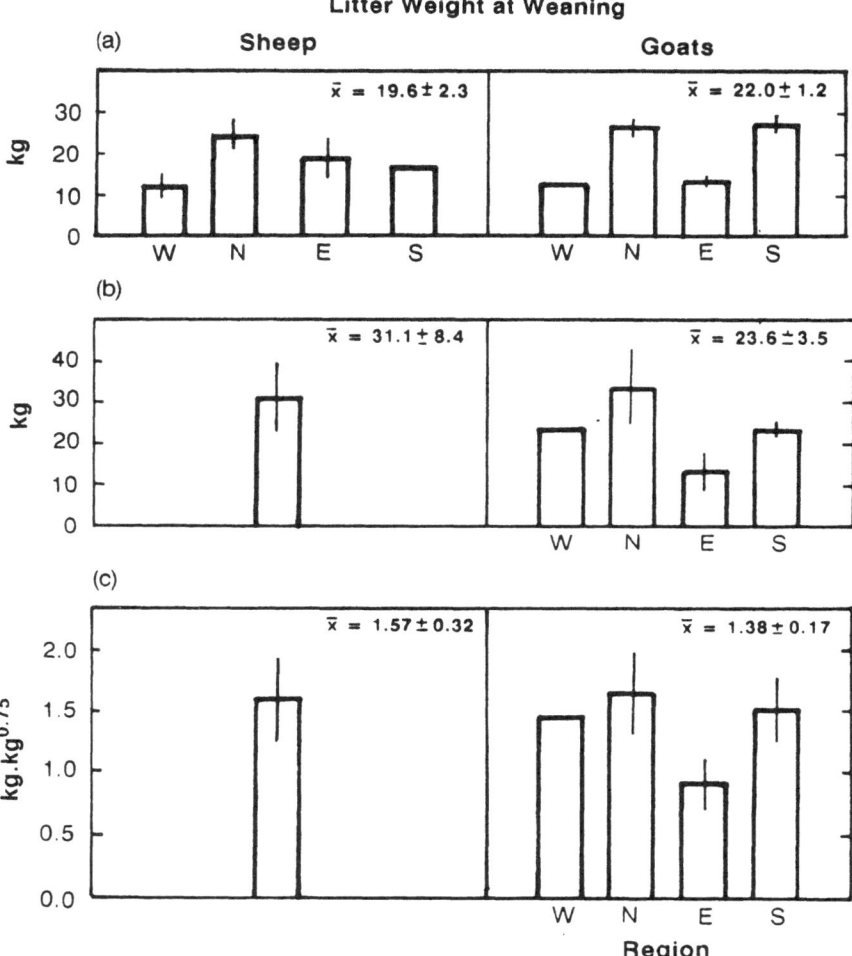

Fig. 1. Results of a survey showing litter weaning performance (a) as recorded, (b) corrected to standard weaning age (75 days) and for parturition interval, and (c) biological productivity (adjusted litter weaning weight per annum and mature metabolic dam weight) in the western (W), northern (N), eastern (E), and southern (S) Mediterranean regions.

strate the influences of genotype and environment on small ruminant productivity.

Establishment of gene banks

Evaluation should precede genetic conservation. Not all currently available genotypes can be actively preserved indefinitely for economic reasons. However, those populations that are characterized by either high general productivity or specific, potentially valuable adaptive traits should be protected and preserved in animal or gamete banks. Conservation is cheap relative to the production value of small ruminants in West Asia (Awa and Abdullahi 1986) and to the potential benefits that can be expected from superior, more diversified genetic materials. The cost-benefit ratios are favourable for the evaluation and conservation of genetic stock in the form of pure breeds, which is necessary if their special performance characteristics are to be preserved (Smith 1984). Live animal banks would permit conservation by management and the continuous screening and evaluation of the maintained population. In addition to domesticated sheep and goats, special attention should be given to preserving and maintaining the genetic integrity of endangered populations of wild sheep and goats (Goodland et al. 1984).

Improvement of sheep and goat populations

Contrary to evaluation, breeding methods are well established for sheep and goat improvement. Frequently the choice of a particular method e.g., crossbreeding or selection, may be questionable and there may be doubt whether or not the breeding objectives have been appropriately defined and harmonized with production goals and the target production systems.

Production goals and production systems

Genetic improvement must take into account target products and dominant production systems. Nomadic herding, horizontal or vertical transhumance, and settled forms of grazing or stall-feeding affect the optimum approach to genetic improvement, as does the combination of products that are the target of improvement or the ecosystem in which the flock is kept. For example, in migratory flocks complex recording or selection and crossbreeding programmes are not feasible.

Selection and crossbreeding

Genetic improvement can be achieved by selection within the autochthonous population or by crossbreeding with either regional or exotic genotypes. The aim is to utilize non-additive genetic effects, combine adaptive and productive traits, and create a new breed following intensive selection or introduction of major genes into indigenous populations.

Selection can be a powerful tool in unselected regional sheep and goat populations that show considerable phenotypic variation. Although the precise additive genetic component is frequently unknown, it is generally believed that it is sufficiently large to make selection programmes successful if a large portion of the population is included in the selection process (Timon 1987). To do this, a multiple-stage selection procedure might be useful, with many animals involved in a simple, population-wide screening process and successively more intense selection procedures up to the level of central nucleus flocks. Consistent and continuous selection within unselected populations will lead to genotype fixation and the formation of a new breed.

Crossbreeding of distant breeds or ecotypes results in heterosis. Estimates of heterosis for small ruminants vary widely (Turner 1982) and the contribution to hybrid vigour in sheep and goat productivity cannot be predicted at present. Moreover, continuous crossbreeding programmes are difficult to manage under the flock husbandry conditions common throughout most of the semi-arid and arid regions. On the other hand, desired traits could easily be combined in nucleus flocks to develop a synthetic, more productive breed. The new self-replacing breed can then be transferred into private flocks following intensive selection under commercial conditions. In a similar way, major genes can be introduced into local flocks. Here too, the unwanted characteristics of the major gene donor breed must be filtered out by subsequent selection.

Biotechnology of gene transfer and genetic engineering

Artificial insemination with frozen semen and embryo-transfer techniques are available for the transfer and storage of genetic material. These techniques are only useful for long-distance gene transfer, nucleus flock development, and where there are import restrictions on livestock. Limitations of infrastructure generally prohibit their use in large-scale breed improvement programmes in the semi-arid regions.

First successes were reported recently (Minhas et al. 1986) on the transfer of genetic material into the visualized pronuclei of sheep embryos. If major genes for specific proteins or increased fertility could be transferred by this method, time-consuming selection procedures could be avoided.

Genetic improvement of private flocks

Essentially all the small ruminants in North Africa and West Asia are kept either on small farms or in migratory flocks, which makes genetic improvement rather difficult. The most promising improvement procedure would involve the establishment of a central sire breeding nucleus flock consisting of 300 effective female breeders (Turner 1982) from which the males are distributed to smaller flocks whose males are castrated or sold. Extension agents visiting each flock at least monthly could supervise the use and rotation of improved males and assist with simple flock recording and selection of females. Intermediate multiplier flocks may be useful in some environments.

Conclusions

Genetic improvement should be the last step in improving small ruminant productivity in arid and semi-arid regions. Improvements in the nutritional status, health, and general flock management should take precedence over breeding. However, the evaluation of genotypes and establishment of nucleus flocks and selection and screening procedures are time-consuming. Moreover, the danger of losing potentially valuable genetic material is imminent, so genetic evaluation and improvement of the region's sheep and goat populations should be initiated immediately, thereby supplying progressive flock owners with genetic material that can give them increased economic returns.

References

Awa, O.A. and Abdullahi, A.N. 1986. Research priorities, coordination of activities and transfer of information. Pages 139–153 in Compte Rendu du Seminaire sur la Coordination de la Recherche pour le Developpement des Petits Ruminants en Afrique, Montpellier, 13–17 Oct 1986. CTA, EC, GTZ, IEMVT.

Boulanger, A., Grosclaude, F. and Mahe, M.F. 1984. Polymorphisme des caseines α_1 et α_2 de la chevre (*Capra hircus*). Genetic Selection and Evolution 16: 157–176.

CSIRO (Commonwealth Scientific and Industrial Research Organization). 1982. Goats for meat and fibre in Australia. Report of the Expert Panel appointed by the Animal Production Commission SCA, Canberra, Australia.

Cunningham, E.P. 1981. Selection and crossbreeding strategies in adverse environments. Pages 279–288 in Animal Production and Health Paper 24. FAO, Rome, Italy.

Davis, G.H., Montgomery, G.W. and Kelly, R.W. 1982. Estimates of the repeatability of ovulation rate in Booroola cross ewes. Mimeograph.

Finch, V.A., Dmi'el, R., Boxmann, R., Shkolnik, A. and Taylor, C.R. 1980. Why black goats in hot deserts? Effect of coat colour on heat exchanges of wild and domestic goats. Physiological Zoology 53: 19–25.

Goodland, R.J.A., Watson, C. and Ledec, G. 1984. Conserving biological and genetic diversity. Pages 207–216 in Environmental Management in Tropical Agriculture. Westview Press, Boulder, USA.

Mason, I.L. 1969. A World Dictionary of Livestock Breeds, Types and Varieties. Commonwealth Agricultural Bureaux, Farnham Royal, UK.

Minhas, B.S., Capehart, J.S., Bowen, M.J. and Kraemer, D.C. 1986. Developing methods for gene transfer in sheep. Research Report CPR 4377. College Station, Texas A & M University, USA.

Peacock, C.P. 1987. Measures for assessing the productivity of sheep and goats. Agricultural Systems 23: 197–210.

Smith, C. 1984. Economic benefits of conserving animal genetic resources. Animal Genetic Resources Information 3: 10–14. FAO, Rome, Italy.

Steinbach, J. 1987a. Evaluation of indigenous and exotic breeds and their crosses for production in unfavourable environments. Pages 625–641 in Proceedings of the Fourth International Conference on Goats, 8–13 March 1987, Brasilia, Brazil.

Steinbach, J. 1987b. The characterization of the reproductive potential of sheep and goats. Paper presented at the Symposium on the Evaluation of Mediterranean Sheep and Goats "Philoetios", Santarem, Portugal.

Timon, V. 1987. Genetic selection for improvement of native highly adaptive breeds. Paper presented at the Fourth International Conference on Goats, 8–13 March 1987, Brasilia, Brazil.

Turner, H.N. 1982. Basic considerations of breeding plans. In Small Ruminant Breed Productivity in Africa (Gatenby, R.M. and Trail, J.C.M., eds). ILCA, Addis Ababa, Ethiopia. 96 p.

Van Soest, P.J. 1981. Impact of feeding behaviour and digestive capacity on nutritional response. Pages 140–161 in Animal Production and Health Paper 24. FAO, Rome, Italy.

Willingham, T., Shelton, M., Spiller, D. and Thompson, P. 1986. Increasing ovulation rate in Rambouillet ewes through inclusion of the Booroola genotype as compared to other prolific breeds. Research Report CPR 4372. College Station, Texas A & M University, USA.

E.F. Thomson and F.S. Thomson (eds), Increasing Small Ruminant Productivity in Semi-arid Areas
© 1988 ICARDA . ISBN 978-94-010-7086-7

New Technologies for Animal Improvement and Developing Countries

R.B. Land

Introduction

Livestock are a principle source of food in developed and developing countries. Their value is related to the efficiency with which they are able to meet the requirements of the local society. Society sets the ethical and economic framework of animal production systems but it is the responsibility of the scientist to develop appropriate technologies to enhance livestock production.

Traditionally, farm animals have been selected over many centuries to be well adapted to local conditions. Livestock husbandry has developed to increase the efficiency of production by reducing costs and increasing the value of the output. Genetic and husbandry improvements are not alternatives but should be considered integral parts of a single strategy. Much has been written on improved husbandry so this paper will address the new technologies that can be used in animal breeding so that genetic selection might best complement husbandry and make a greater contribution to improved animal production. Particular emphasis is given to methods which are not dependent upon sophisticated local or national infrastructures.

New technologies

Genetic selection, husbandry, and health are the traditional technologies of animal production. During the past decade, several new techniques have become available, including the use of growth promoters, partition agents, protein hormones, biotechnology and immunological modulation of performance.

Doubts have been cast over the acceptability of steroidal growth promoters and partition agents. Equally, despite considerable promise, protein hormones have not yet been accepted. The immunological modulation of performance has, however, been successfully developed for reproduction. The biological basis and benefits of this process have been reviewed by Scaramuzzi and Hoskinson (1984). The procedure is simple and requires only an initial vaccination followed by a booster 3 weeks before mating. Examples of the benefits of vaccination are given in Table 1 for two experiments in which Merino ewes were immunized against androstenedione.

Table 1. Effect of immunization against androstenedione on reproductive performance of Merino ewes.

	Experiment 1		Experiment 2	
	control	treated	control	treated
No. of sheep	50	50	48	49
Mean no. of ovulations	1.46	1.82	1.14	1.43
Percent mated	98	98	96	98
Percent lambing	94	96	87	79
Lambs/ewe mated	1.25	1.51	0.91	0.92
Lambs/ewe lambing	1.33	1.57	1.05	1.16

Source: Scaramuzzi and Hoskinson (1984).

The technique clearly works, and is ideal for increasing the normal litter size to take advantage of an anticipated increase in nutrient supply. In this way, the productivity of breeds which normally produce single lambs in extensive conditions could be increased to take advantage of, for example, the better conditions of irrigated agriculture.

More recently, immunization has been used against fat cell membranes to reduce the proportion of fat and improve carcass quality. This introduces a new principle as the immunization is actually against a component of the unwanted tissue rather than a circulating hormone. It was first demonstrated by Dr D. Flint of the Hannah Research Institute and is being commercially developed. Another development in immunology which could have far-reaching implications is the discovery that antibodies to antibodies, anti-idiotypes, can have the properties of the original antigen. This can provide a ready supply of antigen and be the basis for producing a protein with the properties of, for example, a steroid.

New technologies to manipulate animals directly will always have a place. However, it is simpler for the farmer if the genetic makeup of livestock directly determines appropriate characteristics. The attractiveness of genetic methods is related to the rate of change that can be achieved and the difficulty of controlling the environment or improving husbandry. New developments in animal breeding have been considered in general by Land (1985). In the rest of this paper, genetic selection will first be considered in general to give a framework within which the new opportunities can be judged and applied.

Genetic selection

The substitution of a superior population, be it a different species or breed, is well recognised as an effective first step in any programme of genetic improvement. Once the superior population has been established, however, improvement by selection is slow compared with the rapid improvements that might be made through, for example, controlling particular diseases by vaccination or improving the food supply by irrigation. However, environmental improvements are often expensive and require continued inputs. Genetic selection is cumulative, with each year's progress being added to that of earlier years. Thus, it is not necessarily dependent upon greater inputs and once achieved it is maintained without further effort. Many of the advantages of genetic improvement apply particularly to developing countries.

In assessing the role of genetic change, it is important to appreciate that progressive selection over several years can achieve dramatic results. Taking examples from the UK, the growth rate of poultry has increased by 50% over the past 12 years as a result of genetic change and although the high reproductive rate of poultry has contributed to the speed of this change, significant improvements have also been made in other species. In pigs, for example, growth rate has increased by 4% and efficiency by 6% in the UK over the past 10 years. This improvement has been accompanied by an improvement in the quality with leanness increasing by 14% over the same period. The crucial factor in an effective programme of genetic improvement is the rigorous use of objective criteria of performance. The need to first set appropriate criteria for selection and then adhere to them strictly cannot be overemphasized.

The improved growth of pigs and poultry clearly illustrates the benefits of genetic selection, but the opportunity to improve other traits and other species is also apparent. The potential to improve the reproductive performance, growth rate, and carcass quality of cattle, sheep, and pigs has been assessed by Smith (1985). The estimated annual rates of response to genetic improvement in cattle, sheep, pigs, and poultry are shown in Table 2. Most traits can be improved by about 3% per generation and while this might seem small, the cumulative effects are substantial. The opportunity to improve the characteristics of livestock by 25% in eight generations is very significant.

Despite the magnitude of the response, genetic selection has not been effectively harnessed as a means of improving most of the world's livestock. Eight generations is a long period for investors or administrators and this tends to discourage investment. Over a long period, the benefits of investment in animal breeding are considerable. For example, annual benefits to the UK of 100 million GBP are often cited for an annual expenditure of 2 million GBP (HM Treasury 1985).

Table 2. Annual rates of genetic response of various traits in several species.

Trait	Species			
	cattle	sheep	pigs	poultry
Growth	1.0	1.5	2.0	5.0
Leanness	0.5	0.8	1.0	2.0
Milk production	2.0	–	–	–
Litter size	–	1.5	1.5	–
Egg production	–	–	–	2.0

Source: Smith (1984).

Genetic selection would be used more frequently for improvement if the potential rate of change were greater. Fortunately, recent developments in animal breeding show that this is possible and many of these developments are appropriate for developing and developed countries. Two examples are the multibreed approach to choosing among populations and the use of multiple ovulation and embryo transfer (MOET) to accelerate genetic progress within the chosen population.

Selecting an appropriate population for further improvement

It is very effective to choose the best of available populations, but this can be difficult especially if there are many populations. Sufficient resources must be allocated to characterise each of the breeds for the particular environment and samples should not be limited to the offspring of a small number of sires which themselves must be representative. Furthermore, it is often possible that a cross might meet requirements better than any of the individual breeds available and it might be important to know the proportion of the two parents that should be used. With limited testing facilities, the choice of a base population can be simplified to one of two basic approaches, multibreed selection or the choice of a particular cross with an exotic breed.

Where there are many populations, it would be difficult to ensure that the best breed or cross was chosen and so a simpler concept of multibreed selection has been put forward by Taylor and Thiessen (1984). The aim of this approach is to ensure that the best of the available populations are represented and then pooled to form the new base for continued selection. Individual breeds need not be characterised precisely as the choice or omission of one marginal population is unimportant. Samples of each of the populations are assessed in the local system of husbandry and the best third or so are chosen to make up the new population.

Where it is not clear whether an imported breed itself might have superior performance or improvement might best be gained by crossing imported with local breeds, it is important to consider how best to choose the most suitable breed or cross. Ideally, several should be evaluated, but this is often impractical. If there are several candidate breeds for importation, multibreed selection based on pure and crossbred types would be appropriate.

The pragmatic choice of the base population is a compromise between the gain that would be achieved if the best population were chosen and the cost of the resources required to do so. Other populations will continue to be available and should be introduced later if it is clear that they would confer an advantage.

The use of multiple ovulation and embryo transfer (MOET)

In sheep and cattle, the rate of response to genetic selection is restricted by the rate of female reproduction. Females are chosen at the expense of increasing the duration of the generation interval. The reproductive rate can now be increased using gonadotrophins to stimulate the ovulation of additional eggs which are then transferred to surrogate mothers.

The benefits of multiple ovulation have been best quantified for dairy cattle, most recently by Woolliams and Smith (1987). They showed that with four male and four female offspring per cow, the rate of response to selection could be 30% greater than that achieved with progeny testing. This is relevant to both developed and developing countries, for it is much easier to ensure that strict objective selection is practised in a single herd than in a large-scale progeny testing programme. It is particularly relevant to developing countries because it does not require a sophisticated infrastructure. The level of technology required for MOET is higher than that for progeny testing, but the requirement is restricted to a single location.

MOET technology allows developing countries to select livestock according to local requirements. Once the choice has been made between a local breed or a cross to an exotic breed for the base population, selection can be made in the local environment with no requirement to continually import and evaluate exotic stocks.

Using MOET in beef cattle, the rate of genetic improvement can be increased by 50% or more (Land and Hill 1975). Woolliams and Smith (1987)

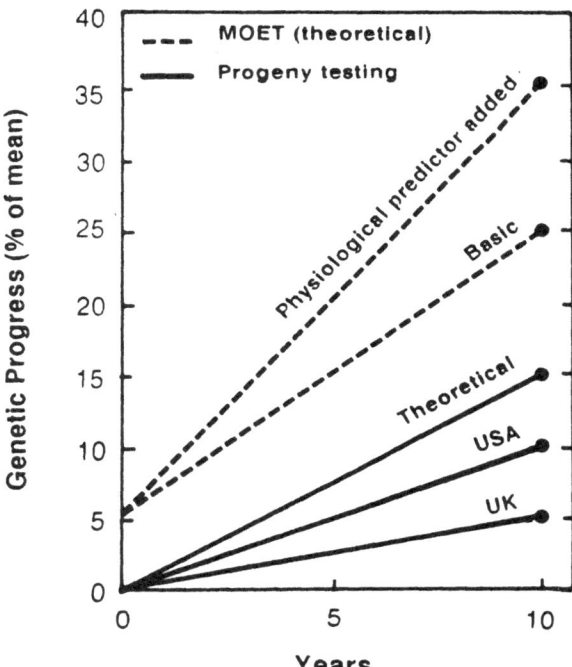

Fig. 1. The potential benefits of applying biotechnology to the genetic improvement of dairy cattle.

showed that combining MOET with a physiological predictor of genetic merit, such as the concentration of blood urea nitrogen (BUN), could double the rate of response to selection for milk production compared to progeny testing if the coheritability ($h_1 h_2 r_g$) of the predictor with yield is 0.27 (Fig. 1). New physiological technologies are directly relevant to genetic improvement, particularly in developing countries.

Future developments

The use of MOET accelerates genetic progress by increasing the selection differential. Looking further ahead, recombinant DNA technology will allow the direct introduction of desirable genetic variation. Isolated genes from one animal are multiplied or cloned and introduced into another animal of the same or a different species. Genes are presently transferred by injecting several hundred copies into the pronucleus of the egg during fertilisation. In some cases, the gene is incorporated into the chromosome and in a proportion of these the gene is expressed, so that about 1% of injected embryos develop into transgenic livestock.

An important step in the application of this technology is the identification of suitable genes. This is discussed by Land and Wilmut (1987). Generally, traits can be changed by about 10% in 5 years using selection alone, which sets a formidable baseline for the application of transgenics. The technique is therefore first likely to be applied in the improvement of traits where genetic variation is presently limited, such as the production of pharmaceutical proteins (medicines) by the mammary gland, disease resistance, and twinning in cattle.

With novel traits, the identification of genes coding for the new proteins is likely to be important while conventional traits are likely to be improved through the identification of control sequences which allow the expression of a gene to escape normal feedback control. The ability to turn off genes is likely to have a greater impact than the addition or turning up of genes.

The place of gene transfer in animal improvement has yet to be established. Like MOET, it does not depend upon a sophisticated infrastructure and it could be seen as a logical extension of the laboratory, animal testing, and statistical resources established for MOET.

Conclusions

Resources are always limited and it is important that those available are deployed to the best advantage. Genetic improvement has an important role to play, facilitated by new technologies such as MOET. Potentially greater rates of gain are possible in genetic selection programmes using MOET, so the timescale of return on investment is shortened and genetic improvement of livestock becomes a more attractive option for investors. The rates of improvement that can be achieved in cattle with MOET are substantial when applied to a properly structured programme of genetic improvement.

To date, most embryo transfer has been used for short-term financial gain and has not been linked to planned long-term genetic improvement programmes. With limited resources, national and international funds must be used for the long-term benefit of the community, not the short-term financial gain of the entrepreneur.

References

H.M. Treasury 1985. The government's expenditure plans 1985–86 to 1987–88. Cmnd. 9428, 11: 57.

Land, R.B. 1985. Knowledge for animal breeding. Philosophical Transactions of the Royal Society of London B 310: 243–289.

Land, R.B. and Hill, W.G. 1975. The possible use of superovulation and embryo transfer in cattle to increase response to selection. Animal Production 21: 1–12.

Land, R.B. and Wilmut, I. 1987. Gene transfer and animal breeding. Theriogenology 27: 169–179.

Scaramuzzi, R.J. and Hoskinson, R.M. 1984. Active immunization against steroid hormones for increasing fecundity. Pages 445–474 in Immunological Aspects of Reproduction in Mammals (Crighton, D.B., ed.). Butterworths, London, UK.

Smith, C. 1984. Rates of genetic change in farm livestock. Research and Development in Agriculture 1: 79–85.

Taylor, St. C.S. and Thiessen, R.B. 1984. Multibreed designs for breed testing and selection. Pages 547–564 in Proceedings of the 2nd World Congress on Sheep and Beef Cattle Breeding, South Africa.

Woolliams, J.A. and Smith, C. 1988. The value of indicator traits in the genetic improvement of dairy cattle. Animal Production . In press.

E.F. Thomson and F.S. Thomson (eds), Increasing Small Ruminant Productivity in Semi-arid Areas
© *1988 ICARDA . ISBN 978-94-010-7086-7*

Selection for Lamb Growth in Libyan Barbary Sheep

R.J. Lightfoot

Introduction

In 1974, the Western Australian Department of Agriculture commenced a series of two 5-year contracts with the Libyan Ministry of Agriculture to provide managerial and technical supervision for a "Cereal Project" to be commissioned by the Geffara Plains Authority. The project involved the development of nine low rainfall sites totalling 50000 ha for cereals and sheep production using the dryland legume pasture/cereal crop ley farming system used in Western Australia.

The project was located within a 150 km radius from Tripoli. Seven project sites were on the Geffara Plain which extends approximately 100 km to the east, south, and west of Tripoli and is bounded by a major scarp leading up to an elevated plateau. Two of the nine sites (Gendoubah and Tarhuna) were on the plateau. The climate is typically Mediterranean with hot, dry summers and mild winters. Average annual rainfall (90% of which falls in winter) declines from around 250 mm near the coast to 150 mm in the south and on the scarp.

In the initial years the Cereal Project concentrated on land clearing, levelling, establishing medic pasture/cereal crop rotations, and training Libyans. Carrying capacity rose from approximately one sheep per 5 ha on unimproved native pastures to one sheep per ha on the medic pastures. Flocks of the Libyan Barbary sheep (Mason 1967), the dominant local breed, were established and by 1978 when the author was appointed to advise on flock policy there were about 10000 breeding ewes.

Materials and methods

Flock management

The ewes were grazed in flocks of 300–500 under the supervision of shepherds. All sheep were corralled each night with the shepherds sleeping nearby. Rams were joined to ewes (1 to 20) in the first week of June for 8 weeks to lamb in November or December. All lambs were reared on their mothers and the ewes were not milked. Supplementary feeding (hay and grain) was practiced for flock maintenance through the autumn/early winter and in poor seasons. All lambs were weaned in one group about 110 days after the start of lambing. Shearing was in March/April.

Breeding goals

Available information suggested a continuing trend towards increased per capita consumption of red meats, with sheep meat the first choice of the Muslim community. Of the available breeds, the local Barbary sheep were preferred, particularly young, well grown ram lambs which commanded substantial premiums in the market when compared with imported breeds. In view of this preference and because of the proven adaptation of the Barbary to the local environment, the project focused on improvement through management and selection of the local breed rather than by importing new genotypes.

Because of the very high economic value of lamb meat compared with wool in Libya and comparatively minor use of the Barbary sheep for milking, it was decided that the breeding goals should emphasize meat production. Given very high market returns from 4–6 month old rams at 40–50 kg off medic pastures in spring, it was agreed that "reserves" would be selected initially on corrected rate of liveweight gain to weaning with final selection on liveweight at 18 months of age. The initial culling on rate of liveweight gain to weaning enabled the early sale of excess stock to maximise numbers of breeding ewes and therefore lambs available for sale. Although genetic parameters were not available for the Libyan Barbary, corrected lamb growth and, in particular, 18 month liveweight are usually moderately to highly heritable and can be measured in the field relatively simply.

In basing initial selection on rate of liveweight gain to weaning, it was essential that appropriate corrections for birth rank (twin or single), date of birth, and environment (flock, farm, etc.) were made to improve the accuracy of selection and guard against any negative effects that use of uncorrected weight could have on fertility. While no direct selection for either fleece weight or fibre diameter was proposed, the Libyan advisers felt that some restrictions on colour were warranted to limit black or brown in the body fleece. However, it was agreed that relatively little selection pressure should be expended on wool characteristics as these were economically insignificant compared with meat.

The breeding plan

The initial plan proposed a total flock of 15000 breeding ewes, 2000 of which were to form an elite ram breeding nucleus. The nucleus and associated selection programme were established in three stages.

Stage 1: initial nucleus formation (April 1978)

This involved the selection of 2000 breeding ewes plus rams and replacements in April 1978 (Table 1) and their relocation to a single project site for mating

Table 1. Initial nucleus formation–April 1978.

Class of stock	Total available sheep	Selected for nucleus		Selection criteria [2]
		number	% of available sheep	
Breeding ewes	9507	1558 [1]	16	L, W, C
Ewe hoggets	1043	442 [1]	42	W, C
Ewe lambs	3706	465	13	W, C
Rams	714	–	–	W, C
Ram hoggets	325	100 [1]	31	W, C
Ram lambs	3669	105	3	W, C
Total	18964	2670		

[1] For joining in June 1978.
[2] L = lambed; W = liveweight; C = fleece colour.

in June. Ewes and rams were selected proportionately within age groups on the basis of liveweight. As far as could be determined, all selected adult ewes had reared a lamb in 1977/78 and had no black or brown patches on the main trunk of the body.

Stage 2: open nucleus–genetic upgrading (1978–81)

Throughout the first 28 days of lambing sequentially numbered sets of ear tags were given to the shepherds who, each morning, tagged all lambs born during the previous 24 h before the flocks went to graze. Single lambs received one tag, twin lambs two. The tag numbers used in each flock were recorded by the sheep supervisors on a daily basis. By this means, full documentation of date of birth, birth rank, and flock or site of origin was obtained for all lambs born in the first 4 weeks.

Each year, immediately following weaning (late February) about 650 ewe and 350 ram lambs were selected as reserves for the nucleus. After an initial culling for physical deformity and excessive colour on the body trunk (scores 3 and 4, Table 5), all tagged lambs were weighed and selection then based entirely on corrected rate of liveweight gain from birth, assuming 3 kg average birth weight to weaning. The individual values were then adjusted by additive/deductive correction factors to account for variation in average performance for flocks within sites, between sites, and for birth rank.

The ewe and ram reserves were run as separate flocks and weighed again in May the following year at approximately 18 months old. Final selection using 18 month liveweight, corrected for birth rank and flock, reduced numbers to approximately 440 ewes which entered the nucleus as two-tooth replacements and 100 rams for mating the nucleus in June. The nucleus of 2000 breeding ewes was managed as five separate flocks, one for each age group from 1.5 years to 5.5 years. Rams were used only once in the nucleus, always as two-tooths. The 250 reserve rams not selected for the nucleus together with the (then) four-tooth rams joined to the nucleus the previous year, were used to join the Project's general flocks.

Stage 3: closed nucleus (1982 onwards)

The nucleus of 2000 breeding ewes was "closed" in 1982 and annual screening for selection from the general flocks was discontinued. The nucleus was managed as a self-regenerating elite flock, breeding rams and ewes for its own replacements and rams for the general flocks. This provided the opportunity to calculate improved estimates of breeding value based on both individual performance and that of relatives.

Results

Reproductive performance

A total of 77161 ewe records were made from 1977 to 1983 inclusive (Table 2). Overall figures show moderate levels of fertility for ewes lambing (87%) and ewes twinning (10%) and exceptionally low lamb mortality (2.8%). There was highly significant ($P < 0.001$) variation between years in the proportion of ewes lambing (range 75–94%), ewes twinning (3–16%), and lambs dying (1.2–4.1%).

Within years, there was also highly significant variation ($P < 0.001$) between the nine sites in all components of flock fertility. This was most marked for the proportion of ewes twinning, which in 1981 (Table 3) varied from 7 to 31%.

Table 2. Variation between years in components of flock fertility.

Lambing Nov-Dec	Number of ewes joined	Ewes lambing /ewes joined (%)	Ewes twinning /ewes lambing (%)	Lambs born /ewes joined (%)	Lambs dead /lambs born (%)
1977	9661	75	3	77	2.6
1978	9777	94	5	99	3.5
1979	10920	91	10	101	2.4
1980	11445	91	12	102	4.1
1981	11486	88	16	103	3.1
1982	14446	86	8	93	2.4
1983	12426 [2]	86	14	98	1.2
Overall	77161	87 [1]	10 [1]	96 [1]	2.8 [1]

[1] Mean %.

[2] Excluding Gendoubah which was transferred from the Cereal Project in 1983.

Table 3. Variation between project sites in components of flock fertility (November–December 1981).

Project site	No. of ewes joined	Ewes lambing /ewes joined (%)	Ewes twinning /ewes lambed (%)	Lambs born /ewes joined (%)	Lambs dead [2] /lambs born (%)
Abu Ayesha	710	94	14	108	2.2
Abu Shaybah	1913	82	17	96	2.6
Ajeylat	1346	91	19	108	2.0
Al-Hira	838	95	11	105	2.3
Bir El Ghanam [1]	2249	91	17	107	3.6
Diga	580	86	24	106	2.1
Gendoubah	1509	88	8	87	1.1
Tarhuna	1071	92	7	99	4.4
Wadi Athel	1270	88	31	115	6.5
Overall	11486	88	16	103	3.1

[1] Nucleus flock.
[2] Birth to weaning.

Table 4. Lambing performance in the nucleus flock, Bir El Ghanam, 1983.

Year of birth	Number of ewes joined (1/6/83)	Ewes lambing /ewes joined (%)	Ewes twinning /ewes lambed (%)	Lambs born /ewes joined (%)	Lambs dead /lambs born (%)
1981	543	89	13	99	0.4
1980	376	88	32	115	0.1
1979	447	88	40	123	0.4
1978	349	79	33	105	1.4
Pre-1978	146	66	34	89	0.8
Overall	1861	85	28 [1]	108	0.5

[1] Includes six ewes producing triplets.

Table 5. Percentage distribution of lambs born Nov–Dec 1981 according to colour score.

Lamb group	Colour score					Total no. of lambs
	0	1	2	3	4	
All lambs born [1]	0.7	14.7	56.5	27.0	1.1	8869
Lambs born in nucleus	0.2	26.9	60.8	11.7	0.7	1796

[1] Lambs born in first 28 days.
Score 0 All white, no coloured patches or spots.
Score 1 Standard breed type, black or brown head or head and neck with no coloured patches or spots on the body or legs.
Score 2 Modified standard type, colour may extend from the head and neck onto the shoulder. There may also be patches of colour on the belly, knees, and/or hocks.
Score 3 Patches or spots, may be similar to scores 1 or 2, but will also display separate coloured patches or spots on the trunk or tail.
Score 4 Coloured, completely, or almost completely (greater than 75%) black or brown.

Data on reproductive performance according to age of ewe were available only from the nucleus flock. Results for 1983 show highly significant differences (Table 4; P < 0.001) in the proportion of ewes lambing (oldest, pre-1978, ewes 66% v remainder 86%) and of ewes twinning (2 year old 13% v 3 years and older 35%).

Fleece colour

The policy of rejecting all lambs with colour scores of 3 or 4 for entry into the nucleus resulted in the nucleus being noticeably more uniform in colour than the general flocks. More significantly, the effect was also apparent in the progeny of the nucleus flock as illustrated for the 1981/82 lambing (Table 5) showing a significantly smaller (P < 0.001) proportion of lambs with scores 3 or 4 in the nucleus (12.1%) than in the general flock (28.1%).

Colour scores for lambs born in 1979 were examined to test for any relationship with lamb growth rate. The results (Table 6) suggest that growth rate may be slightly depressed for white lambs (238 g/hd/d) compared with lambs with some fleece colour (scores 1–4, 249 g/hd/d), although the effect was relatively small.

Growth rate

Lamb growth rates varied considerably, both between years and between sites within years. The latter is illustrated for lambs born in November and December 1980 (Table 7) when overall flock means for individual sites ranged from 141 g/hd/d at Gendoubah to 269 g/hd/d at Bir El Ghanam. This highlights the need to correct for such environmental effects when selecting lambs. Nine percent of available ram lambs were selected as reserves with a mean advantage of 52 g/hd/d (+23%) over the unselected flock. For ewe lambs, the proportion selected as reserves was somewhat higher at 21% and the mean advantage of 31 g/hd/d (+16%) correspondingly lower.

The 1980 data also illustrate the effect of birth rank on growth rate with overall means for single versus twin lambs of 218 and 190 g/hd/d, respectively, or −13%. In 1982, when seasonal conditions were better, single lambs

Table 6. Relationship between colour score and lamb growth rate, birth to weaning. Lambs born Nov/Dec 1979.

Observation	Colour score					Overall
	0	1	2	3	4	
Number	86	1612	3570	1523	162	6953
%	1.2	23.2	51.3	21.9	2.3	
g/hd/d	238	248	250	249	245	249

Table 7. Effects of site, sex of lamb, and selection on mean lamb growth rate. Lambs born Nov–Dec 1980.

Site	Ram lambs				Ewe lambs			
	total flock		selected for nucleus		total flock		selected for nucleus	
	no.	mean g/hd/d	no.	mean g/hd/d	no.	mean g/hd/d	no.	mean g/hd/d
Abu Ayesha	320	242	29	302	313	207	62	240
Abu Shaybah	1051	201	95	253	1026	178	258	216
Ajeylat	776	245	68	297	733	224	148	254
Al-Hira	555	258	47	319	453	232	92	254
Bir El Ghanam	165	283	13	359	195	257	37	281
Diga	146	244	12	299	160	206	38	246
Gendoubah	611	147	55	191	555	134	110	164
Tarhuna	470	200	42	255	508	184	104	219
Wadi Athel	439	280	34	333	461	241	92	277
Overall	4533	223	395 (9)[1]	275 (+23)[2]	4404	200	942 (21)[1]	231 (+16)[2]

[1] Percent of total flock.
[2] Percent increase over total flock.

born in the nucleus averaged 297 g/hd/d compared with 243 g/hd/d (−18%) for twins.

Final selection of rams and ewes from the reserves for entry into the nucleus was based on corrected liveweight at 18 months of age. For rams born in 1980 relatively small corrections were required for site of origin, with mean liveweight varying from 58 kg for rams from Tarhuna to 63 kg for those from Wadi Athel (Table 8). Corrections for type of birth were also carried out with

Table 8. Liveweight of rams born Nov–Dec 1980 at 18 months of age (May 1982).

Site of origin [1]	All reserve rams		Rams selected for nucleus	
	no.	kg	no.	kg
Abu Ayesha	21	62	9	67
Abu Shaybah	75	60	32	64
Ajeylat	48	59	15	65
Al-Hira	29	61	12	66
Bir El Ghanam	10	60	4	61
Diga	8	62	4	65
Gendoubah	34	60	11	66
Tarhuna	34	58	12	63
Wadi Athel	13	63	2	69
Overall	272 [2]	60.1	101	64.9 (+8%)

[1] Born and reared to weaning at this site.
[2] Original selection reduced due to mortality, lost tags, and further culling for colour and skeletal deformity.

Table 9. Selection of reserves from the nucleus flock. Lambs born Nov–Dec 1982.

	Ewe flock/year of birth				Overall
	pre-1978		1978	1979	1980
Ram lambs					
No. lambs weaned	160	164	163	212	215	914
Mean wt. at weaning (kg)	33.8	36.7	33.1	31.8	32.0	33.3
Growth to weaning (g/hd/d)	322	335	300	293	286	308
No. selected	34	70	79	82	84	349 (38) [1]
Ewe lambs					
No. lambs weaned	162	168	165	203	190	888
Mean wt. at weaning (kg)	29.8	32.5	27.9	28.3	28.4	29.3
Growth to weaning (g/hd/d)	262	284	254	253	247	259
No. selected	89	84	97	140	142	552 (62) [1]

[1] Figures in parentheses are percent of lambs weaned.

overall means for single versus twin born rams of 60.5 and 58.8 kg, respectively. The 101 rams finally selected averaged 64.9 kg, about 8% above the mean for all available reserves. With the commencement of Stage 3 (closed nucleus, 1982 onwards) all reserves were selected only for lambs born within the nucleus. The results for 1982 (Table 9) show that quite substantial corrections were necessary for variation due to flock/age of dam, especially for lambs born in the youngest age groups where growth rates were relatively depressed.

Discussion

The Cereal Project's sheep breeding programme provided a unique opportunity to implement a package of staff training, flock performance recording, and objective selection procedures directed towards genetic improvement of the Libyan Barbary breed. Six years of intensive selection based on corrected rate of growth to weaning and hogget liveweight established an elite ram breeding nucleus with the capacity to produce superior sheep for use both within the project and for upgrading elsewhere. The Cereal Project's scale of operations, well structured staffing arrangements, and commitment to improved agricultural technology provided the essential foundations for success.

Because of the large numbers of sheep and numerous project sites, the overall success of the sheep improvement programme depended heavily on the development of a simple yet effective lamb tagging system. This provided virtually automatic documentation of date of birth, birth rank, and flock or site of origin for all lambs born within the first 28 days of lambing. Without this, it would have been impossible to correct individual performance data for major environmental bias, thereby seriously reducing the effectiveness of subsequent "objective" selection procedures.

The results of 6 years performance recording demonstrated that, given sound husbandry and adequate nutrition, the Libyan Barbary was capable of very satisfactory lamb production. While it could not be classed as highly fecund, the Barbary had the capacity to respond to good seasonal conditions when twinning frequently rose to 25–35%. The more modest levels of twinning (5–15%) that characterised poor to average seasons were undoubtedly quite appropriate for the extensively managed dryland farming systems developed within the project.

While not entirely definitive, an average of only 2.8% lamb deaths suggests that the Barbary is quite exceptional with respect to perinatal lamb mortality. The traditional practice of corralling the flock each night and providing individual attention to lambing ewes undoubtedly reduced lamb mortality but, even so, this figure is very low compared with the 10% or more usually cited in the international literature.

Lamb growth rate to weaning was markedly affected by seasonal conditions and pasture availability which varied considerably between years and between sites within years. Nevertheless, under average conditions, overall growth rates were generally 220–280 g/hd/d. Given the considerable variation between individuals, the best rams usually achieved 400 g/hd/d, weighing up to 50 kg when weaned. The 350 nucleus ram reserves were usually about 25% above the overall mean for all eligible ram lambs each year. On the basis of its potential for high lamb growth rates and relatively good conformation, the Libyan Barbary must be ranked highly for lamb production under dryland farming conditions such as those experienced by the Cereal Project.

There were problems that required considerable attention and warrant some comment here. The first and perhaps most basic problem concerned the credibility of lambs selected objectively on corrected performance data. When selecting reserves post-weaning, some sheep supervisors had great difficulty in accepting that a relatively small lamb (probably late born, twin reared, and/or on a poor site) could be genetically superior to physically larger lambs. This required close supervision initially to ensure the correct procedures were followed. Subsequent training in genetic principles provided a long-term solution.

The second problem arose from the widespread belief that young 18 month old rams were relatively infertile. This was important as the breeding plan called for the exclusive use of two-tooth rams to mate the nucleus and a mix of two- and four-tooth rams for the general flocks. The problem was finally resolved by demonstrating that flocks joined only with two-tooth rams (1 ram to 20 ewes) lambed as well as those joined with older rams.

Thirdly, there was a problem with ram control generally in the early years of the project. Some shepherds, and even some supervisors, wanted to use their favourite rams year after year. A policy of strict supervision to ensure that all rams were removed from each project site after joining and training in genetic principles helped to overcome the problem.

In conclusion, I believe that the systems developed for the Cereal Project with the Libyan Barbary breed provide a model for the introduction of performance recording and objective selection procedures elsewhere. With appropriate changes in breeding objectives it should be ideal for establishing a ram breeding nucleus within a large-scale intensive sheep breeding unit. It could also provide the basis for a regional or national flock improvement programme based on screening a large number of participating project or Bedouin flocks.

Acknowledgements

I wish to acknowledge the support and enthusiasm of Bashir El-Wahashi, Director of the Cereal Project and the assistance of his Senior Sheep Supervisors, Magdi Mustafa Fituri, Mohammed Zawia, and Abdulsalam Krayem throughout my consultancy. I am also indebted to the Senior Project Consultant, Norman Halse, for his encouragement and the Australian Officers in Charge, John Allen, Mike Ewing, Pierre Fievez, Geoff Collins, Andrew Watson, John Richardson, and John Peirce for their skilled supervision throughout their respective terms.

References

Allen, J.M. 1979. Ley farming in Libya – North Africa. Wool Technology and Sheep Breeding 27: 5–9.
Mason, I.L. 1967. Sheep Breeds of the Mediterranean. Published by arrangement with FAO by the Commonwealth Agricultural Bureaux, Edinburgh, UK. 215 p.

E.F. Thomson and F.S. Thomson (eds), Increasing Small Ruminant Productivity in Semi-arid Areas
© 1988 ICARDA . ISBN 978-94-010-7086-7

The Awassi Sheep Breeding Project in Syria

R. Kassem

Introduction

The fat-tailed Awassi is indigenous to West Asia. In Syria it is the main source of milk, meat, and wool, accounting for about 69% of total meat production, 17% of milk production, and 40% of milk products. The value of sheep production is about 25% of total agricultural production.

In 1974, a large project was initiated by the Ministry of Agriculture and Agrarian Reform (MAAR) and the Arab Centre for the Study of Arid Zones and Dry Lands (ACSAD) at the Kraim Centre, 40 km east of Hama in west Syria. The objectives were to develop three strains of Awassi sheep with above average production of milk, meat, and wool, respectively, and ultimately combine the three lines to produce an Awassi strain of all-round excellence, to assess the increase in production achieved, to study the adaptability of the specialized strains for production under various environmental conditions, and to multiply improved sheep and test selected rams in privately owned flocks in various environmental zones.

Management

Animal performance data were collected annually from the main flock of 500–600 ewes at the Kraim Centre. The management system applied at the centre was similar to traditional sheep husbandry in the region, with some improvements. The production year starts with the mating season during July and August. Ewes are mated or inseminated with fresh semen as required and lambing is in December and January, sometimes extending into mid-February. Ewes are culled when they are not in lamb for two successive seasons, they have chronic mastitis, or are too old. Lambs are weaned at about 60 days.

Milk yield

Milk recording started when lambs were 2 weeks old. The lambs were separated from their dams for 12 h during the night and in the morning the milk weight was recorded. The individual weights were multiplied by two to give an estimate of total milk yield of each ewe for a 24 h period . After weaning the ewes were milked twice daily and the total weight of the two milkings recorded. The procedure was repeated every fortnight until the ewes dried off to calculate total milk yield for the different stages of lactation. All the data were analysed using the SPSS statistical package, except those for heritability for which the Harvey programme was used.

Hossamo et al. (1985) described the results in relation to the genetic and non-genetic factors influencing milk yield and meat and wool during 1975–81. The milk line was superior in milk yield to the control line (160.3 ± 1.32 (SE) kg and 132.8 ± 1.80 kg obtained in 179 and 169 days for milk and control lines, respectively) and ewe body weight at lambing was greater in the meat than in the control line (63.0 ± 0.16 and 59.1 ± 0.21 kg, respectively).

Milk yield, particularly total milk yield, had moderately high heritability as estimated from data from 2 year olds or from age-corrected data of 2–9 year olds (0.53 ± 0.169 and 0.60 ± 0.137). Phenotypic correlations were positive between the various measures of lactation (0–30 days, 30–60 days, and 0–90 days) and between the maximum daily yield and the other measures. There was a low positive correlation between milk yield and ewe weight at lambing but a low negative correlation with shearing weight. Lactation length was positively correlated with milk yield, particularly total lactation yield, with a lower correlation for yield measured in early lactation. Milk yield was positively correlated with lamb weaning weight but there seemed to be no phenotypic association with greasy fleece weight.

The genetic correlations showed a high positive relationship between the various measures of milk yield, particularly between maximum daily yield and total lactation yield. Genetic correlations of milk yield with ewe weight at lambing were generally positive and rather higher than the corresponding phenotypic values, while those with ewe weight at shearing were less consistent and smaller. The genetic and phenotypic correlations of lactation length with milk yield were strongly positive.

The important lactation traits of the Awassi could be rapidly improved. The high correlation between maximum daily yield and total milk production for phenotypic (0.82 and 0.99) and for genetic (0.84 and 0.98) correlation of 2 and 2–9 year old Awassi sheep, respectively, indicates that a simplified recording system, possibly involving only one visit to a flock, could be used to screen a large number of flocks to select superior ewes for a major sheep improvement programme.

Body condition score and production under range conditions

Descriptions of body condition are useful for management and marketing, or for genetic improvement. Descriptive terms such as poor, fairly good, or fat are often used but they have different meanings for different people. Therefore, Hossamo et al. (1986) have adapted the British system of body condition scoring for use with fat-tailed breeds such as the Awassi. Six grades are used from 0 (extremely emaciated and near death) to 5 (moderately covered with fat).

There are important associations between ewe condition score at mating and lambing and the subsequent reproductive performance of single bearing ewes. Body condition score could be used as an easily measurable trait to aid selection of superior animals, and the differential supplementation of ewes according to body condition score might help to reduce variations in milk yield, lamb growth, and fleece weight. Under semi-arid conditions grades 1, 2, and 3 have the greatest practical implications.

Interactions between genotype and feeding level

The management system adopted at the Kraim Centre was similar to the traditional system of sheep production. To determine whether selection would be more accurate under normal than under ideal nutritional conditions, two levels of supplementary feeding were imposed on a flock during pregnancy and early lactation for 2 consecutive years (Hossamo et al. 1987). The flock was fed and managed exactly as the other flocks at the centre but the concentrate part of the diet was reduced to 60% of that of the normally fed ewes. Milk yield increased with increased feeding, but the other productivity traits studied were only slightly and insignificantly better with normal feeding than with poor feeding. There was no interaction between feeding level and selection line.

These results show that adequate nutrition during pregnancy and early lactation can improve milk production and lamb traits up to weaning and maintenance of ewe body weight. Therefore, until further evidence is available, selection for milk and meat traits in the Awassi under feeding conditions similar to those in the arid or semi-arid areas should be possible.

Age at puberty, level of feeding, and presence of rams

Breeding from ewe lambs may extend the productive life of the ewe and can shorten the interval between generations, so speeding up genetic improvement. Ewe lambs can be mated successfully at puberty i.e., the age at which the animals become capable of reproduction (Kassem 1986). Certain thresholds of liveweight (the average liveweight at first mating in ewe lambs expressed as a percentage of the adult weight) must be met before puberty is reached. Therefore, ewe lambs that grow slowly may not be sufficiently developed for normal sexual function in their first year. Thus, puberty may be delayed or advanced by varying the plane of nutrition. Also, introducing rams to ewe lambs may stimulate and hasten the onset of oestrus activity.

The effect of ewe nutrition and presence of rams was studied using 197 and 165 single ewe lambs of approximately 75 days of age in 1982 and 1984, respectively. The animals were weighed and randomly divided into three equal groups. These groups were given a low, normal, and high (L, N, H) plane of

158

Table 1. Effect of level of feeding on reproduction of Awassi ewes.

	1982			1984		
	H [1]	N	L	H	N	L
Ewe lambs showing oestrus (%)	86	74	40	89	68	43
Mean age of first oestros (d)	257.1	267.5	280.8	247.1	254.8	268.2
	(2.33) [2]	(2.54)	(3.54)	(2.31)	(2.72)	(3.40)
Mean age of conception (d)	256.6	269.5	281.6	252.2	257.9	268.2
	(2.37)	(2.63)	(3.94)	(2.84)	(3.13)	(4.12)

[1] H = high; N = normal; L = low plane of nutrition.
[2] Standard error of mean.

nutrition to produce gains of 100, 130, and 160 g/day, respectively, by the age of 7–9 months. The ewe lambs from 1984 had the same nutrition and management as those in 1982 but they were divided into four sub-groups: the first, second, and third had continuous access to vasectomized rams from the age of 175, 200, and 230 days, respectively, while the fourth group (control) did not have access to vasectomized rams.

For visual detection of oestrus, rams were run with ewe lambs from day 175 onwards for half an hour at 07.00 h and half an hour at 18.00 h. A ewe was considered to be on heat when she stood and accepted service. The proportion of ewe lambs that showed oestrus was higher in the H and N groups than in the L group, while the mean ages of first oestrus were lower (P < 0.01) for H and N than for L (Table 1). The mean ages of conception were also lower (P < 0.01) in H and N than in L.

The introduction of rams to ewes at different ages reduced the age to first oestrus (P < 0.01) with mean ages at first oestrus of 249.4 ± 3.48, 253.4 ± 2.93, 258.5 ± 3.26, and 265.4 ± 2.39 days for the first, second, third, and control groups, respectively. The mean age at first oestrus was reduced by 15.9 days when rams were introduced to ewe lambs at 175 days compared with ewe lambs only in contact with rams for a short time daily.

These results suggest that improving the level of nutrition after weaning and the continuous access of rams from the beginning of the breeding season may increase the proportion of ewe lambs reaching puberty during the first breeding season.

Post-partum interval to oestrus and conception

Increasing lambing frequency may be one method of increasing lamb production. With a post-partum interval of 3 months between pregnancies, ewes will lamb at 8-month intervals. To lamb twice a year, ewes must conceive a month after lambing. Most breeders in Syria run the rams with the flock all year round and since some ewes are mated about 60–90 days post-partum, it is possible for ewes to lamb three times in 2 years.

Three studies on the factors affecting post-partum interval were carried out at Kraim Centre. In the first, 98 adult Awassi ewes were used to study the interval from parturition to first oestrus in relation to previous and current lactation and age of the ewe. Post-partum oestrus was visually determined by running mature vasectomized rams with ewes in the morning and evening from the first day after parturition until the end of May. In the second study, 60 mature ewes of proven fertility were divided into three equal groups and sponged at 14, 44, and 74 days, respectively, after parturition. Fertile rams were introduced 48 h after the withdrawal of the sponges and remained with the ewes for 2 days. After 10 days one ram per group was turned out with the ewes for 1 week to cover the returns to oestrus. In the third study, 28 ewes were run with fertile rams from just after parturition to the end of March and were allowed to mate naturally.

In all the studies, lambs had continuous access to dams and the ewes were hand milked once a day pre-weaning and twice a day post-weaning. The management system was as close to the traditional system of husbandry as possible with some additional improvements.

Of the ewes in the first study, 61 exhibited oestrus at an average interval of 83.4 ± 31.89 days, ranging from 1 to 170 days. The number of ewes showing oestrus within 30, 60, 90, 120, and 150 days of parturition was 5, 7, 24, 22, and 2, respectively. Neither the age of the ewe nor the previous or current lactation had any significant effect on the time of occurrence of oestrus.

In the second study, there were differences ($P < 0.01$) between the groups sponged at different times in terms of the interval to post-partum oestrus and conception. Out of each group 7, 12, and 15 ewes exhibited oestrus at an average of 29.1 ± 1.68, 67.7 ± 5.26, and 91.4 ± 3.31 days and 5, 9, and 14 of them conceived at an average of 40.2 ± 9.60, 73.9 ± 9.80 and 93.6 ± 5.23 days, respectively. All the ewes lambed.

In the third study, 14 out of 28 ewes showed oestrus at an average of 56.4 ± 23.67 days, ranging from 33 to 113 days. Thirteen of the ewes conceived at an average of 70.3 ± 32.95 days, ranging from 33 to 133 days, while 9, 4, and 1 ewes showed oestrus within 60, 90, and 120 days, respectively.

Since in most cases post-partum oestrus and conception occurred between the second and third month after parturition, lambing three times in 2 years would be possible.

Gestation length, litter size, age of ewe, and sex of lambs carried

The effect of litter size, age of ewe, and sex of lamb carried on the duration of pregnancy was studied over 5 years using 1997 lambing ewes. The overall average gestation period was 151.7 ± 2.17 days. Litter size had no significant effect on the length of gestation, but single males were carried longer than single females. Ewes bearing a male with a female twin had longer gestations than those bearing all male or all female twins, and ewes bearing all male twins had longer gestations than those bearing all female twins. In ewes carrying single lambs, gestation was longer (P < 0.01) in older ewes. These results suggest that variations in gestation length due to litter size, age of ewe, or sex of foetus carried are of minor biological importance.

Lambing rate in relation to ewe age and pre-mating body weight

Lambing rate in relation to ewe age and body weight pre-mating was examined using over 2500 ewe records obtained from the Kraim Centre during 1979–85. The overall mean number of lambs born per ewe lambed ranged between 1.11 ± 0.014 and 1.19 ± 0.017. The mean number of lambs born increased (P < 0.01) with the age of the dam up to 5 years old then declined slowly at 6 years old and over. The number of lambs born also increased significantly (P < 0.01), ranging from 0.007 ± 0.0029 to 0.013 ± 0.0029 for each kg increase in body weight before mating.

In this study the ewes over 6 years old were combined with the 6 year olds because only a few ewes over 6 years were kept in the flock each year. Therefore it is not clear whether this age group has been influenced by the over 6 year olds and consequently showed a lower average lambing rate than the group of 5 year olds.

The overall mean percentage of ewes lambing per ewe mated ranged between 67.4 ± 2.11 and 93.0 ± 1.20. The mean percentages of fertile ewes were not significantly affected by either age or ewe body weight pre-mating, but they increased slightly from 3 to 4 years of age then declined at 6 years and over. However, culling for barrenness, environmental factors causing fertilization failure, early embryonic death, and abortion may have distorted the results and the limited breeding season of 60–70 days may have meant that some fertile ewes were not mated when they returned to service.

Lamb survival, type of birth, lamb birth weight, and lambing season

During 1979–85 over 3000 lamb records were used to determine lamb survival (lambs weaned/lambs born alive) from birth to weaning at 60 days in relation to birth weight, type of birth (single or twin), and lambing season (early, medium, and late).

Overall mean survival ranged between 0.91 ± 0.012 and 0.98 ± 0.007 and increased (P < 0.01) at the rate of 0.043 ± 0.022 to 0.094 ± 0.021 for each kg increase in lamb birth weight. Neither season of birth nor type of birth affected lamb survival which may be due to the special shepherding given to twins and to the good nourishment of dams during pregnancy and after lambing which in turn produced vigorous lambs and sufficient milk for twins. Also, ewes and their lambs were kept inside when it was raining or snowing which would affect lamb survival. The results suggest that a high survival rate can be obtained by good management during pregnancy and after lambing.

The length of the oestrous cycle and duration of oestrus

The length of the oestrous cycle was studied in relation to age of ewe from 1979 to 1982 and involved 424 recordings. The oestrous cycle averaged 17.3 ± 1.63 days.

Duration of oestrus was also studied in relation to ewe age. Forty ewes were divided into three groups according to age (1.5, 3.5, and 5.5 years) and treated with vaginal sponges to synchronize oestrus. Recordings were taken when oestrus was synchronized and when ewes returned for the next oestrus without synchronization. The mean duration of oestrus was 40.0 ± 2.85 and 34.6 ± 2.01 h. There were no observable effects of ewe age on the duration of oestrus or on the length of the oestrous cycle.

Ovulation rate

Ovulation rate, determined from the number of corpora lutea counted at laproscopy, was studied in the ewes used for studying the duration of oestrus. Ovulation rate was measured 24 h after oestrus detection when oestrus was synchronized and when ewes returned for the next oestrus without synchronization.

In both cases, the mean ovulation rate tended to increase with ewe age (1.00 ± 0.153, 1.11 ± 0.153, and 1.40 ± 0.147 in the first measurement and 1.00 ± 0.144, 1.11 ± 0.152, and 1.55 ± 0.137 in the second for 1.5, 3.5, and 5.5 year old ewes, respectively).

Since there is an association between ovulation rate and litter size (Hanrahan 1980), ovulation rate could be used at the earliest possible ages as a selection criterion in breeding programmes to increase litter size.

Economics of sheep production under different suckling regimes

This study (Fadel 1988) was carried out to investigate five milking regimes: partial milking or milking the residual up to 60 days when the lamb was weaned and hand milking to the end of lactation (approximately 150 days post-lambing); no partial milking with lambs weaned at 60 days followed by hand milking; no partial milking with weaning at 90 days followed by hand milking; no partial milking with weaning at 120 days; and no partial milking and no hand milking with ewes suckled by the lamb for the full lactation period (lambs weaned at 150 days).

Time of weaning had no effect on lactation performance, but it affected the milk available for sale. Lamb weight increased as the amount of milk suckled from birth to weaning increased and ewe body loss from lambing till weaning was small when the ewe was adequately fed. The largest profit was obtained from the first system.

Factors affecting milk quality

Fat, total solids, and solids not fat percentages were not affected by ewe age but increased with advancing lactation. Milk from the evening milking was richer in fat than that from the morning milking in spite of equal milking intervals (Fadel 1988).

The shape of the lactation curve

The shape of the lactation curve was studied in relation to various environmental factors to find methods for predicting milk yield, which would simplify recording systems (Fadel 1988).

In the pre-weaning stage of lactation, the curve was inconsistent suggesting that no useful general equation for selection could be determined from this stage. In the post-weaning stage milk yield increased with age of ewe from 2 years up to 3 years and over. Milk yield of 2 year old ewes started at a lower level with higher persistency than that of older ewes which have a higher initial level with low persistency. Ewes that lamb early in the lambing season have a lower initial milk yield and a flatter lactation curve compared to those lambing late. The general shape of the lactation curve for the post-weaning stage is more consistent and slightly curvilinear.

Ewes can be selected for milk production ability on the basis of one daily record i.e., morning and evening weighings, taken on 1 day in one flock shortly after the lambs are weaned at approximately 2 months old. There was a high correlation (Spearman's Rank Correlation Coefficient) between the ranking of all the ewes in the group based on their performance on the recording day and the ranking based on their total milk yield recorded every 14 days. The correlation of approximately 0.9 was not significantly improved by correcting for the stage of lactation in ewes where the range in lambing date was 8–10 weeks.

If these findings are applicable to other flocks in this and other areas it suggests that extensively managed, nomadic flocks can be efficiently screened for ewes with high milk production without individual identification of sheep. Flocks could be visited by arrangement 1 day shortly after weaning and milk production recorded for each ewe, which would be temporarily identified. High performance ewes could be identified by ranking on milk yield, possibly correcting for any known major age effects.

Future work

These studies have led to the establishment of a new project for producing improved Awassi rams in Syria by ACSAD and MAAR. The project aims to extend the basis of genetic selection using a much larger number of sheep and conducting further studies on reproduction, nutrition, and management systems.

References

Fadel, I. 1988. Economic and Technical Aspects of Lactation in Awassi Sheep. PhD thesis. University College of North Wales, UK.

Hossamo, H.E., Owen, J.B. and Farid, M.F.A. 1985. The genetic improvement of Syrian Awassi sheep with special reference to milk production. Journal of Agricultural Science, Cambridge 105(2): 327–337.

Hossamo, H.E., Owen, J.B. and Farid, M.F.A. 1986. Body condition score and production in fat-tailed Awassi sheep under range conditions. Research and Development in Agriculture 3, 2.

Hossamo, H.E., Kassem, R. and Fadel, I. 1987. The interaction between genotype and feeding level. The effect of the level of supplementary feeding on the productivity of Awassi sheep. Paper presented at the 27th Science Week, 7–12 Nov 1987, Damascus. ACSAD and MAAR, Damascus, Syria.

Hanrahan, J.P. 1980. Ovulation rate as a selection criterion for litter size in sheep. Proceedings of the Australian Society of Animal Production 13: 405–408.

Kassem, R. 1986. Reproduction in Awassi ewe with particular preference to increasing efficiency under semi-arid conditions. PhD thesis. University College of North Wales, UK.

E.F. Thomson and F.S. Thomson (eds), Increasing Small Ruminant Productivity in Semi-arid Areas
© *1988 ICARDA . ISBN 978-94-010-7086-7*

Past Experiences of Sheep Improvement in Egypt and Future Directions

A.M. Aboul-Naga and A.M. El-Serafy

Introduction

Egypt can be divided into three regions with different sheep production systems and breeds. In the Nile Delta region agriculture is intensive and 1 million sheep are raised either on small holdings or in commercial village flocks managed by specialized shepherds. Lamb production in this region could be intensified to fit the prevailing intensive conditions.

The second region is Upper Egypt, where agriculture is less intensive and the 1.5 million sheep are raised mainly in mixed flocks with goats as scavengers. The number of sheep per acre of cultivated land is 0.76 and 0.26 in Upper Egypt and the Nile Delta region, respectively, with 1.43 and 0.67 sheep per farm owner in the two regions, respectively (Galal 1987).

The third region is the extensive rangelands of the northwest coastal zone of the desert where rainfall averages 140 mm/year. Here, 1 million sheep and over 0.5 million goats are raised extensively. Sheep and goat populations have doubled in this area over the past 2 decades in spite of the degradation of the range (Aboul-Naga 1987).

Distribution of local sheep breeds

The local sheep breeds, the Rahmani, Ossimi, and Barki, are fat-tailed and have coarse wool. They are raised mainly for meat with carpet wool as a secondary product. Milk is of very minor importance.

Rahmani sheep are found in the North and Mid-Delta region, while Ossimi are dominant in the Southern Delta and in Mid and Upper Egypt. Barki sheep are raised in the coastal zone of the Western Desert. Another minor breed, Seidi, is raised in the northern part of Upper Egypt. The origin and description of these breeds have been reviewed by Mason (1967), Ghanem (1980), and Galal (1987).

Aboul-Naga (1976; 1977) found that Rahmani sheep are specifically adapted to the conditions of the North Delta while the Ossimis are more generally adapted to conditions in the valley (Table 1). The intensive agriculture in the Delta has not improved the performance of the Barki sheep which are well adapted to the arid conditions of the desert. When different flocks of the three breeds were raised at one location (Mid-Delta), they had similar reproductive

Table 1. Reproductive performance of the three main Egyptian local sheep breeds (Ossimi, Rahmani, and Barki) under the management system of one crop/year (c/y) and 3 crops/2 years (3 c/2 y) at different locations.

Classification	No. of records	Conception rate	Lambs born/ewe joined	Lambs weaned/ewe joined	Lambs born/ewe lambed	Lambs weaned/ewe lambed	Kg weaned/ewe lambed
Ossimi							
Overall mean ± SE							
c/y	4269	0.83±0.01	0.95±0.01	0.83±0.01	1.14±0.01	0.99±0.01	22.8±0.17
3c/2y	3222	0.73±0.01	0.88±0.01	0.71±0.01	1.22±0.01	0.99±0.01	18.8±0.28
Deviation for location (%)							
Mid Delta	1588 (1091)	-1.2(-17.6)	1.0(-20.7)	3.6(-23.0)	28.6(-2.5)	5.0(-3.3)	0.0(-2.6)
South Delta	1292 (1142)	3.6 (2.3)	-2.1(-2.8)	1.2 (2.8)	-42.8(-4.9)	-2.0(-5.7)	-7.5(-9.8)
Middle Egypt	665 (1089)	4.8 (15.2)	11.6 (23.0)	10.8 (26.3)	42.8 (7.4)	5.0 (9.1)	33.3 (12.4)
Upper Egypt	724	-7.2 –	-10.5 –	-15.6 –	-28.6 –	-8.0 –	-25.8 –
Rahmani							
Overall mean ± SE							
c/y	3567	0.86±0.01	1.06±0.01	0.93±0.01	1.23±0.01	1.08±0.01	24.6±0.19
3c/2y	2905	0.77±0.01	1.01±0.02	0.80±0.02	1.33±0.02	1.10±0.02	22.7±0.28
Deviation for location (%)							
Mid Delta	2086 (1491)	-4.6 (0.4)	-4.7 (0.0)	-9.7(-5.8)	0.0(-0.2)	-5.6(-5.7)	-10.4(-6.4)
North Delta	1482 (1414)	4.6 (0.4)	4.7 (0.0)	9.7 (5.0)	0.0 (0.2)	5.6 (5.7)	10.4 (6.4)
Barki							
Overall mean ± SE							
c/y	937	0.88±0.01	0.92±0.01	0.83±0.02	1.05±0.05	0.94±0.01	20.6±0.26
3c/2y	1023	0.71±0.02	0.76±0.02	0.66±0.02	1.07±0.01	0.93±0.02	18.2±0.32
Deviation of location (%)							
Mid Delta	592 (492)	-4.5 (1.4)	-3.3 (-3.1)	-6.0 (3.9)	0.0 (2.3)	-3.2 (1.9)	-0.2 (4.8)
North Coast	345 (531)	4.5 (-1.4)	3.3 (3.1)	6.0 (-3.9)	0.0 (-2.3)	3.2 (-1.9)	0.2 (-4.8)

Source: Aboul-Naga et al. (1976; 1977).

performance and averaged 0.82, 0.87, and 0.83 lambs/ewe joined for Rahmani, Ossimi, and Barki, respectively (Aboul-Naga 1976; 1977). The only significant differences were in the incidence of multiple births; 21, 17, and 7% for Rahmani, Ossimi, and Barki, respectively.

Variation in climate from one location to another does not seem to be the main factor determining the natural distribution of the local breeds (Shalaby 1985).

Genetic improvement

Crossing with exotic temperate breeds

Several trials have been carried out to improve lamb production by crossing local with European breeds. These trials, started early in the 1940s, used Suffolk, Hampshire, Fleisch Merino, Hungarian Merino, Finnish Landrace, and more recently Romanov breeds. Other minor trials were also carried out using Merino, Texel, and Ile-de-France.

The results have been reviewed by Aboul-Naga and Aboul-Ela (1985), Galal (1987), and Aboul-Naga et al. (1987a) and are summarized in Table 2. From these results, it can be concluded that the crossbreds can reproduce more than once per year and so compete with the local breeds in annual lamb production.

The best crossbreds were generally the 1/4 temperate 3/4 local crosses which are able to reproduce more than once per year and are more adapted to the prevailing subtropical conditions than other crosses. They are also more marketable and can be easily reproduced in large-scale development programmes utilizing crossbred rams.

One trial used a prolific Finn sheep. The 1/4 Finn ewes had the best fertility and lamb survival and gave birth to 0.43 and 0.21 more lambs than the local Rahmani and Ossimi, respectively. This represents an advantage of 81.5 and 103.3% over the Rahmani and Ossimi, respectively, in annual lambs produced per ewe exposed. The preliminary results of the Romanov cross are encouraging, showing an improvement of 20% in prolificacy over the local Rahmani ewes (Aboul-Naga et al., unpublished data).

Adaptation of imported temperate breeds and their crosses to the prevailing hot, dry climate has also been studied (El-Sheikh et al. 1981; Shalaby et al. 1986; Aboul-Ela et al. 1986; 1987; Fawzy 1986). Heat tolerance in the crossbreds was closer to the local than the exotic temperate parents.

Crosses between native and other subtropical breeds

Asker et al. (1954) crossed Rahmani and Ossimi local breeds and while the results were inconclusive they were promising. Crossbred lambs from Rahmani

Table 2. Reproductive performance (as % of local breed) of temperate sheep breeds and their crosses (as blood %) when bred once a year.

Trait [1]	Temperate breed grade (%)			
	100	75	50	25
Suffolk % Ossimi				
EL/EE	103	115 (104)	117	
LW/EE	86	109 (112)	111	
LB/EL	98	103 (101)	104	
Ann. LW/EL	76	96 (112)	103	
Hampshire % Ossimi				
EL/EE	42	68	95	
LW/EE	36	58	82	
LB/EL	93	112	98	
Ann. LW/EL	69	79	84	
Fleisch Merino % Ossimi				
EL/EE	105 (90)	110	121	98
LW/EE	99 (96)	116	125	112
LB/EL	105 (94)	105	105	100
Ann. LW/EL	93 (95)	108	107	112
Fleisch Merino % Barki				
EL/EE	102	111	115	
LW/EE		115	120	
LB/EL	118	110	107	
Ann. LW/EL	99	100	103	
Hungarian Merino % Barki				
EL/EE	66		93	101
LW/EL	53		100	103
LB/EL	106		101	104
Ann. LW/EL	67		98	99
Finn % Ossimi				
EL/EE	84		101	132
LW/EE	130		142	170
LB/EL	204		134	
Ann. LW/EL	167		135	129
Finn % Ossimi				
EL/EE	75		108	114
LW/EE	119		141	157
LB/EL	188		147	132
Ann. LW/EL	157		130	133

Source: Aboul-Naga and Aboul-Ela (1985).
[1] EL/EE = ewe lambed lambing/ewe exposed; LW/EE = lamb weight/ewe exposed; LB/EL = lambs born/ewe lambing; Ann. LW/EL = annual lamb weight/ewe lambing.

ewes performed significantly better than their reciprocal. In another trial, heterosis estimates of 5–9% were found in crosses between the two native breeds for growth performance, with a greater advantage for the cross resulting from Rahmani dams (El-Said 1983).

In a diallel cross experiment between Ossimi and Barki local breeds and the imported Fleisch Merino, Galal et al. (1972) found that the Ossimi-Barki cross exhibited the highest specific combining ability. Aboul-Naga et al. (1987a) investigated a crossbreeding system utilizing the desert Barki (B) ewes and Ossimi (O) valley breeds to increase lamb production. The results were encouraging with Barki but not with Ossimi. Improvements over Barki in kgs lamb weaned/ewe lambed were 16.8, 39.7, and 48.0% for O.B, O.(OB), and O.(O.OB) matings, respectively. They suggested that crossbred ewes should be tested under the extensive conditions in the desert before recommendations for application could be made.

When Awassi sheep were imported from Syria and crossed with local Barki under desert conditions, their lambs were heavier at birth than the local breed, but this weight difference declined with age (Fahmy et al. 1969). The Awassi–Barki crossbred ewes weaned significantly fewer kgs of lambs/ewe exposed than the local Barki but milk production was slightly better (El-Shahat 1970). A trial is now underway using Chios from Cyprus and the local Ossimi.

Selection

Because of the long-term planning required and the high cost, no well controlled, long-term selection programmes have been initiated for improving local sheep. Long-term selection is practiced in many flocks by different organizations but no control flocks have been kept to evaluate the genetic improvement due to selection. However, genetic progress has been estimated in the Barki flock of the Desert Research Institute as 0.02, 0.25, 1.02, and 0.27 per generation for birth, weaning, and yearling and first fleece weights (Mansour et al. 1977). Genetic progress in Ministry flocks is currently being estimated following long-term selection for body weight, multiple births, and conception rate.

Estimates of genetic parameters for different traits have been widely reported. Heritability estimates have been recorded of 0.05–0.22 for birth weight, 0.08–0.45 for weaning weight, 0.08–0.41 for yearling weight, and 0.15–0.28 for greasy fleece weight (Galal 1987). Aboul-Naga et al. (1985) estimated heritabilities of 0–0.11 for different reproductive traits in Rahmani and Ossimi breeds, with estimates from the first record of 0.15–0.47 for Ossimi and 0.02–0.27 for Rahmani. Heritability of date of first oestrus has been estimated to be 0.08 in Rahmani ewes (Aboul-Naga et al. 1987).

Improved management

Improving reproductivity

Like most subtropical breeds, Egyptian sheep can breed at different times of the year (Aboul-Naga 1985) and this can be used to improve lamb production. In 1970, a system of one crop of lambs every 8 months was applied to Ministry flocks. Details of the management system and preliminary results have been reported by Aboul-Naga (1983). The annual number of lambs born/ewe exposed was increased by 32.5, 35, and 21.6% for Rahmani, Ossimi, and Barki, respectively (Table 1). There were highly significant differences between season of mating (September, May, and January) for almost all reproductive traits in the three breeds. September mating consistently resulted in the best performance in different reproduction traits, followed by May (the common breeding season in Egypt), with January mating resulting in poorest performance (Table 3).

The oestrous and ovarian activities of local breeds at different times of the year have also been investigated in an attempt to utilize their potential to produce more than one crop per year. These studies, which were reviewed by Aboul-Naga et al. (1987b), indicated that local breeds showed oestrous activity all year round with a decline in spring and early summer. This decline is greater in Ossimi (March–May) than in Rahmani (May-June). There was also large variation in flocks and individuals for oestrous activity, especially in the Ossimi breed. Ovarian activity, as measured by endoscopy or hormonal assay, showed less seasonal variation. Ovulation rate averaged 1.5 for Rahmani and 1.3 for Ossimi and was lowest in May. The seasonality in reproductive performance of the local breeds corresponds more with ovarian than with oestrous activity (Table 3) and breeding activity in these breeds seems to be more precisely predicted by ovarian than oestrous activity.

Table 3. Fertility, prolificacy, and oestrous and ovarian activities of Rahmani and Ossimi sheep at different mating seasons.

Mating season	Fertility (EL/EE)	Prolificacy (LB/EL)	Ewes in oestrous (%)	Ewes ovulated (%)
Rahmani				
Sept	0.80	1.48	90	100
May	0.78	1.29	77	95
Jan	0.68	1.27	90	62
Ossimi				
Sept	0.87	1.29	81	100
May	0.78	1.24	34	78
Jan	0.74	1.16	94	53

Source: Aboul-Naga et al. (1987a).
EL = ewe lambed; EE = ewe exposed; LB = lambs born.

Increasing fertility and prolificacy using hormonal treatment (progesterone and PMS) has been tried but there have been no conclusive results for commercial application (Aboul-Naga and Abdel-Rahman 1981). Recently, immunization against endocrines has been used to increase prolificacy in Rahmani and 1/4 Finn ewes and resulted in an increase in litter size of less than 15% (unpublished data), which is insufficient for commercial application of the technique.

Lamb performance

Pre-weaning

Proper management and feeding of newly born lambs to weaning might affect post-weaning performance. Some studies have been conducted to investigate the effect of different nutrients in milk or milk replacers on lamb performance from birth to weaning. Early weaning, the effect of starter quantity and quality, and the suitability of different roughages have also been investigated.

El-Serafy et al. (1976) found that either cow or buffalo milk could be used as a substitute for ewes' milk for rearing Ossimi lambs from 2 days to 8 weeks. The energy stored in the fat tail was positively correlated ($r = 0.89$, $P < 0.01$) with energy intake. In formulating milk replacers for Ossimi lambs, either lupine termis or soyabean meal can provide 30% of the milk proteins (Tawilla 1984). Early weaning of local breeds is successful at 6–8 weeks and/or 8–10 kg liveweight (Swidan et al. 1979a; 1979b). However, early-weaned lambs must be carefully managed to reduce mortality.

In intensive lamb production systems, the proper starter should be used for newly born lambs to ensure high growth rates. The three main native breeds and some of their crosses have been successively reared on a starter containing 20% skimmed milk powder plus berseem hay (Hassona 1980). All lambs were weaned at 8 weeks or 10 kg liveweight. Average daily gain was 115–145 g and there were no significant differences in performance among local breeds.

Post-weaning

The Ossimi and Rahmani breeds usually graze berseem (*Trifolium alexandrinum*) after cattle or buffaloes in winter and the aftermath of summer crops. Ewes are commonly given 0.5 kg of concentrates in late pregnancy and for 4–6 weeks post-partum. Flushing, by giving ewes the same amount of concentrates 2 weeks before and 2 weeks after the start of breeding is not uncommon in large, commercial Delta flocks.

The Barki breed is extensively grazed on range plants native to the dry region along the northwest coast. They are given concentrates in summer and during the breeding season.

Since 1950, studies with native breeds have investigated the effect of different feeding practices on post-weaning performance. The proper roughage to concentrate ratio (R : C) for growing lambs to 12 months was found to be 60 : 40 on a dry matter (DM) basis, and ewe-lambs could be reared successfully on green forages. For fattening, the R : C ratio is 40 : 60. The daily maintenance energy and protein requirements for growing and mature sheep were reported to be 29.35 and 26.59 g TDN and 5.06 and 1.38 g $DP/W^{0.75}$. Sugarcane molasses at 300 g/h/d was recommended as a good nutrient in fattening rations, while ensiled or dry dairy cattle manure and dry poultry litter were used safely in rations at up to 20% of the DM (El-Serafy et al. 1980; El-Ashry et al. 1985; Khattab et al. 1982). Urea and ammonia were used to improve the nutritive value of rice straw.

Estimates of maintenance requirements for Ossimi and Rahmani sheep were between 450 g TDN and 809 g DP (Soliman 1968) and 465 g TDN and 90 g DP (Abou-Raya et al. 1969). The proper R : C ratio was 40% berseem hay (50% TDN; 81% DCP): 40% concentrate mixture (65% TDN; 11% DCP) for rearing ewe lambs from 28 to 50 kg liveweight (Ali et al. 1982; El-Serafy et al. 1981). Lambs fed the 100 : 0% ratio had the poorest gains. Overall average daily gains (ADG) over 300 days of lambs fed 100, 80, 60, 40, and 20% roughage were 80, 95, 98, 115, and 118 g, respectively.

The Ministry of Agriculture has developed a concentrate feed formula (53–57% TDN; 10.5–11.5% DCP) for the northwest region of Egypt as a supplement for mature Barki ewes during summer and gives ammonia-treated rice straw during the mating season.

Fattening and carcass evaluation

Ossimi and Rahmani sheep are usually fattened to 10–12 months. Fattening operations are also very active a few months before the Eid-Al Adha feast.

A number of studies have investigated the effect of different management practices on ADG, fat deposition, and fat : lean ratios in local breeds and their crosses with exotic breeds. The results gave indicators of the feeding/management system which gives high ADG with low carcass fat. The Ossimi yearlings had lower ADG during fattening, lighter carcasses, higher dressings, more lean, fewer prime cuts, and poorer carcass conformation than the Ossimi-Suffolk cross (El-Shobokshy and Aboul-Naga 1978). Fattening and carcass performance data of local lambs in different age categories (Table 4) indicate that the most economic system was fattening for 4 weeks at 6 months old (Riad 1985).

Sugarcane molasses has been used successfully in rations for fattening Ossimi lambs from 25 to 45 kg (El-Serafy et al. 1981). High, medium, and low energy levels resulted in values of ADG and fat tail weight of 157 g and 5.6% of body weight, 138 g and 4.8%, and 120 g and 4.6%, respectively. Liquid

Table 4. Fattening and carcass performance of local lambs under different systems of fattening.

Fattening period according to age (weeks)	Final weight (kg)	Average daily gain (kg)	SE Intake /kg gain (kg)	Internal fat (kg)	Tail wt. (kg)	Carcass conformation score	Fat in carcass (%)
8–16	29.8	0.168	2.87	0.203	1.83	2.84	17.50
8–24	39.1	0.179	3.00	0.263	2.85	4.17	20.40
4–32	47.7	0.197	2.88	0.348	4.41	4.50	24.70
8–32	54.2	0.204	3.05	0.294	5.50	5.60	25.60

Source: Riad (1985).

Table 5. Feed resources ($\times 1000$ t) in Egypt for 1982 and 2000.

Item	1982		2000	
	TDN	DCP	TDN	DCP
Available feed resources	9625	1536	13629	2235
Requirement	12730	1367	18132	2173
Balance	− 3105	169	− 4503	62
Self-sufficiency (%)	75.6	112	75.2	103

Source: Hathout (1987).

molasses supplements and ammonia-treated rice straw are recommended by the Ministry and the Animal Production Research Institute (Hathout 1987).

Feedstuff resources and needs

Abou-Akkada et al. (1984) and Hathout (1986; 1987) compared the existing nutrition of livestock and projected needs. They showed a feed gap of 3.1 million t of TDN which is expected to increase to 4.5 million t by the year 2000 (Table 5). Hathout (1987) has suggested a number of strategies to increase the availability of feedstuffs, including utilization of non-conventional resources, increasing forage and maize production, and efficient utilization of feed resources.

Ongoing and future research (1985–2000)

On-farm trials to evaluate productivity of native sheep under local conditions will be continued. These trials aim to evaluate the productivity of local sheep breeds under breeding conditions, characterize prevailing sheep production systems and determine how they interact with livestock and crop production in general, and provide production parameters for analysis of existing or proposed production systems.

On-going trials will continue to improve the lamb production system based on the introduction of 25% prolific sheep blood to local sheep. The main object is to confirm the results of intensive lamb production studies under the intensive conditions in the Delta. Selection trials for the Ministry's Rahmani flock will be planned to improve reproductive performance on the basis of indirect selection for early oestrous activity. Investigations into the different physiological and management factors affecting reproductive performance of Rahmani sheep will continue and possible bottlenecks in the reproductive cycle from puberty to weaning will also be identified.

The role of the fat tail in feed utilization will be studied and in particular the feed energy and fat mobilization in the body as a whole. Finally, studies on the utilization of roughages improved by ammonia or urea treatment under intensive and extensive systems will continue. The utilization of feed formulas based on non-conventional agroindustrial residues and poultry wastes and of liquid molasses supplements will also be studied.

References

Abou-Akkada, A.R., Youssef, A.M., Abou-Raya, A.k., Hathout, M.K., El-Ashry, M.A., Abdel Aziz, A.S., Makky, A.M. and Kassem, M.H. 1984. Policy for development of feed resources until the year 2000. Report submitted to the National Council for Production and Economic Affairs, Egypt. Ministry of Agriculture, Cairo, Egypt.

Abou-Raya, A.K., El-Samman, S., Raafat, M.A. and Soliman, I.M. 1969. The maintenance of energy for mature sheep in prolonged feeding trials. Pages 51–52 in Proceedings of the Third Conference on Animal Production, 19–21 September 1969, Cairo. Cairo University Press, Giza, Cairo, Egypt.

Aboul-Ela, M.B., Aboul-Naga, A.M., Shalaby, T.H. and Maijala, K. 1987. Physiological response to climatic change in Finnish Landrace ewes imported to Egypt and their half-sibs in Finland. Livestock Production Science 17: 179–185.

Aboul-Ela, M.B., El-Nakhla, S.M. and Aboul-Naga, A.M. 1986. Serum progesterone, prolactin and LH concentration as affected by season and light treatment in fat-tailed Rahmani sheep. Animal Reproduction Science. In press.

Aboul-Naga, A.M. 1976. Location effect on the reproductive performance of three indigenous breeds of sheep under the subtropical conditions of Egypt. Indian Journal of Animal Science 46: 630–636.

Aboul-Naga, A.M. 1977. Location effect on the lamb performance of the indigenous breeds of sheep raised under the semi-tropical conditions of Egypt. Indian Journal of Animal Science 47: 29–33.

Aboul-Naga, A.M. 1983. Lamb crop every eight months from subtropical fat-tailed sheep. Pages 147–148 in Proceedings of the Fifth World Conference on Animal Production, 14–19 August 1983, Tokyo, Japan. Japanese Society of Zootechnical Science, Tokyo, Japan.

Aboul-Naga, A.M. 1985. Crossbreeding for fecundity in subtropical sheep. Pages 55–62 in Genetics of Reproduction in Sheep (Land, R. and Robinson, D., eds). Butterworths, London, UK.

Aboul-Naga, A.M. 1987. Extensive flock management in arid range land: case study of north western coast of Egypt. Pages 853–866 in Proceedings of the Fourth International Conference on Goats, 8–13 March 1987, Brazil. Departmento de Difvsao of Technologia-DDT Brazilia, Brazil.

Aboul-Naga, A.M. and Abdel-Rahman, H. 1981. Hormonal control of fertility in Ossimi and Rahmani ewes. Menoufia Journal of Agricultural Research 16: 100.

Aboul-Naga, A.M. and Aboul-Ela, M.B. 1985. The performance of Egyptian breeds of sheep, European breeds and their crosses. II. European breeds and their crosses. Paper presented at the 36th Annual Meeting of the European Association for Animal Production, Kallithea, Halkidiki, Greece, 30 Sept–3 Oct 1985.

Aboul-Naga, A.M., Aboul-Ela, M.B. and Mansour, H. 1987a. Crossbreeding system utilizing desert and valley native sheep breeds. Paper presented at the Second International Conference on Desert Development, 25–31 Jan 1987. In press.

Aboul-Naga, A.M., Aboul-Ela, M.B. and Mansour, H. 1987b. Seasonality of breeding activity in subtropical Egyptian sheep breeds. Paper presented at the 38th Annual Meeting of the European Association for Animal Production, 28 Sept–1 Oct 1987, Lisbon, Portugal. In press.

Aboul-Naga, A.M., Ferial Hassan and Aboul-Ela, M.B. 1987. Reproductive performance of local Egyptian sheep and goat breeds and their crosses with imported temperate breeds. Paper presented at the 38th Annual Meeting of the European Association for Animal Production, 28 Sept–1 Oct 1987, Lisbon, Portugal. In press.

Aboul-Naga, A.M., Mansour, H. and Afifi, A. 1985. Genetic aspects of reproductive performance in two local fat-tailed breeds of sheep. Egyptian Journal of Genetics 40: 100.

Ali, H.M., El-Serafy, A.M., Soliman, H.S., El-Ashry, M.A. and Sawsan, M. 1982. The effect of feeding different roughage to concentrate ratios on the performance of yearling Rahmani lambs. Egyptian Journal of Animal Production 22 (1): 73.

Asker, A.A., Ragab, M.T. and Bastawisy, A.E. 1954. Effect of crossing Egyptian sheep on growth and development of lambs. Empire Journal of Experimental Agriculture 22: 256–260.

El-Ashry, M.A., Khattab, H.M., El-Serafy, A.M. and Soliman, A. 1985. Feeding value of poultry wastes for sheep. International Wastes 14: 51.

El-Said, A.I. 1983. Studies on some production traits in sheep. MSc thesis. Zagazig University, Egypt.

El-Serafy, A.M., El-Ashry, M.A. and Khattab, H.M. 1980. The nutritive value of wastelage containing rations. Alexandria Journal of Agricultural Research 27 (3): 561.

El-Serafy, A.M., El-Ashry, M.A. and Zaki, A. 1976. Growth performance, feed efficiency and carcass characteristics of lambs fed buffalo or cow milk. Indian Journal of Animal Science 46–87.

El-Serafy, A.M., Soliman, H.S., El-Ashry, M.A. and Khattab, H.M. 1981. Effect of replacing dietary maize with grading amounts of sugarcane molasses. Egyptian Journal of Animal Production 21 (2): 221.

El-Shahat, A.A. 1970. Study of some factors affecting milk production in native, imported and crossbred sheep under coastal desert conditions. MSc thesis. Ain Shams University, Egypt.

El-Sheikh, A.S., Salem, M.H., Ibrahim, I.I., Mohamed, A.A., El-Sherbiny, A.A. and Yousef, M.K. 1981. Relative adaptability of some local and foreign breeds of sheep to Sahara desert. Egyptian Journal of Animal Production 21: 109–120.

El-Shobokshy, A.S. and Aboul-Naga, A.M. 1978. Using Suffolk sheep for improving lamb production from subtropical Egyptian sheep. 2. Lamb and fattening performance. Journal of Agricultural Science, Cambridge 90: 131–137.

Fahmy, M.H., Galal, E.S.E., Ghanem, Y.S. and Khighin, S.S. 1969. Crossbreeding of sheep under semi-arid conditions. Animal Production 11: 351–360.

Fawzy, S.A. 1986. Physiological studies on sheep. PhD thesis. Mansoura University, Egypt.

Galal, E.S.E. 1987. Sheep and goat production research and development in Egypt. Pages 117–156 in Small Ruminants in the Near East. FAO, Rome, Italy.

Galal, E.S.E., Aboul-Naga, A., El-Tawil, E.A. and Khishim, E.S. 1972. Estimates of combining abilities and maternal influence in crosses between Merino, Ossimi, and Barki sheep. Animal Production 15: 47–52.

Ghanem, Y.S. (ed.). 1980. (Encyclopaedia of Animal Wealth. Part I: Arab Sheep Breeds.) In Arabic. Arab Organization for Education, Culture and Sciences, Arab Centre for the Studies of Arid and Dry Lands, Syria.

Hassona, E.A.E. 1980. Some studies on sheep performance fed different levels of feeding. MSc thesis. Zagazig University, Egypt.

Hathout, M.K. 1986. Feed resources for livestock in Egypt. In New Techniques in Sheep Production (Marai, I.F.M. and Owen, J.B., eds). Butterworths, London, UK.

Hathout, M.K. 1987. Animal population and feed resources in Egypt. Pages 17–28 in Proceedings and Recommendations of the Egyptian-Dutch Workshop on Husbandry and Veterinary Care, 30–31 March 1987, Cairo, Egypt. Ministry of Agriculture and Fisheries, The Hague, The Netherlands.

Khattab, H.M., El-Ashry, M.A., El-Serafy, A.M. and Zaki, A. 1982. Wood shaving duck litter in rations for growing lambs. Agricultural Wastes 4: 25.

Mansour, H.M., Galal, E.S.E., Hassan, G.H. and Ghanem, Y.S. 1977. Estimation of genetic trend in field records of a flock of Barki sheep. Egyptian Journal of Genetics and Cytology 6: 12–20.

Mason, I.L. 1967. Sheep Breeds of the Mediterranean. FAO and Commonwealth Agricultural Bureaux, Edinburgh, UK. 215 p.

Riad, M.M. 1985. Studies on carcass evaluation in lambs. MSc thesis. Zagazig University, Egypt.

Shalaby, T.H. 1985. Performance and adaptation of local sheep to varied environmental and managerial conditions. PhD thesis. Cairo University, Cairo, Egypt.

Shalaby, T.H., Aboul-Ela, M.B. and Aboul-Naga, A.M. 1986. Physiological responses of Barki desert goats, Damascus, Zaraibi and their crosses to heat stress under the semi-arid conditions of the western desert. In New Techniques in Sheep Production (Marai, I.F.M. and Owen, J.B., eds). Butterworths, London, UK.

Soliman, H.S. 1968. A study on the level of maintenance ration for sheep with regard to the energy and digestible protein. MSc thesis. Ain Shams University, Egypt.

Swidan, F.Z., Aboul-Naga, A.M., El-Shobokshy, A.S. and Abbas, A.M. 1979a. Rahmani male lambs weaned at six or eight weeks of age. Egyptian Journal of Animal Production 19: 159.

Swidan, F.Z., Aboul-Naga, A.M., El-Shobokshy, A.S. and Abbas, A.M. 1979b. Fattening performance and carcass traits of early weaned Rahmani lambs. Egyptian Journal of Animal Production 19: 169.

Tawilla, M.A.M. 1984. Utilization of different protein sources in milk replacers by the newly born ruminant. MSc thesis. Ain Shams University, Egypt.

E.F. Thomson and F.S. Thomson (eds), Increasing Small Ruminant Productivity in Semi-arid Areas
© 1988 ICARDA . ISBN 978-94-010-7086-7

Genetic Improvement of Sheep in Turkey

B. Ankarali

Introduction

Sheep have an important role in the agricultural economy of Turkey and in the nutrition of its people. They convert otherwise unusable vegetation on poor grazing land to meat, milk, fiber, and skins. Eastern, southeastern, and central Turkey are arid and semi-arid. The vast native grazing land and steppe in these regions are more suitable for sheep and goats than dairy cattle. In the more productive western regions agriculture is becoming increasingly intensified, but sheep production continues to be profitable.

This paper summarizes efforts to improve the native sheep breeds of Turkey by crossing and selection carried out since 1934. Yalcin (1986) has reviewed the Turkish sheep breeds in detail.

Improvement of wool

Efforts to improve the wool of native breeds started in 1934 when a flock of German mutton Merino (Merino-Fleisch-Schafe) ewes and rams were imported to Karacabey state farm in the south Marmara region. The imported rams and their male progeny were used to improve the purebred native Kivircik breed of private breeders interested in improving their flocks. Initially, the effect of environmental conditions was not considered and lamb mortality increased as the proportion of Merino genes increased. The milk yield fell as the lambs suckled longer and the animals could not cope with the walk to and from summer and winter pastures. Also, the crossbreeds were less acceptable to consumers who considered the native breed had the best quality meat. As a result, only one fifth of the planned number of improved sheep were obtained in the first 20 years. However, the Merino population in this region still supplies rams to projects in other regions, especially in Middle Anatolia.

In 1950, the crossing project was moved to Middle and East Anatolia where the native sheep breeds are White Karaman and Red Karaman, respectively. They are both fat-tailed with mixed coarse wool. Because the Merino rams could not mate freely with the fat-tailed ewes, an extensive program of artificial insemination was introduced. The same methods were used and some heterosis was removed in the first generation (Duzgunes 1961) which helped the project to be accepted by the breeders. In later generations, lamb mortality increased to 35%, growth rate fell, and wool quality declined. The breeders reacted against this project even though the government applied a large subsidy to the fine wool.

The Ministry of Agriculture then introduced two strategies to solve these problems. The main goal was to develop new local types and breeds. The strategy first involved keeping one or two flocks of native Karaman on each state farm and applying selection programs to improve the uniformity of the coarse wool. The second involved stopping backcrossing and using spotless lambs from the first backcross as they were found to be as effective as purebred Merino rams in eliminating the spots on the crossbreds (Duzgunes et al. 1960).

There are now four new types of sheep with different proportions of Merino blood. One, the Malya, has a small fat tail. The rams can naturally mate the fat-tailed Karaman ewes, thus making it easier to improve the native breed. The second type, the Middle-Anatolian Merino, is 70–80% Merino and has a long tail, while the third, the Konya Merino, contains even more Merino blood and has a finer and heavier fleece and a larger body. The fourth type, the Ramlic, was obtained by selection from the crosses of native Daglic ewes and Rambouillet rams. The characteristics of these new types are given by Duzgunes (1975), Yalcin (1972), Yalcin et al. (1972), Yalcin et al. (1977), Cangir (1977), and Bayraktaroglu (1977).

Improvement of meat production

The early attempts to improve the meat production of native sheep used Ile de France rams imported from France. Several crossbreeding experiments were carried out on Konya-Eregli state farm (Oznacar 1971; Akcapinar 1974; Gonul 1974; Yalcin and Aktas 1976). Further attempts to improve meat production in Kivircik sheep used Texel rams. But the animals died for no apparent reason, leaving only a few F_1 offspring.

In 1986, meat breeds were imported from England (Border Leicester, Dorset Down, Hampshire Down, and Lincoln Longwool), France (Ile de France), and West Germany (Schwarzkopfiges-Fleisch-Schafe) to the Marmara, Middle Anatolia, and East Anatolia regions. They are being used in crosses on state farms to improve new breeds and by some breeders to produce commercial lambs.

Improvement of milk production

The first attempt to improve milk yield used Awassi sheep raised on Ceylanpinar state farm in southeast Anatolia. One elite flock reached 175–205 kg in two generations and the average milk yield of the farm is reported to be three times the country average. Some sheep from this flock have been exported to Saudi Arabia, Libya, and Cyprus.

Awassis have also been used to improve the milk yield of fat-tailed native Karamans (Yalcin and Aktas 1971; Pekel 1973). The F_1 ewes yielded twice as much milk as their dams. This result interested farmers who then wanted Awassi rams for their flocks. Another experiment has been started at Ege University in the province of Denizli to improve the milk yield and body weight of the Daglic breed using Awassi rams.

There are about 30000 Chios sheep in Turkey. This milk breed has high fertility and a large body. The average milk yield under normal conditions was reported to be 210–220 kg by Bulgurlu (1960) and Sonmez (1963). These sheep are raised in small groups of 2–4 by the farmers growing vegetables along the Aegean coast. In 1986 the Ministry of Agriculture established a flock on Kumbale state farm to improve milk production by selection.

In Thrace, southern Marmara, and along the Aegean coast, where the price of sheep milk is higher than that of cows' milk, an important breed is the Kivircik. According to studies made on two state farms in Thrace and on some private flocks, the average milk yield of this breed is 62–119 kg (Alpbaz 1970; Ozcan 1975; Sonmez et al. 1975). In these regions agriculture is becoming increasingly intensive and costs of production are increasing so attempts are being made to improve the genetic potential of the native animals. One project, developed by the Turkish Scientific and Technical Research Organization, involved crossing Kivircik ewes and East Friesian rams. This resulted in the Tahirova breed. The project has been closely followed by the Kivircik breeders near to the state farm and, having realized the advantages of the new type, they have asked for rams for their own flocks. Thus, a large nucleus of breeding material has been established in this area.

References

Akcapinar, H. 1974. Ile de France × Turk Merinosu Melezlemesi ile Kaliteli Kesim Kuzulari Elde Etme Imkanlari. Lalahan Zootekni Arastirma Enstitusu Yayinlari No. 37.

Alpbaz, A.G. 1970. Bati Anadolu ve Trakyada yetistirilen saf ve cesitli melez kivircik koyunlarinin bazi onemli verimlerle ilgili ozellikleri uzerinde mukayeseli arastirmalar. Doctoral thesis, Ege University.

Bayraktaroglu, E. 1977. Orta-Anadolu Devlet Uretme Ciftliklerinde yetistirilen Anadolu Merinoslarinda verimle ilgili bazi ozelliklere ait fenotipik ve genetik parametreler. Doctoral thesis, Ankara University.

Bulgurlu, S. 1960. Rasyonel Besleme ve Itinali Bakim Sartlarinda Ivesi ve Sakiz Koyunlarinin Sut Verimleri Uzerinde Arastirmalar. Ege Universitesi, Yayin No. 48.

Cangir, S. 1977. Orta Anadolu Uretme Ciftliklerinde yetistirilen Anadolu Merinoslarinda yapagi verimi ile ilgili bazi ozellikere ait fenotipik ve genetik parametreler. Doctoral thesis, Ankara University.

Duzgunes, O. 1961. Heterosis in crossings between Merino-Fleisch-Schafe and the native Karaman sheep in Middle Anatolia. Zeitschrift fur Tierzuchtung und Zuchtungsbiologie 75 (3): 207–208.

Duzgunes, D. 1975. Improving Karaman Sheep of Middle-Anatolia by using German Merino, 1973. Pages 27–34 in Yearbook of the Faculty of Agriculture, University of Ankara, Turkey.

Duzgunes, O. Yarkin, L. amd Sonmez, R. 1960. A study on the variation in colour in the fat-tailed White Karaman sheep, Merino-Fleisch-Schafe and their crosses. Zeitschrift furTierzuchtung und Zuchtungsbiologie 74 (1): 36–47.

Gonul, T. 1974. Kasaplik Kuzu Uretimi icin Daglic Koyunlari Uzerinde Melezleme Denemeleri. Ege Universitesi, Yayini No. 236.

Ozcan, H. 1975. Kivircik Koyunlarinin Onemli Verim Ozelliklerinin Gelistirilmesinde Texel Irkindan Faydalanma Imkanlari. Project Final Report. TBTAK-VHAG 51k.

Oznacar, K. 1971. Ile de France×Akkaraman melezlerinin yapagi ozellikleri uzerinde arastirma. Lalahan Zootekni Arastirma Enstitusu Derg. 11 (3–4): 56–71.

Pekel, E. 1973. Akkaraman koyunlarinin sut verimlerinin arttiril-masinda Ivesilerden yararlanma imkanlari. Ankara Universitesi, Yayin No. 43/3.

Sonmez, R. 1963. Breed characters and different productions in the Sakiz sheep (Chios Schafe) of Turkey. Zeitschrift fur Tierzuchtung und Zuchtungsbiologie 78 (3): 281–286.

Sonmez, R., Alpbaz, A.G. and Kizilay, E. 1975. Kivircik koyunlarinin Texel'le melezleme yolu ile islahi imkanlari. TBTAK V. Bilim Kongresi, VHAG tebligi.

Yalcin, B.C. 1972. Konya Merinoslarinda onemli bazi dolverimi ozelliklerinin fenotipik ve genetik parametreleri ve bu ozelliklerin seleksiyonla islahi uzerinde arastirmalar. (English summary.) Ankara Universitesi Derg. 19 (3): 349–363.

Yalcin, B.C. 1986. Sheep and Goats in Turkey. FAO Animal Production and Health Paper 60. FAO, Rome, Italy. 168 p.

Yalcin, B.C. and Aktas, G. 1971. Ivesi ve Akkaraman koyunlari ile bunlarin melezlerinin sut verimi ve diger verim ozellikleri yonunden karsilastirilmasi. TBTAK III. Bilim Kongresi, 25–27 October 1971, Ankara. VHAG Tebligleri 48–49.

Yalcin, B.C. and Aktas, G. 1976. Ile de France ve Akkaraman koyunlari ile bunlarin melezlerinin verimle ilgili ozellikleri uzerinde karsilastirmali arastirmalar. (English summary.) Istanbul Universitesi Derg. 2 (1):21–40.

Yalcin, B.C., Ayabakan, S. and Koseoglu, H. 1977. Daglic koyunlarinin et ve yapagi verimi ozelliklerinin gelistirilmesinde Rambouillet irkindan yararlanilma olanaklari TBTAK VHAG-51 g No. 1u projenin kesin raporu.

Yalcin, B.C. Muftuoglu, S. and Yurtcu, B. 1972. Orta Anadolu Merinoslarinda onemli verim ozelliklerinin seleksiyonla gelistirilme imkanlari 1. Cesitli ozellikler bakimindan performans seviyeleri. (English summary.) Ankara Universitesi Derg. 19 (1–2): 227–255.

E.F. Thomson and F.S. Thomson (eds), Increasing Small Ruminant Productivity in Semi-arid Areas
© 1988 ICARDA . ISBN 978-94-010-7086-7

Sheep Breeding in Jordan and a Proposed Awassi Breed Improvement Programme

I.G.H. Goddard

Introduction

The tradition of keeping semi-nomadic flocks of small ruminants extends back to the start of civilization in the Middle East. As population and living standards have increased, farming practices and values have also changed, with increasing pressure to improve productivity in all sectors of agriculture including animal production.

It is not easy to improve production in areas with high summer temperatures and limited winter rainfall and any programme aiming to improve productivity through selective breeding must first improve nutrition, disease prevention and control, and flock management practices (Goddard 1982).

A number of local organizations are working with a variety of donors on integrated development programmes. The Jordan Cooperative Organization (JCO) is involved in five main programmes:

- rangeland improvement and lamb fattening with the World Food Programme (WFP),
- forage production with the Australian Dryland Farming Project (ADFP) and WFP,
- sheep health and management with the United Kingdom Assistance Programme and ADFP,
- control of external parasites with West German Government support, and
- Awassi sheep improvement projects supported by the European Economic Community and the European Investment Bank.

Many of these programmes were established or have been maintained as a result of the recommendations of the Sheep Production Workshop held at the University of Jordan in October 1982 (Harb and Goddard, unpublished data). One of the major requirements identified at that workshop was the need to increase the number and quality of selected breeding stock available within Jordan and sheep owners stressed the importance of Awassi sheep and Shami goats. The results from the first four of these programmes have already clearly demonstrated the financial benefits of improved productivity and the possible financial returns when farmers adopt the recommended practices.

Basic objectives of the cooperative programme

The small ruminant improvement programme established by the JCO aims to maintain the present production characteristics valued by the semi-nomadic pastoral flock owners. These include disease resistance, climatic tolerance, hardiness, and carcass characteristics such as fat tails. It also hopes to improve average flock productivity, especially for red meat and milk, and so increase national production from local resources, and raise real farm incomes per unit flock size.

Jordanian data on breed improvement

The comparative data available for Awassis (Table 1) show clearly that in 1982 there had been little change in productive traits in well managed flocks on government stations and the results suggest that government sheep should not be considered an improved strain. In 1985, only 41 sheep were issued to commercial farmers. The same applies to Shami goat breeding (Table 2) with around 30-50 animals being issued annually to commercial farmers.

In 1982 the University of Jordan's flock, with ewes selected from local farm flocks, had been established for less than 2 years so had no selective breeding

Table 1. Awassi production data, Jordan.

Parameter		University of Jordan 1982/83 Average ± S.D.		Commercial Flocks 1982/84 Average ± S.D.		Ministry of Agriculture 1982 Average
Adult liveweight	Ewes	59.48	4.58	43.70	7.91	N.A.
(< 2 years, kg)	Rams	74.00	8.19	71.23	5.92	N.A.
Body length (cm)	Ewes	75.60	2.13	69.82	4.75	N.A.
	Rams	82.70	8.63	80.40	8.61	N.A.
Adult shoulder height	Ewes	69.84	3.94	56.18	4.12	N.A.
(cm)	Rams	77.60	4.27	75.13	4.49	N.A.
Birth weight (kg)	Female	3.85	0.404	3.94	0.375	5.8
	Male	4.32	0.622	4.28	0.412	5.9
Pre-weaning growth rate	Female	299.8	61.5	207	57.8	197
(g/day)	Male	324.3	73.9	232	59.6	236
Post-weaning growth rate	Female	168	49	N.A.	N.A.	N.A.
(g/day) over 60 days	Male	235	49	210	74	N.A.
Average lactation length	Commercial	N.A.	N.A.	120	N.A.	100
(days)	Nomadic	N.A.	N.A.	65	N.A.	N.A.
Milk yield, post-weaning (kg/lactation)		N.A.	N.A.	45–90	70	N.A.
Wool yields (kg/head)	Ewe	2.41	1.01	1.83	0.84	1.65
	Ram	3.21	0.79	2.57	0.86	N.A.

Source: Goddard (1982).
N.A. = not available.

Table 2. Government Shami goat breeding results.

Parameter	Year		
	1982/83	1984	1985
Fertility (%)	93.3	100.0	95.5
Kid mortality (%)	9.25	3.5	6.9
Birth rate (%)			
male	53.4	35.6	56.3
female	44.3	61.1	37.0
hermaphrodite	2.3	3.3	6.7
Multiple births(%)			
twins	59.2	50.0	46.6
triplets	1.9	5.5	4.6
Average birth weight (kg)			
twins male	4.5	3.8	4.0
female	3.5	3.7	3.5
singles male	4.5	4.5	4.1
female	4.0	4.2	3.5
Average weaning weight (kg)			
twins male	17.5	16.4	13.6
female	14.5	14.6	11.5
singles male	17.5	16.2	14.6
female	17.5	20.2	13.1
Average age at weaning (days)	74	73	76
Average daily milk production (kg)	1.5	1.1	1.0

Source: Goddard (1982).

programme. The main improvements in flock performance were considered to be the result of good management practices, especially feeding and disease prevention.

For the assessment of any of the current breeding programmes for sheep or goats in Jordan, a higher standard of record keeping and data processing and retrival would be necessary. This is one of the major management improvements being stressed under the JCO scheme.

Changes in breeding units and stock

Since the workshop in 1982 there have been a number of changes in Awassi and Shami goat breeding and stock availability. More commercial farmers now keep better records of their semi-intensive flocks and are slowly improving stock selection.

Two large commercial units have been established with recorded flocks of Awassis from Turkey, and Chios and Shami from Cyprus. Both groups are recording productivity and plan to maintain closed flocks and select for meat and milk production. Surplus stock will be sold.

The University of Jordan also maintains a closed breeding flock and has started a selection programme based on ewe performance records and lamb growth, while the University of Science and Technology at Irbid is establishing a sheep research unit which will select and evaluate different breeds. A major programme for sheep development was started in 1987, including the establishment of an Awassi Breed Improvement Unit financed by the JCO, the government, and the EEC as well as five farmer service and fattening units financed by the JCO, the government, and the EIB. The six units will be fully operational by the end of 1989.

The JCO is also committed to the establishment of a new Shami Goat Breeding Unit in the current 5-year plan. There has been little change in the government's closed Awassi flock at Kanassri which disposes of limited numbers of sheep each year and one of the Ministry of Agriculture's Awassi breeding flocks has been disbursed. There have been no significant improvements in the government's Shami goat flock at Wadi Walla due to the management constraints of limited land, capital, and quality of inputs.

Planned breeding and selection for the joint JCO / EEC breeding unit

The designs and equipment specifications for the JCO/EEC breeding unit have been based on the need to establish good performance records which allow for the measurement of phenotypic and genotypic performance. Adjustments will have to be made for the effect of major environmental factors on phenotypic performance to evaluate repeatability and heritability estimations for genetic selection.

A number of general characters are considered to be important, including total lamb production per ewe per annum as a combined effect of prolificacy and lambing frequency, total and sellable milk production per ewe, efficiency of feed conversion in the ewe, meat production efficiency based on growth rate, feed conversion, and carcass quality, and adaptability to the environment. This last character is very important due to the probable differences in management systems between the breed improvement unit and the normal commercial flock and it will be difficult to assess accurately.

One of the initial problems in attempting to rapidly improve the Awassi is its fertility. It has been assumed that, initially, the heritability of litter size at first lambing will be very low so selection should be based on the results of the third lambing rather than the first or pooled values for the first three. Also, measures of prolificacy based on number weaned can be seriously affected by pre-weaning losses and other traits such as ewe liveweight (Young et al. 1963; Pursar 1965) and time of mating (Reeve and Robertson 1953; Bowman 1966). However, it is well established that the Awassi has an extended breeding season which can increase total lamb production by a breeding frequency period of under 1 year. This must be related to feed availability for commercial flocks and so initial plans are based on one lambing per year.

Measurement of milk production using pre-weaning lamb weights and measurements of milk taken for sale are good measures of performance but

185

selection must allow for environmental effects. The method proposed by the JCO is to rank groups lambing at the same time and managed under similar conditions. Current selection plans do not include a major component based on feed conversion due to problems of measurement of intake, and selection will be based more on associated factors such as output of meat and milk.

In evaluating characteristics important for meat production, emphasis will be placed on high reproductive rates and high weaning weights with corrections for birth type and age of ewe and lamb (Turner 1979). The JCO plans to establish a breeding flock based on an open nucleus structure to maintain contact with the semi-nomadic flocks and environmental effects.

The present approach to improving breeds is based on the purebreeding system. This was selected because as a pure type, the Awassi has a very strong commercial appeal both locally and within the region so all animals will be suitable for commercial production and no 'by-product' animals will be produced which could affect the market. This system allows the design of relatively simple selection programmes in which animals from all levels of the population can be used, so helping to increase selection pressure. Also, results from comparisons of pure and crossbreeding have shown that selection within a breed can be more beneficial, especially when there is wide variation within the pure breed (Turner 1979). Finally, each producer can be encouraged to produce most of the required replacements, and to buy mainly males. This reduces disease risks and capital requirements.

The decision by JCO to develop a centralized open nucleus breeding system for purebreds was an attempt to overcome the problems of a lack of farm records, failure to develop an organization for supervising and conducting data analysis, small average flock size, low reproductive rate and high loss rates allowing mainly limited male selection, and poor, uncontrolled dissemination of improved stock. The JCO breeding farm, with a final flock of 2000 breeding ewes and good recording and analysis, aims to overcome the first three of these problems. Other development programmes currently operating in Jordan are also increasing and improving farm records from commercial owners.

The long-term aim of breed improvement is to help increase reproductive rates which will help increase production and possible selection pressure. The JCO plans for stock distribution and total numbers are based on Bowman (1979) and Owen (1971) and aim to improve dissemination through the specialist sheep breeding co-operative societies. Recipients of improved stock will be encouraged to improve their record keeping.

Breeding plans to improve the Awassi

In developing the initial plans for an open nucleus type flock system for breed improvement based on the approaches of Parker (1979), Shepherd (1979), Jackson and Turner (1972), Knight and Rae (1970), and James (1977), the major problems to be overcome are the lack of farm flocks with suitable records and initial farmer participation.

It was decided that for the early stages of the scheme the main breeding flock would be divided into an elite central nucleus with a maximum of 200 ewes and nine sub-flocks of equal size for breeding. This would allow the development of a nucleus scheme within the main co-operative breeding flock.

All rams retained for breeding and 50% of the ewe replacements for the nucleus would be produced by the nucleus flock. The other 50% of ewe replacements would be taken from the offspring of superior ewes in the other flocks.

The plans are to initially replace elite ewes after the third lambing and so improve selection rate and generation turnover. Early ewe selection and rapid turnover have been shown by Turner (1979) to maximize annual genetic gain, assuming accurate selection, and to give better results than crossbreeding without selection.

Ewes culled from the elite flock will be transferred to the sub-flocks. Ewe selection pressure will be maintained within the sub-flocks and ewes culled for low performance will be sold or slaughtered depending on age and reason for culling. The ram breeding policy will be based on the selection of the best male lambs of each generation from those produced by the elite flock for use within the main breeding flock.

In the first 3 years, only the number of ram replacements initially required by the main unit will be selected and there will be no major external sales. The number of ram replacements kept will be increased from the third year onwards to produce stock for sale to members of co-operative societies. After 5 years the unit should produce around 300 rams annually for sale as breeding stock. Depending on improvements achieved and demand patterns, it would be possible to sell more by selling animals that are not of the best quality. The current recommendation is that at least 60% of all ram lambs produced should be transferred to a fattening centre after weaning for sale as meat and not for breeding.

Initial planning allows for transfer of stock between other top breeding flocks to ensure wide blood lines are maintained and the spread of quality stock. This will be related to disease status and management standards of the flocks concerned.

In the future, stock exchange or inputs from other flocks which are operated as commercial semi-intensive flocks by members will be developed. This is currently assumed to be selection of ewe lambs from good range ewes and their transfer into the main breeding flock in return for equal numbers of yearling to four-tooth ewes. This is considered to be important in maintaining the locally important characteristics related to environmental factors.

The basic concept is to develop a short generation interval within the main breeding flock to maximize genetic gain, associated with transfer of improved animals to farmers by selling extra lambs and culling breeding stock on age not performance failure.

Workers must be aware of the type of animals which are suitable for the clients. For example, large increases in average body weights and therefore feed maintenance requirements should be avoided in semi-nomadic flocks. This is an example of the need to relate the breed selection unit to the requirements of commercial owners.

One of the future considerations in the management of this flock will be whether or not selection for adaptation to summer conditions will be an advantage in terms of economic selection. Hopkins et al. (1979) reported that it is possible to identify adapted animals within a genetic pool based on rectal temperature and respiration rate in summer. This may help in improving breeding results. Stephenson et al. (1979) showed that improved breeding in hot climates depended on improved husbandry techniques as well as genetic selection, especially for lamb survival. This re-emphasizes the importance of the current projects combining nutrition and flock health with a successful breeding programme, especially in semi-arid zones with hot summers.

Evaluation of the results to maintain the long breeding period of the Awassi will be important to ensure widespread lambing to stabilize local meat supply and milk for processing. Management of breeding programmes to achieve this is possible in flocks where supplementary feeding is practiced.

The ram lamb selection programme

This programme is based on the growth rate of lambs, as fast growth is normally the prime indicator of efficient meat production and of good ewe milk production. Early selection based on corrected weaning weights will be used to rank all available ram lambs and the choice confirmed later from body weights and body characteristics before first mating. Weaning weights will be corrected using birth weight, age at weaning, age of dam, and litter size.

Rams will be ranked according to adjusted weaning weights for each lambing period. Other factors, such as body conformation and parental performance, can then be included in the selection process. The inclusion of multiple births in this process is important in selecting good rams, as farmers require high reproductive performance, good milk yields, and rapid growth rates to raise flock performance.

References

Bowman, J.C. 1966. Meat from sheep. Animal Breeding Abstracts 34: 293–319.

Bowman, J.C. 1979. Breeding for Improvement. Management and Diseases of Sheep. British Council (ed.). Commonwealth Agricultural Bureaux, UK.

Goddard, I.G.H. 1982. Improvement of sheep production in Jordan. Proceedings of a Workshop on Sheep Production in Jordan. Faculty of Agriculture, University of Jordan, Amman.

Hopkins, P.S., Pratt, M.S. and Knight, G.I. 1979. The impact of environmental factors on sheep breeding in the semi-arid tropics. Pages 131–134 in Sheep Breeding (Tomes, G.J., Robertson, D.E., and Lightfoot, R.J., eds). Second edition. Butterworths, London, UK.

Jackson, N. and Turner, H.N. 1972. Optimal structure for a co-operative nucleus breeding system. Proceedings of the Australian Society of Animal Production 9: 55–64.

James, J.W. 1977. Open nucleus breeding systems. Animal Production 24: 287–305.

Knight, G.K. and Rae, A.L. 1970. Large scale sheep breeding, it's development and possibilities. Pages 73–85 in Australian Sheep Farming Annual.

Owen, J.B. 1971. Performance recording in sheep. Technical Communication 20. Commonwealth Agricultural Bureaux, UK.

Parker, A.G. 1979. Advantages of group breeding schemes. Pages 231–234 in Sheep Breeding (Tomes, G.J., Robertson, D.E., and Lightfoot, R.J., eds). Second edition. Butterworths, London, UK.

Pursar, A.F. 1965. Repeatability and heritability of fertility in hill sheep. Journal of Animal Production 7: 75–82.

Reeve, E.C.R. and Robertson, F.W. 1953. Factors affecting multiple births in sheep. Animal Breeding Abstracts 21: 211–224.

Shepherd, J.H. 1979. The Australian Merino Society nucleus breeding scheme. Pages 235–246 in Sheep Breeding (Tomes, G.J., Robertson, D.E., and Lightfoot, R.J., eds). Second edition. Butterworths, London, UK.

Stephenson, R.G.A., Tierney, M. and Hopkins, P.S. 1979. Husbandry and genetic considerations affecting sheep breeding in the semi-arid tropics. Pages 135–138 in Sheep Breeding (Tomes, G.J., Robertson, D.E., and Lightfoot, R.J., eds). Butterworths, London, UK.

Turner, H.N. 1979. Methods of improving production in characters of importance. Pages 93–112 in Sheep Breeding (Tomes, G.J., Robertson, D.E., and Lightfoot, R.J., eds). Butterworths, London, UK.

Young, S.S.Y., Turner, H.N. and Dollings, C.H.S. 1963. Selection for fertility in Merino sheep. Australian Journal of Agricultural Research 14: 460–482.

E.F. Thomson and F.S. Thomson (eds), Increasing Small Ruminant Productivity in Semi-arid Areas
© 1988 ICARDA . ISBN 978-94-010-7086-7

Genetic Improvement of Sheep in Cyprus by Selection and / or Crossbreeding

A.P. Mavrogenis

Introduction

The ultimate goal of any breeding program is undoubtedly the improvement of one or more economically important traits. Choosing a particular program is not easy and depends on the mode of inheritance of particular traits. The first step is to define the program's aims or breeding goals, then to devise measurement techniques. A general outline of a commonly used strategy is presented in Fig. 1.

Because of the importance of milk and meat in Cyprus the three main targets of all improvement efforts have been milk, growth, and prolificacy. The

Fig. 1. General strategy for choosing a breeding program.

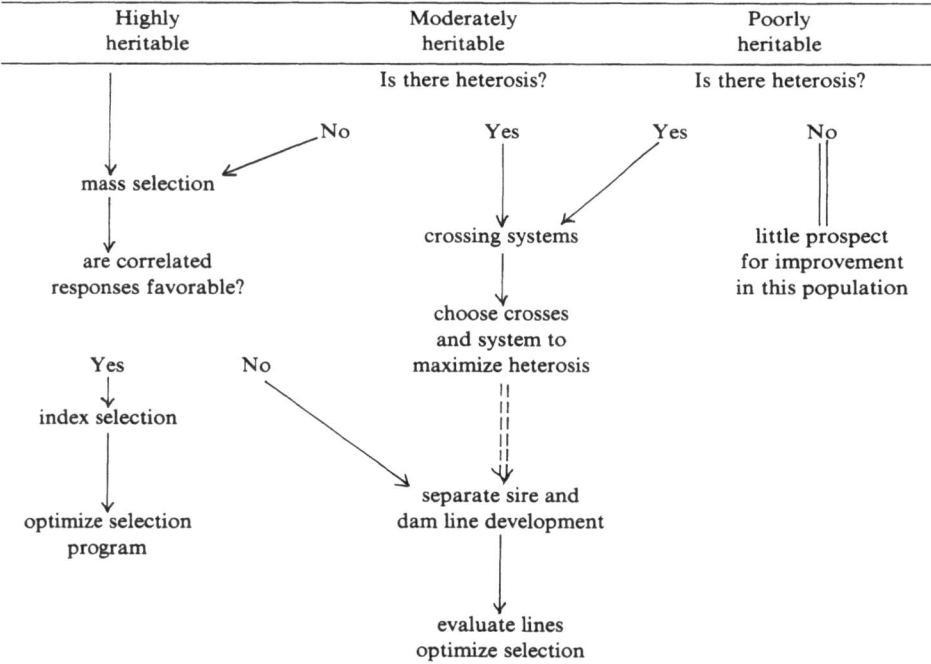

first attempts at animal improvement in Cyprus were initiated in the late 1930s and consisted of characterizing the local population based on external characteristics (Finci 1938).

Until 1972, the policy was to upgrade the local population by using Chios and Awassi improver rams. These breeds were chosen for their greater prolificacy and milk production under semi-intensive conditions and under extensive conditions, respectively. This upgrading was unsuccessful due to the indiscriminate use of the Chios breed in all environments. The simplest solution at the time was to resort to either backcrosses to the local population or to three-way crosses using the Awassi.

Livestock Production Improvement Project

The Livestock Production Improvement Project operated from 1970 to 1974. Its aims were to measure the relative economic and biological value and adaptability of the Chios, Awassi, and local fat-tailed Cyprus breed, improve these breeds through selection, produce sheep in which the favorable traits of the parent breeds were combined and the unfavorable traits were eliminated, test these crosses in various environments, provide commercial breeders with superior (mainly male) stock, and test the applicability of modern breed improvement methods to the existing breeds and breed types.

Three self-contained flocks of Chios, Awassi, and local ewes were established on government farms, totalling 1200 sheep. For the pure breeds, selection pressure was aimed at improving lamb growth rate and milk yield. Selection for growth in all three breeds was made on the basis of growth of the ram lambs to be used as sires in the following generation.

For genetic improvement of milk yield in the Chios breed, a system of sib testing was practiced. Since generation turnover in the Awassi and local breeds is slower than in Chios, selection for milk yield in these breeds was based on the dam's yield only. In the Awassi, sib or progeny tests were carried out to evaluate a different basis for selection.

Breed comparisons were made on the basis of whole flock performance over 2 or more years at three levels of nutrition (or two in the case of local) over the whole production cycle. Lambs and ewes of all breeds and crosses were constantly observed for the occurrence of heat to establish breed differences in the patterns of sexual maturity and seasonal sexual activity.

Several different crosses of the three main breeds were made to test their suitability under the various environmental conditions. To determine whether it was possible to increase prolificacy, growth, and meat quality, crosses were also made with Finn sheep and French Merinos.

Special flocks of 100 breeding ewes were established to study how the three main breeds may perform under very intensive management. These were managed so as to allow for more lambings per year.

Research after 1975

The main activities after 1975 concentrated on building up the number of animals required for research and development. Several studies were initiated to estimate genetic parameters on which to base decisions for the breeding program. Summaries of these parameters are shown in Tables 1–4.

Most methods and objectives in this period were the same as those in 1972–74. In addition, selection procedures in purebred Chios populations were improved and index selection was used. The index included milk production and lamb liveweight. Milk production was based on the dam's 90-day yield after weaning and lamb liveweight on individual performance at 105

Table 1. Estimates of heritabilities of Chios ewes.

Trait	h^2	SE
Litter size at birth (LSB)	0.27	0.07
Litter size at birth (live only) (LSBL)	0.20	0.07
Litter weight at birth (LWTB)	0.21	0.07
Litter size at weaning (LSWN)	0.19	0.07
Litter weight at weaning (LWTWN)	0.13	0.06
90-day milk yield (MLK 90)	0.18	0.06
Total days in milk (DAYS)	0.22	0.07
Total milk yield (TOTMLK)	0.30	0.08
Fat percent (FAT)	0.64	0.11
Fat yield (FATKG)	0.33	0.08
Fat corrected milk yield (6% fat) (FCM)	0.31	0.08

Table 2. Estimates of genetic and phenotypic correlations in Chios ewes.

Trait	MLK90	DAYS	TOTMLK	FAT	FATKG	FCM
MLK90		0.58	0.99	−0.24	0.87	0.96
DAYS	0.52		0.78	0.39	0.88	0.86
TOTMLK	0.80	0.78		−0.05	0.91	0.97
FAT	−0.07	0.08	−0.04		0.37	0.20
FATKG	0.74	0.79	0.95	0.22		0.99
FCM	0.77	0.79	0.98	0.11	0.99	

Table 3. Estimates of heritabilities of Chios lambs.

Trait	h^2	SE
Birth weight (BWT)	0.13	0.07
Weaning weight (WWT)	0.36	0.12
Body weight at		
5 weeks (WT5)	0.34	0.12
10 weeks (WT10)	0.63	0.16
15 weeks (WT15)	0.73	0.17
20 weeks (WT20)	0.66	0.16
Preweaning growth rate (ADG1)	0.35	0.12
Postweaning growth rate (ADG2)	0.56	0.15

Table 4. Estimates of genetic and phenotypic correlations in Chios lambs.

Trait	BWT	WWT	WT5	WT10	WT15	WT20	ADG1	ADG2
BWT		0.21	0.19	0.17	0.18	0.19	0.16	0.19
WWT	0.42		0.23	0.24	0.24	0.25	0.22	0.25
WT5	0.47	0.88		0.22	0.21	0.22	0.25	0.19
WT10	0.40	0.75	0.80		0.24	0.24	0.21	0.24
WT15	0.38	0.67	0.70	0.88		0.25	0.21	0.25
WT20	0.36	0.59	0.62	0.78	0.89		0.22	0.24
ADG1	0.18	0.87	0.92	0.76	0.66	0.58		0.19
ADG2	0.15	0.16	0.13	0.42	0.64	0.83	0.08	

days old. Weaning weight was not considered because of the complex nature of the trait.

Crossbreeding studies were restricted to crosses between Chios and Awassis and investigations of the effects of crossbreeding using a breed from a temperate environment (East Friesian). The crossbreeding programs with Chios and Awassi sheep aimed to improve the ability of the Chios or locally improved populations to withstand adverse management conditions. The second program aimed to further improve the milking capacity and growth potential of the locally improved population, with minor emphasis on udder conformation.

It was estimated that the expected genetic progress per year from index selection is approximately 6.7 kg of milk and 1.8 kg of liveweight. These estimates were possible because estimates of genetic parameters were available and selection indices for purebred populations were developed (Mavrogenis et al. 1980; Mavrogenis 1982).

Table 5. Effects of crossbreeding and estimates of heterosi in Chios × Awassi lambs.

Breed or cross	Trait				
	BWT	WWT	WT15	ADG1	ADG2
Chios (Ch)	4.0	13.5	27.5	0.215	0.230
Awassi (A)	4.9	16.8	30.7	0.257	0.238
Ch × A	5.1	17.1	30.1	0.260	0.220
A × Ch	4.2	16.2	31.9	0.250	0.274
Heterosis (%)	4.5	10.9	6.5	8.1	5.6

Table 6. Reproductive traits of Chios × Awassi ewes.

Breed or cross	Trait				
	LSB	LSBL	LWTB	LSWN	LWTWN
Chios (Ch)	1.73	1.61	6.6	1.50	20.3
Awassi (A)	1.12	1.10	5.4	1.07	17.0
Ch × A	1.42	1.39	6.7	1.34	21.2
A × Ch	1.25	1.24	6.1	1.20	19.6
Heterosis (%)	neg.	neg.	6.67	neg.	9.38

Table 7. Milk production of Chios × Awassi ewes.

Breed or cross	Trait					
	MLK90	DAYS	TOTMLK	FAT	FATKG	FCM
Chios (Ch)	130	161	174	6.4	11.1	179
Awassi (A)	113	173	173	7.3	12.7	194
Ch × A	131	133	167	6.5	11.0	175
A × Ch	119	118	150	6.5	9.8	157
Heterosis (%)	2.88	neg.	neg.	neg.	neg.	neg.

Table 8. Lamb traits of Chios × East Friesian crosses.

Breed or cross	Trait				
	BWT	WWT	WT15	ADG1	ADG2
Chios	4.0	13.5	27.5	0.215	0.230
EF × Ch (F₁)	4.7	16.7	31.0	0.247	0.250
EF × Ch (F₂)	4.2	14.8	31.3	0.246	0.266
(EF × Ch) × Ch	4.4	14.2	30.8	0.231	0.267
Ch × (EF × Ch)	4.4	14.6	31.4	0.240	0.269

Table 9. Reproductive traits of Chios × East Friesian ewes.

Breed or cross	Trait				
	LSB	LSBL	LWTB	LSWN	LWTWN
Chios	1.73	1.61	6.6	1.50	20.3
EF × Ch (F₁)	1.91	1.83	8.5	1.70	25.6
EF × Ch (F₂)	1.69	1.60	7.2	1.48	21.6
(EF × Ch) × Ch	1.83	1.80	7.9	1.63	24.3
Ch × (EF × Ch)	1.58	1.54	6.9	1.49	23.4

Table 10. Milk production of Chios × East Friesian ewes.

Breed or cross	Trait					
	MLK90	DAYS	TOTMLK	FAT	FATKG	FCM
Chios	130	161	174	6.4	11.1	179
EF × Ch (F₁)	155	161	215	5.9	12.6	212
EF × Ch (F₂)	126	143	164	6.1	10.0	165
(EF × Ch) × Ch	131	144	169	6.1	10.2	170
Ch × (EF × Ch)	123	140	165	6.1	9.9	166

Estimates of heterosis showed that in some cases crossbreeding was not the best method of improvement and that much more work is needed to understand the mode of inheritance and effects of crossbreeding (Tables 5–10). For example, estimated heterosis in Chios × Awassi reciprocal crosses was between 4.5% for birth weight and 10.9% for weaning weight and estimates of litter size and weight were negative for size but positive for weight.

The crossbreeding studies, particularly those involving the East Friesian, indicate that there may be important maternal effects but further studies are required (Mavrogenis and Constantinou 1986).

The three tier breeding program

As a result of all these studies a three tier national breeding program was initiated on government farms. About 1200 Chios sheep form the elite flock, which is a closed flock. The second tier (multiplier flocks) is formed by selecting private flocks with a total population of about 3500 Chios and East Friesian × Chios sheep. These flocks are an integral part of the National Improvement Program which is assisted by the extension services of the Ministry of Agriculture. The traits recorded and the average performance of these flocks in 1985/86 are presented in Tables 11 and 12. Assistance is given during milk recording and selection of males and females for replacement and disposal (to other farmers for breeding or slaughter) and advice given on management and feeding. The third tier is formed by the sale of rams or other breeding stock from the multiplier flocks to farmers. In the second and third tiers there is a two-way flow of genes.

Table 11. Ewe traits of purebred and crossbred [1] sheep in private flocks participating in the National Breeding Program.

Trait	Yearling	Adult
Total no. of animals	1136	2017
No. of animals lambing	552 (48.6) [2]	1600 (79.3)
No. aborted	24 (1.8)	16 (0.8)
Barren	230 (20.3)	128 (6.4)
No. of animals sold	340 (30.9)	396 (14.7)
No. of animals recorded	462	1349
90-day milk yield (kg)	128	138
Litter size at birth	1.51	1.85
Litter size at weaning	1.16	1.50

[1] Crossbred sheep refer mostly to EF × Chios crosses.
[2] Figures in parentheses are percentages of the total.

Table 12. Ewe traits of purebred and crossbred [1] sheep in private flocks participating in the National Breeding Program.

Trait	Ewes of all classes [2]
Birth weight (kg)	4.0
Weaning weight (kg)	14.0
Days to weaning	48.0
105-day weight (kg)	29.5

[1] Crossbred sheep refer mostly to EF × Chios crosses.
[2] Averaged over sex, type of birth, and parity of ewe.

Conclusion

There is no doubt that milk and meat production have been improved. But this may not be solely genetic improvement as non-genetic factors may also have been improved, such as management and feeding practices. The extent of genetic progress over the past 10 years can only be determined after more generations have elapsed.

Acknowledgements

The author wishes to acknowledge the valuable cooperation and assistance of his colleagues at the Agricultural Research Institute and the Department of Agriculture.

References

Finci, M. 1938. The relation between body-conformation and productivity in the Cyprus fat-tailed sheep. Empire Journal of Experimental Agriculture 6: 25–37.

Mavrogenis, A.P. 1982. Environmental and genetic factors influencing milk production and lamb output of Chios sheep. Livestock Production Science 8: 519–527.

Mavrogenis, A.P. and Constantinou, A. 1986. Performance evaluation of purebred and crossbred lambs. Agricultural Research Institute Technical Bulletin No. 77. Agricultural Research Institute, Nicosia, Cyprus.

Mavrogenis, A.P., Louca, A. and Robison, O.W. 1980. Estimates of genetic parameters for pre-weaning and post-weaning growth traits of Chios lambs. Animal Production 30: 271–276.

Part III

Health

E.F. Thomson and F.S. Thomson (eds), Increasing Small Ruminant Productivity in Semi-arid Areas
© 1988 ICARDA . ISBN 978-94-010-7086-7

Studying Husbandry and Health of Awassi Sheep in Bedouin Flocks: Evaluation of Methodology Using Initial Results

J.M. King, S.R. McArthur, D.J. Pike and A.J. Woods

Introduction

In 1985 the United Kingdom Overseas Development Administration, the Jordan/Australia Dry Land Farming Project, and the Amman District Sheep Co-operative set up a Sheep Husbandry and Health Programme with the Jordan Co-operative Organization. Although conceived as an advisory and extension project, none of the expatriate advisers had previous experience of Awassi sheep production. Review papers (Epstein 1982; Thomson and Bahhady 1983; Goddard 1984) provided useful information but were no substitute for first hand experience. Therefore, 1 year was spent studying the performance and management of the sheep by the local Bedouin farmers, and 2 years collecting data on lambing intervals.

This paper describes the research strategy and methods devised to obtain information on the constraints to sheep production. Some preliminary results are also presented and used to evaluate the methodology. The constraints identified and their effect on production will be published later together with recommendations for improvements in flock management.

Research strategy

The rationale behind the research strategy is outlined below. It was influenced by the long history of the fat-tailed Awassi sheep in the region and the nature of the Bedouin flock management system.

Because the Awassi has probably been bred in the area for at least 5000 years (Epstein 1982), it was assumed that the breed was well adapted to the environment and had become tolerant to many endemic diseases and parasites. Consequently the detection of normally pathogenic organisms (or antibodies against them) would not mean that the organisms were causing the disease unless symptoms were present in the flock. Therefore, a conventional veterinary survey, including the collection of sera, faeces, and nasal swabs, seemed inappropriate. Furthermore, screening of samples was impossible without recourse to overseas laboratories, due to a lack of diagnostic facilities at the Animal Health Institute (AHI).

Husbandry practices along with sheep diseases were included in the study since mis-management and/or malnutrition can be the underlying causes of disease and mortality. Where these practices included routine vaccinations as government policy, for example against sheep pox and more recently brucellosis, the method of implementing the vaccination campaign was studied rather than the incidence of the disease.

Awassi sheep appeared to thrive on neglect. Hence, there seemed little justification to consider exotic breeds until the local husbandry practices, the potential of the breed, and its response to improved husbandry had been quantified and the general standard of flock management in the country had been raised.

Many Bedouin farmers appeared to be more concerned with minimising risk than maximising profit. They needed help to maintain a precarious livelihood by making more efficient use of scarce and sometimes expensive food and water resources, as well as veterinary and other forms of assistance. It was also recognised that increasing the efficiency of production does not always mean producing higher outputs from higher inputs, and that management advice must be simple to be accepted and based on information obtained from the flock with the minimum of disturbance.

The importance of a potentially pathogenic organism or a bad management practice can be judged by its effect on flock production. Therefore, the parameters of production and their determinants should be measured with sufficient precision to detect differences between flocks under different management.

The decision on whether to collect data in quantity, as in a survey, or to go for quality, as in a case study, was influenced by the resources available and the objectives of the study. The resources available were insufficient to mount a major systems study of the type reported by Wilson et al. (1983), which is difficult to justify in terms of costs and benefits. If a large number of flocks were surveyed, one could assume that the sample was representative of the local sheep population, but this would necessitate collecting much of the information by interview rather than direct measurement. Since the data obtained from questionnaires are often unreliable, it was decided that they should only be used when there was no alternative, for example for information on gross margin analysis. The aim of the study was to produce management plans, which were more likely to be practical if they were based on first hand experience of flock management and farming methods. Therefore, the case study approach using direct measurement was chosen. It had the disadvantage that data collection was time consuming; so the sample size was small and not necessarily representative of the majority of Co-operative members' flocks.

Materials and methods

The team and equipment. The field team consisted of a veterinarian, a livestock specialist, two or more assistants, the flock owner, and/or shepherd and his family. It was equipped with an electronic sheep scales [1] (accurate to 0.1 kg) and trailable sheep yards [2]. The yard panels could enclose 500 sheep comfortably, leaving sufficient spare hurdles to make a 7 m race leading to the weigh scales. Standard equipment for tagging, clinical examination, sample collection, and simple treatments was carried, as well as medicines stored in a refrigerator fitted in a Landrover.

Visiting routine. Data were collected on 1 day per week, following a visit to the flock a few days beforehand to alert the farmer. Further time each week was spent preparing for the visit and processing field records afterwards. It was only possible to examine one flock per day, and 5 weeks were taken as a reasonable interval between visits to each flock. Therefore only five flocks could be taken on as case studies.

Selection of flocks. The flock owners were selected from the members of the Amman District Sheep Co-operative by the Co-operative Manager, primarily because they agreed to take part in the study. But they were considered representative of the membership. For example, mean flock size of the sample was 319 (± 135.3 (SD)) compared with 342 (± 246) for the 220 members. The higher figures for the total membership were due to the skewed distribution, with many small flocks and a few large ones (Fig. 1). Most farmers herded a few goats with the sheep, the mean being 25 (± 53). Goats were not studied in detail but were included in flock management practices such as the control of ectoparasites and vaccination against brucella.

Although the sample size was small, the farmers came from different backgrounds and had different approaches to flock management (Table 1).

Selection of subsample. Because it would have taken too long to examine every sheep in each sample flock, a subsample was selected using standard procedures (Cochran and Cox 1957; Cochran 1963). The subsample size varied from 47 ewes for the flock of 172, to 56 for the flock of 493. To obtain sufficient lambs in the subsample, the ewe subsample was increased to between 78 and 96, assuming a weaning percentage of 65 and subsequent losses of 10% (Goddard 1984).

Ewes were selected by enclosing the flock in the portable yards and catching at random. Young ewes were more elusive and this could have biased the age of the subsample. After capture, the ewes were eartagged and mouthed to obtain the dentition age and the proportion of bad mouths in the flock. The ageing technique was tested in one flock by re-mouthing the subsample a year later, and when it was found to be reasonably precise, the age structure of the

---

[1] E.H. Rudd & Co., 270 Falconer Street, Guyra, NSW 2365, Australia.
[2] Boral Cyclone Ltd., 589 Torrens Road, Woodville, SA 5011, Australia.

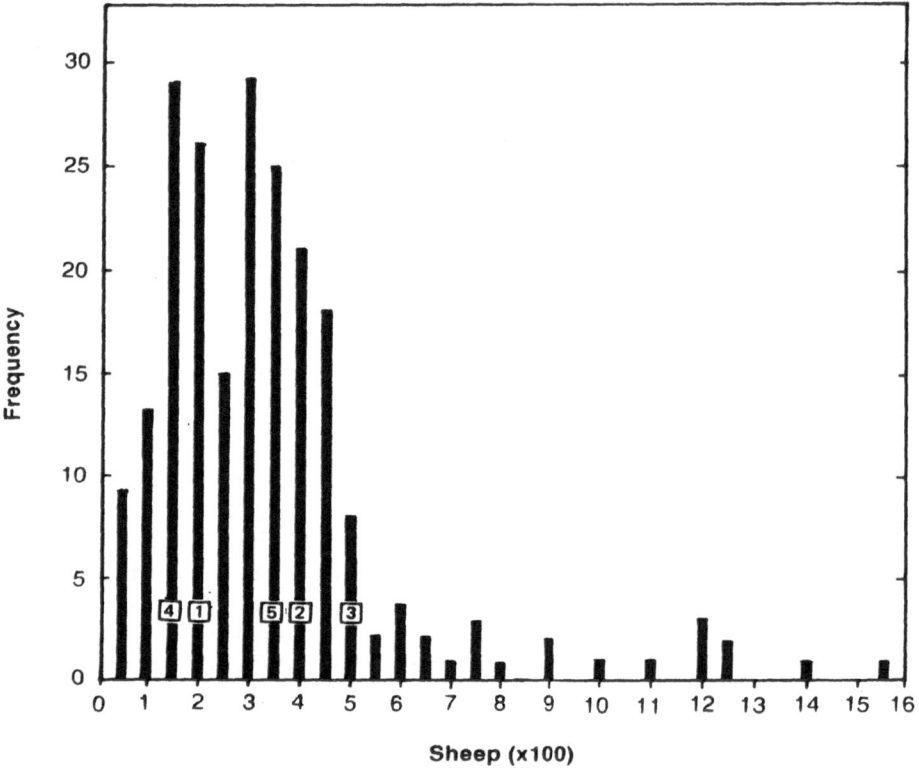

Fig. 1. Frequency distribution of flock size of case-study farmers (5) compared with other co-operative farmers.

subsample was compared with that of the whole flock. Lambs were eartagged at the first visit after birth, on condition that they were removed prior to their sale for Muslim festivals.

Table 1. Characteristics of the five case-study farms.

Farm no.	1	2	3	4	5
Adult sheep	195	393	493	172	340
Adult goats	10	15	20	5	15
Owner's wealth	+	+ + + +	+ + +	+	+ +
Owner's education	+	+ + +	+ + + +	+	+ +
Owner manager	yes	no	yes	yes	yes
Semi-nomadic	yes	yes	no	yes	yes
Lambs sold as weaners	yes	yes	no	yes	yes
Lambs sold after feedlot	no	no	yes	no	no
Lamb selling age (days)	99	83	138	87	77
Supplementary feed	+ + +	+ +	+ + +	+ +	+
Vaccines, antibiotics	no	no	yes	no	no

Recording of production and health data. At each visit, the subsample of ewes and lambs was put through the race, weighed, and condition scored. The standard body condition scoring system was used (MLC 1983) rather than the one which has since been devised specifically for fat-tailed Awassi sheep (Hossamo et al. 1986).

Sick animals, which were brought to our attention as well as those in the subsample, were clinically examined, sampled for suspected diseases, and given appropriate treatment. Samples for laboratory examination were taken to the AHI but, as already indicated, the Institute had very limited diagnostic capability, being unable to do virology, bacteriology, or histology. The AHI tested serum for brucella, using Rose Bengal and serum agglutination tests, examined blood smears for parasites, and identified but would not count parasite eggs and larvae in faeces. Little information was obtained from post mortems, because our visits rarely coincided with a recent death or abortion, and farmers could not be persuaded to take fresh carcasses or viscera to the AHI.

The daily milk yield of eartagged ewes was obtained on three or four occassions after weaning, using a 10 kg Salter spring balance with 10 g calibrations. The ewes were tied head to head to form a herringbone formation and the hand-milkers moved rapidly along each side, rarely returning to milk a ewe a second time. The total flock output was also recorded on these occassions.

Questionnaires were completed at each visit to provide information for flock gross margin analysis (Croston and Pollott 1985), and the construction of flock and bio-economic models and production and health programmes.

Data analysis. Initially the data were sent to the Veterinary Epidemiology and Economics Research Unit at Reading University, and entered onto a micro-computer using a programme designed specifically to collate livestock production and health data. Later the files were transferred to the University's mainframe computer and subsequent field data were entered directly onto it. Data manipulation and analysis were carried out using the SAS package.

Results

The sample was reduced from five to four after 6 months when one farmer cut out all the eartags in his flock, following an outbreak of brucellosis which he attributed to the study.

Dentition-age. A comparison of measurements of the dentition-age of the same ewes, 1 year apart, confirmed that the method could be used as a relative ageing technique, with only 3 wild points out of 63. The anomalies related to ewes with full mouths, at which stage the ageing technique became more difficult. The plot of the remaining 60 ewes is shown in Fig. 2, for which a

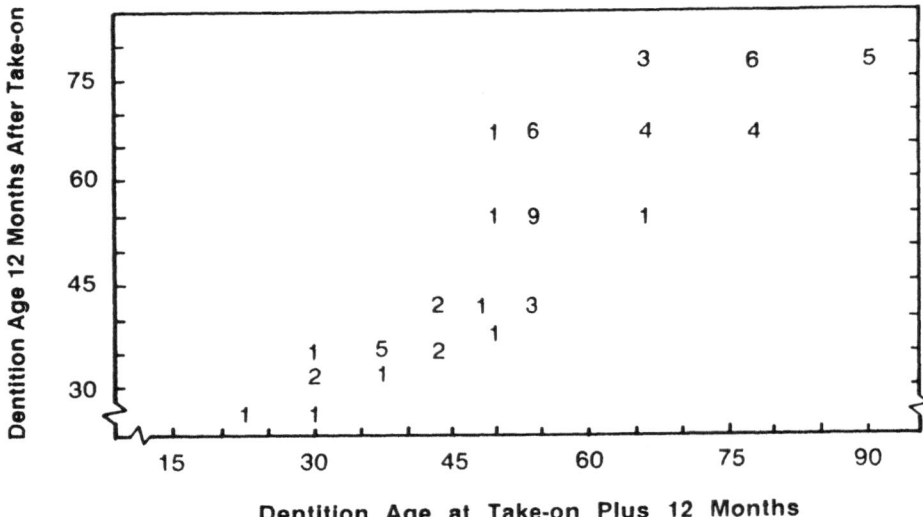

Fig. 2. Dentition-age (months) of a ewe flock sample measured 12 months after take-on, compared with the age calculated by adding 12 months to the dentition-age measured at take-on. The numbers indicate how many points coincide.

regression was obtained with an R^2 value of 0.79. The mean age of the ewe sample in November 1986 was 57 months (± 16.8) compared with 58 months (± 17.4) when 12 months were added to the dentition-age obtained a year earlier.

The frequency distribution of the dentition-age of the ewes sampled was similar to that for the whole flock, indicating that the sampling technique had not given a biased sample even though older ewes were easier to catch.

Nutritional aspects. Nutritional differences between flocks could not be quantified because grazing was sparse and scattered and farmers gave only rough estimates of the amount of supplementary feed they were providing. Therefore, flock nutrition had to be inferred from ewe weight and/or condition score. There were significant differences in the mean post-partum weights between farms (Table 2), but the range (from 30 to 72 kg) exceeded that which

Table 2. Comparison of ewe post-partum weights by farm.

Farm	No.	Mean (kg)	Standard error	Minimum value	Maximum value
1	103	55	0.72	40	72
2	91	52	0.72	30	69
3	113	53	0.56	35	71
4	85	52	0.77	38	68
5	86	47	0.63	35	61

Table 3. Comparison of ewe post-partum condition scores by farm.

Farm	No.	Mean	Standard error	Minimum value	Maximum value
1	95	2.8	0.05	1.5	3.5
2	96	3.2	0.05	1.0	4.0
3	139	2.5	0.05	1.0	3.5
4	88	2.4	0.07	1.0	3.5
5	108	2.1	0.06	0.5	3.0

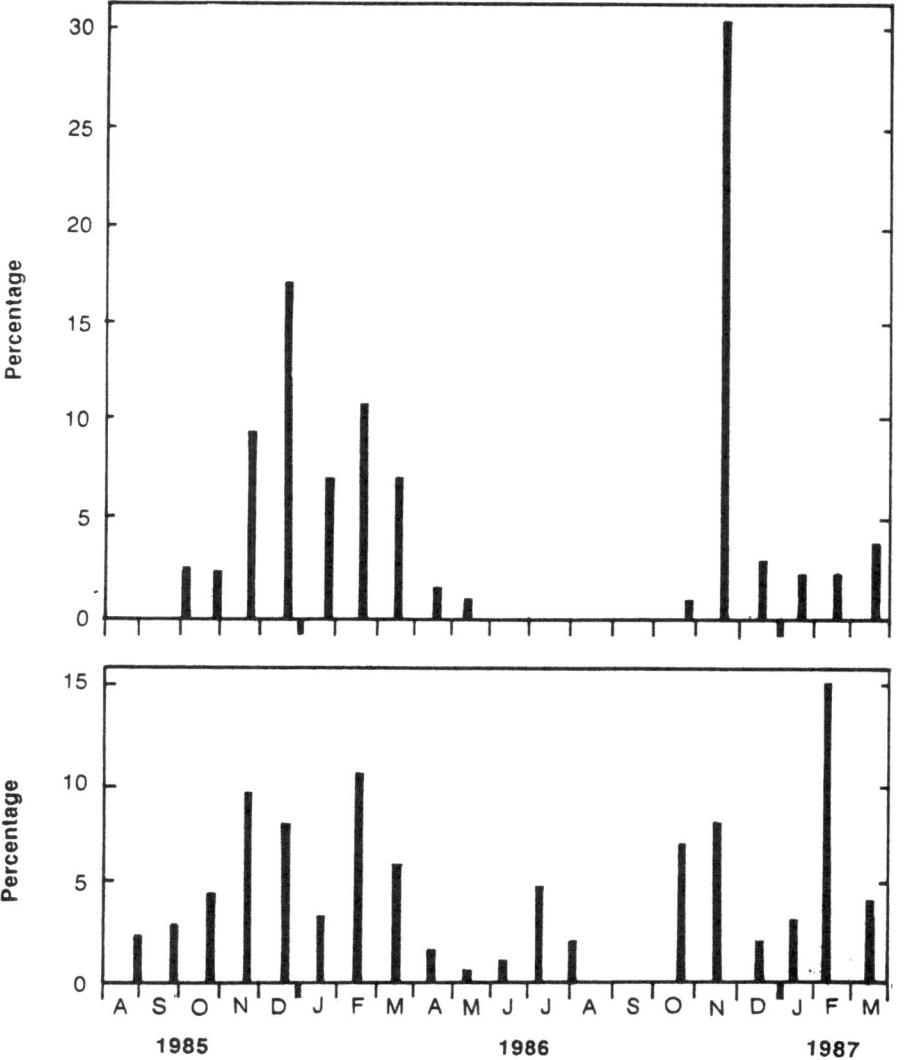

Fig. 3. Percentage bar chart of lambing distribution in two different flocks, with rams all year.

could be attributed to nutritional status corrected for age. Much of the variation in weight was ascribed to differences in structural size, which explained the poor relationship between post-partum weight (W) and condition score (S). The overall equation was:

$$W = 37.94 + 6.50S \ (R^2 = 0.36).$$

Regressions for the individual farms were very similar.

There were significant differences in mean condition score post-partum between all flocks except Farms 3 and 4, which reflected nutritional status (Table 3).

Lambing. There were marked differences between farms in lambing distribution (Fig. 3), lambing percentages (87–126%), and the proportion of barren ewes (4–13%).

Lamb growth. Scatter plots of weight of lamb against age were constructed for each farm, by sex and for single or multiple births. For single births by sex, the regressions gave R^2 values ranging from 0.84 to 0.90 indicating well defined linear relationships for all farms. In addition, those farms which had accurate lambing records could be distinguished from those which had not (Fig. 4).

Lambs were weaned or sold in batches, so the dates when this occurred were easy for the farmer to recall. The accuracy of the weaning and selling ages was affected by the birth records. Weaning ages of males varied from 74 (± 25.6) to 99 (± 19.1) days between farms.

Milk yields. Separate plots of yield against day of lactation were made for each flock and contained three or four records from each ewe (Fig. 5). The regressions never accounted for more than 35% of the total variation in any flock.

Mortality, culling, and bad mouths. Neonatal mortality was negligible except on one farm where it reached 9% and was associated with an outbreak of brucellosis.

Lamb mortality up to selling age varied from 3 to 20% between flocks, the higher figure being associated with an outbreak of pneumonia. Mortality rates approaching 10% due to lamb diarrhoea, occurred on two farms, and would have been higher if antibiotics had not been given.

Adult mortality was much more difficult to define. Out of 65 ewes which went missing, presumed dead, only 27 cases were considered definite and 8 given a cause of death. Consequently it was difficult to make much out of the variation in mortality between farms of 11–24%. A further 6–14% of ewes were culled, or assumed culled.

There were marked differences between flocks in the proportion of bad mouths (5–27%); the largest proportion occurring in a relatively young flock with a median age of approximately 3 years.

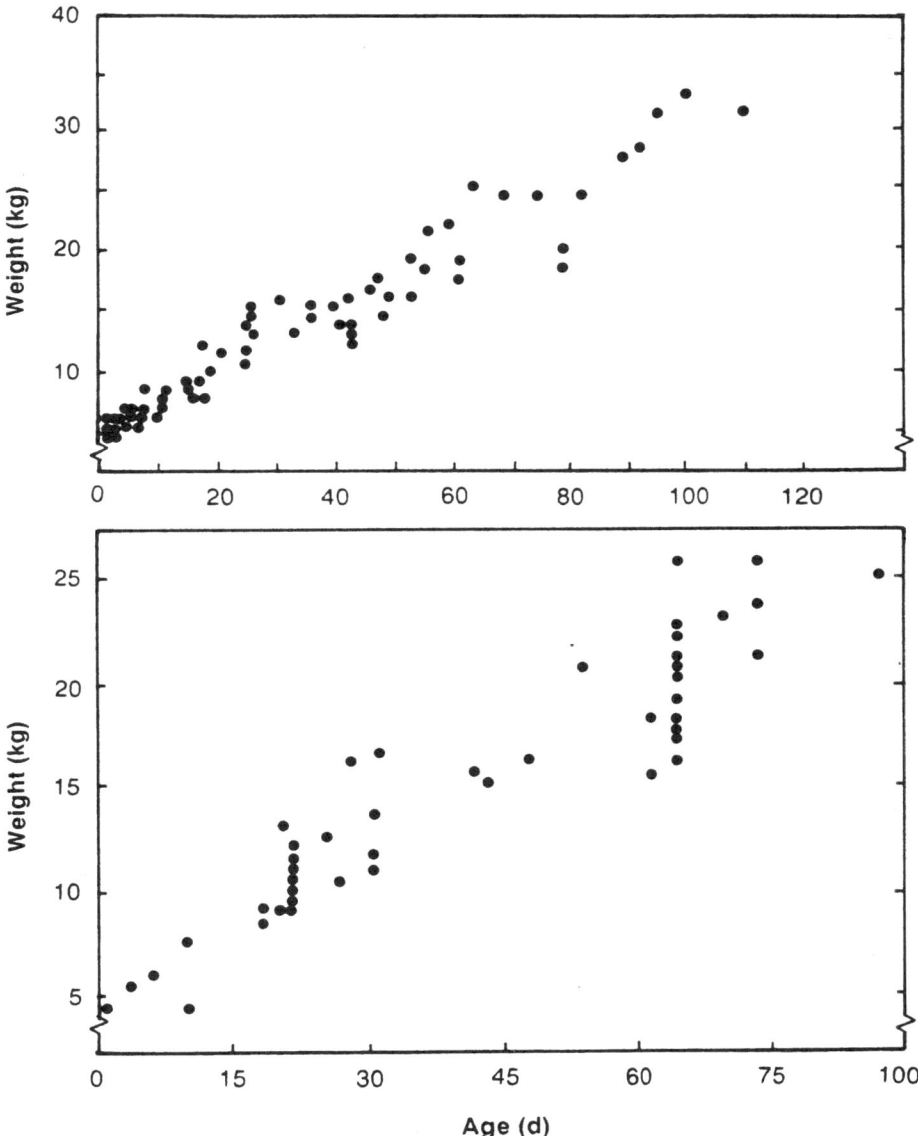

Fig. 4. Plots of weight of single male lambs against age from a farm with accurate lambing records (top) and one without.

Mastitis. The percentage of mastitis varied from 4 to 13 between farms. Gangrenous mastitis was associated with loss of half the udder, but many ewes survived.

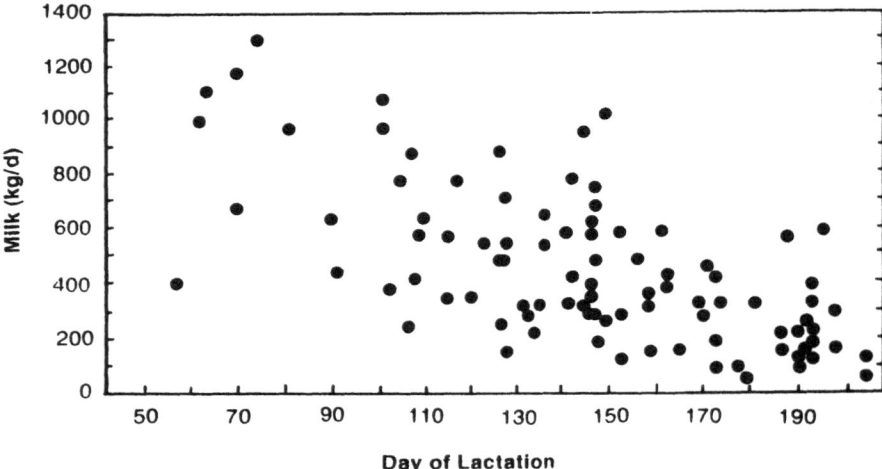

Fig. 5. Plots of daily milk yield against day of lactation for all ewes in a flock sample with good lambing records.

Other clinical diseases. The diseases were grouped into six categories: alimentary, ectoparasites, eye, miscellaneous disorders, and reproductive and respiratory conditions. Of these only three categories had an incidence over the year which exceeded 2% of the ewes examined. They were brucella abortion, ectoparasites (lice) which increased in some flocks during the winter to cause clinical signs in 7% of the ewes, and a chronic respiratory condition characterised by nasal catarrh and occasional pneumonias. The respiratory condition affected 2–40% of the flock at different seasons and may have been related to lungworms (*Muellarius* sp.), and nasal bot (*Oestrus ovis*) larvae which were sometimes found.

Discussion

Frequency of visits. One visit every 5 weeks was not enough to maintain satisfactory records on lamb births, ewe deaths, and milk yields. Monthly visits would have been preferable, but at the rate of one flock per week would have reduced the number of flocks, which was already too low. Therefore, a study of this nature needs visits to two farms each week which would give a sample of eight flocks. The sample would still be too small to be representative of the rest of the Co-operative flocks. However, the results could be compared with those from more general disease surveys such as the Jordan German Veterinary Epidemiology and Ectoparasite Project.

Sample size. The maximum number of ewes that could be examined in detail on one visit was 80–90, which was insufficient to detect many cases of alimentary, eye, and reproductive disease. Such disorders, along with rarer diseases grouped under 'miscellaneous conditions', had a frequency of about 1%, which would not justify prophylactic measures on a flock basis. These cases can be treated individually because of the close shepherding system that is practiced by the Bedouin.

Data collection and analysis. The PANACEA package was efficient at data entry but slow at manipulating data files of any size (e.g., 50000 entries), when the mainframe computer programme was preferred. The files provided a good record of the field work, but were not always in the best form for analysis. It would have been worth spending more time at the outset to consider how the spectrum of diseases should be entered to save problems in the later stages of the data handling.

Nutrition and condition scoring. It was hoped to relate differences in nutrition to flock performance, but it proved impossible to quantify nutrition even when the nomadic flocks were being fed entirely on bought food. The nutritional status was therefore inferred from the condition of the ewe; weight was not considered a reliable indicator because of the big variation in structural size.

The technique of scoring is subjective but reasonably precise, and the operator can improve his accuracy by comparing measurements with visiting sheep specialists, provided both are using the same system. Fortunately, the system recommended by Hossamo et al. (1986) for fat-tailed Awassi is identical to the one described in the MLC (1983) booklet for scoring the lumbar region, as long as the score is less than 4.0.

Lambing dates and lamb growth. Lambing dates and lamb growth proved particularly rewarding production parameters to measure. The visiting scientist should not guess the age of lambs which appear to be more than 1 week old. On the other hand, the inaccurate estimates of the farmer can distort the regression even more.

Milk recording and yields. The milk recording was based on the assumption that milk secretion rate is reasonably constant during the day (Corbett 1968), and that the lactation curve of ewes of the same status (e.g., single bearing ewes in at least their second lactation) would be similar within a flock. These assumptions appeared to be true for milk production prior to weaning, when the growth rates of suckling lambs of the same sex and class could be plotted on a single growth curve for each flock. On the other hand, it may not have been the milk production which was similar, but the growth potential of the lambs given an adequate supply of milk. An additional complication after weaning is that the milk that was available to the lamb is not necessarily available to the milker. Additional factors which influence milk yield include udder conformation, teat location, and the variable proportion of total production that can be obtained at the primary and secondary milkings and the residue which is retained when there is no suckling stimulus (Epstein 1985). These factors, as well as variations in weaning age, result in big differences in the amount of milk that can be taken from each ewe at a single milking. Consequently, it was not possible to detect differences between the post-weaning mean lactation curves of each flock.

Diseases. Information on clinical disease was relatively simple to collect, but obtaining a definitive diagnosis was not. There has always been a need for simple diagnostic kits for use in developing countries and maybe biotechnological research will develop such kits (Caine 1987). Identifying the cause of death is difficult in a study of this sort. For example, Carles (1986) found that the cause of death was unknown in 76% of the deaths in sheep and goats in northern Kenya, and in doubt in a further 13%.

Three disease conditions emerge requiring further attention, but in different ways. The first is caused by *Brucella melitensis* which appears to be an exception to the 'rule' that the Awassi is tolerant of endemic disease; it is more susceptible to brucellosis than, for example, the Maltese sheep (Jones 1981). The explanation could be that the disease has been recently introduced into West Asia, which seems unlikely, but Alton (1987) suggested that it has become more frequent. Alternatively, it may have been endemic for centuries, and differences in susceptibility between individual breeds of sheep may have had little effect on flock productivity in a harsh environment when rams run with the flock throughout the year. In such systems the ewe lambs conceive at the minimum size, and neither they nor their small offspring can be expected to survive a wet, cold winter or lack of grazing in the spring following a dry winter. Aborting the first pregnancy, thereby increasing the yearling ewe's chances of survival, followed by life-long immunity, may be an acceptable way for the Awassi to come to terms with endemic brucellosis. The origin of the disease in Jordan is of secondary importance; it is sufficiently widespread in the small stock population for a national vaccination programme to have been started. It is vital that this programme should succeed because the public now recognises that brucellosis is contracted from sheep and goat dairy produce and there is increasing consumer resistance to these products. There were 450 confirmed cases in Amman district in July 1987 (S.F. al Hussein, personal communication). Therefore the Sheep Husbandry and Health Programme has progressed from studying the occurrence of brucellosis in sheep, to vaccinating Co-operative flocks and observing the effect. This approach will also reduce the risk of brucellosis to members of the team, which is unacceptably high; during the past 18 months two out of the three livestock specialists have contracted the disease.

The second disease complex relates to ectoparasites, a problem at the flock rather than the national level because it has limited public health implications.

Here, research can be directed towards simple and effective ways of applying the best combination of insecticides, and when to apply them.

The third disease condition is a respiratory disease complex characterised by 'snuffles' and occasional pneumonia. It could be the same as that described at ICARDA by Orita et al. (1986), which is caused by protostrongylid nodules in the lungs. The build-up of lesions causes increasing damage to the lungs which predisposes older sheep to pneumonia and death. As the above authors have indicated, the disease could be very difficult to control because the adult worms inhabit fibrous nodules which are relatively impervious to anthelmintics, and the larvae use a snail as secondary host which is active in the autumn and spring. This disease appears to be more refractory to diagnosis and treatment than the others and requires a more detailed epidemiological study (Putt et al. 1986; Thrushfield 1986).

Acknowledgements

We thank Mr Samih Momani of the Amman District Sheep Co-operative for his help in finding and liaising with the case-study farmers, to whom we are also indebted. We were also helped by our relatives and friends, and colleagues in the Jordan Co-operative Organization, Australian Dry Land Farming Project, and European Economic Community Project. We are also grateful to Mr. George Mbadi who entered most of the field data onto the computer, and to Mrs. C.A. King who did much of the field recording, typing, and prepared the illustrations.

References

Alton, G.G. 1987. Control of *Brucella melitensis* infection in sheep and goats–a review. Tropical Animal Health and Production 19: 65–74.

Caine, A. 1987. Rapid progress in diagnostic kits. Veterinary Practice 19 (20): 11–12.

Carles, A.B. 1986. The levels of, and constraints to, productivity of goats and sheep at Ngurunit in Marsabit District. Pages 33–117 in Smallstock and Cattle Productivity, Nutrition and Disease in Northern Kenya. UNESCO/IPAL Technical Report E-8. Nairobi, Kenya.

Cochran, W.G. 1963. Sampling Techniques. John Wiley and Sons, New York, USA.

Cochran, W.G. and Cox, G.M. 1957. Experimental Designs. John Wiley and Sons, New York, USA.

Corbett, J.L. 1968. Variation in the yield and composition of milk of grazing Merino ewes. Australian Journal of Agricultural Research 19: 283–294.

Croston, D. and Pollott, G. 1985. Planned Sheep Production. Collins, London, UK. 211 p.

Epstein, H. 1982. Awassi sheep. World Animal Review (FAO) 44: 9–18.

Epstein, H. 1985. The Awassi Sheep with Special Reference to the Improved Dairy Type. FAO Animal Production and Health Paper No. 57. FAO, Rome, Italy. 282 p.

Goddard, I.G.H. 1984. Performance of Awassi sheep in Jordan. Jordan Co-operative Organization, Amman. 17 p.

Hossamo, H.E., Owen, J.B. and Farid, M.F.A. 1986. Body condition score and production in fat-tailed Awassi sheep under range conditions. Research and Development in Agriculture 3 (2): 99–104.

Jones, L.M. 1981. Brucellosis. Pages 477–480 in Goat Production (Gall, C., ed.). Academic Press, London, UK.

MLC (Meat and Livestock Commission). 1983. Feeding the Ewe. MLC, Bletchley, UK.

Orita, G., Thomson, E.F. and Osman, A.E. 1986. Helminth parasites in sheep. Pages 45–46 in Pasture, Forage and Livestock Program. Annual Report 1985. ICARDA, Aleppo, Syria.

Putt, S.N.H., Shaw, A.P.N., Woods, A.J., Tyler, L. and James, A.D. 1986. Veterinary Epidemiology and Economics in Africa: A Manual of Epidemiological and Economic Techniques for Use in the Design and Appraisal of Livestock Health Policy. VEERU, University of Reading, UK. 178 p.

Thomson, E.F. and Bahhady, F. 1983. Aspects of Sheep Husbandry Systems in Aleppo Province of Northwest Syria. Farming Systems Programme Research Report. ICARDA, Aleppo, Syria.

Thrushfield, M. 1986. Veterinary Epidemiology. Butterworths, London, UK. 280 p.

Wilson, R.T., de Leeuw, P.N. and de Haan, C. (eds). 1983. Recherches sur les Systemes des Zones Arides du Mali: Resultats Preliminaires. Rapport de Recherche 5. ILCA, Addis Ababa, Ethiopia.

E.F. Thomson and F.S. Thomson (eds), Increasing Small Ruminant Productivity in Semi-arid Areas
© 1988 ICARDA . ISBN 978-94-010-7086-7

Emerging Bacterial Diseases that can Affect Small Ruminant Production

A.J. Wilsmore and E.T. EL-Masannat

Introduction

In the low rainfall areas in North Africa and West Asia small ruminants are extensively managed, often by pastoralists. Thus, potentially pathogenic organisms excreted by livestock cannot contaminate the environment to the extent that they would under intensive management. In addition, the lethal effects of sunlight and desiccation on these pathogens decrease their chances of survival. Therefore, with the exception of some classical diseases, such as contagious caprine pleuropneumonia (CCPP) and Malta fever, bacterial diseases have not been a major problem of sheep and goats in dry areas; deficiencies in protein, energy, and macro and micro elements have been more important.

However, certain practices encourage the multiplication of bacteria in the host and result in contamination of the environment. One example is the confinement of small ruminants in a small house or paddock at night to safeguard against loss, theft, or attack by predators. Where necessary, steps can be taken to control disease by providing maximum ventilation and good hygiene. The latter is particularly important during lambing and kidding when the agents of abortion in ewes and does and disease in the neonate are frequently transmitted. Other bacterial diseases can emerge with the development of semi-intensive or intensive systems.

Clostridial diseases

Clostridia are gut commensals and are only locally invasive. When allowed to multiply unchecked, they produce a toxin which causes acute enteritis, for example enterotoxaemias caused by *Clostridium perfringens*, or nervous signs, as in the case of *Cl. tetani*. In some instances, enteritis and nervous signs may occur in the same animal, as in pulpy kidney disease.

Clostridia form resistant spores which can survive well in soil. Those of *Cl. perfringens* types B, C, and D are also found in the faeces of normal animals and can multiply very rapidly in the presence of high levels of carbohydrate. Thus, lamb dysentery is most prevalent in lambs and kids ingesting large quantities of milk from heavily lactating dams, as occurs when nutrition and management are improved. A similar situation exists in pulpy kidney disease.

When small ruminants are suddenly changed from a low to a high plane of nutrition, partially digested food containing carbohydrate reaches the small intestine. This stimulates rapid multiplication of *Cl. perfringens* type D and the accumulation of toxin in the gut which leads to pulpy kidney disease.

The spores of *Cl. tetani, Cl. oedematiens*, and *Cl. chauvoei* are common on intensively stocked and well-manured, cultivated land. In these situations, they are more likely to contaminate cuts and wounds and cause diseases such as tetanus and blackquarter. Therefore, as management and production improve, vaccination against clostridial diseases may be required in areas where the need was not previously apparent.

Neonatal diseases

Sheep and goat mortality is normally highest in the perinatal period and can be divided into three categories; that occurring prior to parturition which is usually associated with infectious causes of abortion, that occurring during parturition and associated with dystokia, and that occurring during the first 2 weeks of life. Major causes of loss in the last category are exposure, mismothering, starvation, and neonatal infectious disease.

As management improves, losses caused by exposure, mismothering, and starvation tend to decrease and the number of lambs or kids produced per breeding female increases. Unfortunately, the intensive indoor lambing and kidding that is usually associated with improved management leads to the build-up of pathogenic bacteria and viruses in the environment. Also, unlike single lambs or kids, twins and triplets may not obtain sufficient colostrum from their dams. Colostrum-derived antibodies are important in protecting neonates against pathogenic bacteria and anything which limits their ingestion, such as competition from litter mates, will jeopardise survival. Insanitary conditions in lambing and kidding pens and buildings may present the newborn animal with such an overwhelming challenge of pathogenic bacteria that it will be infected before it has acquired colostral antibodies. Alternatively, insufficient colostrum may be ingested to prevent the establishment of infection in the alimentary tract or prevent systemic invasion.

Infection of the alimentary system

In addition to *Cl. perfringens*, enterotoxigenic strains of *Escherichia coli*, previously regarded as common causes of diarrhoea in calves and pigs, have become important causes of neonatal diarrhoea in intensively reared lambs and kids. Other bacteria, such as *Salmonella* spp., may also be important. While vaccination of pregnant ewes and does against clostridia is essential to protect offspring where lamb dysentery occurs, and vaccination is possible against enterotoxigenic strains of *E. coli* and rotaviruses, it is also important to control the build-up of pathogenic bacteria in the environment. This can be done by providing lambing and kidding pens with smooth, impervious surfaces which are regularly cleaned. Also, the lambing/kidding period should be short, as this will help to prevent build-up of infection. If lambing or kidding is unavoidably prolonged, the lambing/kidding area should be periodically moved to a new site.

Neonatal polyarthritis

Other organisms which multiply in insanitary lambing and kidding sheds and paddocks can cause neonatal polyarthritis. The commonest are streptococci, *Corynebacterium pyogenes, E. coli, Erysipelothrix rhusiopathae*, and *Fusobacterium necrophorum*. They appear to enter the newborn animal through the umbilicus, which itself often becomes swollen, and then localise in one or more joints, sometimes causing abscesses to form in internal organs. *F. necrophorum*, for example, will often produce necrotic lesions in the liver which may extend through the diaphragm into the thorax.

To control these infections, a clean environment and an adequate supply of colostrum are important. In addition, applying an astringent antiseptic to the umbilicus, such as a solution of iodine in alcohol, as soon after birth as practicable, should be a routine procedure.

Johne's disease

The cause of Johne's disease is *Mycobacterium johnei*. A yellow-pigmented form of the organism is often isolated from sheep although unpigmented strains can also be isolated from small ruminants.

The predominant clinical sign of Johne's disease is loss of body condition caused by reduced absorption of nutrients from the small intestine. In small ruminants, diarrhoea is not a feature of the disease, probably due to the ability to reabsorb water in the large intestine, and the gross thickening of the mucosa of the small intestine is not as apparent as it is in cattle. However, the bright yellow colour of the intestinal mucosa in sheep infected with pigmented strains aids diagnosis.

Infection is spread by faeces and is usually acquired by the newborn animal sucking from a teat contaminated with faeces. Infected sheep may become subclinical carriers and excrete the organism or they may show typical wasting when they are adult.

There is no treatment for clinical cases and they should be culled. Vaccination with killed *M. johnei* in an oil adjuvant prevents the development of the disease but does not eliminate infection.

Johne's disease appears to flourish in hot and arid environments, probably because of the tough nature of the organism and because there is intimate contact between dam and neonate when transmission usually occurs. For example, in a study of mortality in goats conducted in southern India, Johne's disease was the most important cause of loss (Rajan et al. 1976).

Mycoplasma infections

Mycoplasmata are fragile organisms which are highly susceptible to desiccation and can therefore be considered of minor significance in hot, dry environments, although infections by *Mycoplasma* spp. are of great importance in southern Europe, West Asia, and Africa. The practice of keeping stock in small houses and pens at night no doubt facilitates transmission and flies and other arthropods have also been implicated in mechanical transmission.

Classically, the diseases of small ruminants caused by *Mycoplasma* spp. are contagious agalactia and contagious caprine pleuropneumonia (CCPP). The former is caused by *M. agalactiae* which causes fever, mastitis, and agalactia. The syndrome may also include arthritis, keratoconjunctivitis, vulvo-vaginitis, pleurisy, and pneumonia. CCPP is a peracute, acute, or chronic contagious disease of goats, sometimes resulting in devastating epizootics. It is characterised by fibrinous pneumonia, pleurisy, and profuse pleural exudate. Since the causal organism, the F38 strain mycoplasma, was identified, a vaccine has been produced and control is now feasible. Previous outbreaks could only be controlled by treating infected animals with antibiotics, of which tylosine is the most effective.

There are some other species of *Mycoplasma* that may cause syndromes similar to contagious agalactia and CCPP. *M. conjunctivae* is a common cause of keratoconjunctivitis in sheep and goats, often in conjunction with *Bramhamella ovis* and sometimes with *Chlamydia psittaci*.

Pasteurellosis

Pasteurellosis can occur as two distinct syndromes: pneumonic pasteurellosis or pasteurella septicaemia. They are usually caused by *Pasteurella haemolytica* but in some areas *P. multocida* may be involved. There are two biotypes of *P. haemolytica*. Biotype A causes pneumonia in animals of all ages and septicaemia in young animals, while biotype T causes septicaemia in older animals. Both biotypes can be divided into a number of serotypes which in vaccines are not cross-protective. Thus, vaccination is only feasible where the serotypes prevalent in the area the vaccine is to be used are known. This will vary between countries: for example, two new serotypes were first recorded in Ethiopia (Pegram et al. 1979).

Outbreaks of pasteurellosis are often associated with adverse environmental conditions, such as extremes of temperature or windy and wet weather. In

Jordan, the disease is most common in lambs housed in close confinement during winter. There is also evidence that infection with parainfluenza virus type 3 and sheep pulmonary adenomatosis predisposes animals to pneumonic pasteurellosis. Where suitable vaccines are not available, stress and overcrowding should be avoided. Treatment with antibiotics, such as tetracyclines, is effective if carried out early in the disease.

Infectious abortion

Brucellosis

The classical bacterial cause of abortion in small ruminants in southern Europe, North Africa, and West Asia is brucellosis. Sheep and goats are the reservoir of infection for *Brucella melitensis* which can spread from them to cattle and man. *Br. abortus* only infects small ruminants in close contact with infected cattle and, like most causes of infectious abortion, it causes infected animals to abort late in pregnancy. Infected animals have reduced milk production and excrete the organisms in the milk.

Consumption of infected milk and milk products is the most common means by which man is infected by this chronic, debilitating disease. According to Alton (1987), there has been a large increase in the incidence of *Br. melitensis* infection in recent years, especially in West Asia, resulting in disease outbreaks in small ruminants and serious epidemics in humans. Also, the disease is appearing in areas where it was not previously known. Alton ascribes these changes to intensified sheep and goat production, increased trading and movement of small ruminants, and the movement for sale of contaminated dairy products, especially cheeses.

There are reliable serological tests for identifying brucellosis in sheep and goats, the simplest of which is the plate agglutination test using stained antigen, while the most accurate is the complement fixation test.

Except for small areas with effective natural barriers to disease spread, such as islands where test and slaughter policies can be implemented, control measures usually rely on vaccination programmes. The most suitable vaccine currently available is a modified, live vaccine containing the REV 1 strain of *Br. melitensis*. But vaccination is not enough to control infection and the hygienic measures used to control infectious abortion and perinatal loss should be employed.

Campylobacter abortion

Abortion in small ruminants caused by *Campylobacter fetus* subsp. *intestinalis*, or *C. fetus* subsp. *jejuni* has been reported in many parts of the world, including southern Europe and West Asia. Sporadic abortion storms occur, affecting animals in late pregnancy by causing placentitis. Microscopic examination of smears from the cotyledons and stomach contents of freshly aborted fetuses reveals the characteristic, small, comma-shaped bacteria. In some cases macroscopic examination of affected fetuses reveals circular, pale areas of necrosis in the liver.

The disease can be spread from flock to flock through the faeces of carriers and scavenging birds that become infected by consuming contaminated fetuses and afterbirths.

The disease is self-limiting in that after an abortion storm the flock becomes solidly immune to further infection. Vaccination is feasible but there are a number of serotypes of the organism. Those present in the region where vaccination is to be used should be identified and incorporated into a vaccine. Good hygiene at lambing and kidding will reduce the spread of the disease.

Salmonella abortion

Salmonellae have been associated with abortion in many parts of the world. While *Salmonella abortus ovis* is host-specific and only causes abortion in sheep, others, such as *S. typhimurium* and *S. dublin*, are potentially pathogenic to all species including man.

In sheep, *S. abortus ovis* only causes abortion and is spread from flock to flock by infected carriers. Sheep and goats can be infected by other salmonellae by a variety of means, for example through contaminated supplementary feeds, especially when these are inadequately sterilised animal proteins, or from adjacently housed calves or poultry. Abortion can be controlled by isolating aborting animals and treating them parenterally with suitable antibiotics.

In addition to abortion, other species of salmonella can cause pyrexia, diarrhoea, and septicaemia, sometimes leading to the death of the animals. Species such as *S. dublin* and *S. typhimurium* are more important in intensively managed flocks.

Listeriosis

Listeria monocytogenes causes abortion and encephalitis in small ruminants. It can survive in moist soil, faeces, and fodder for many months and is more important where small ruminants are intensively managed.

Q fever

The causal organism of Q fever is *Coxiella burnetii*, a rickettsia with exceptional resistance to desiccation, sunlight, and chemical agents. The rickettsiae, including *Coxiella*, are arthropod-transmitted infections. Ticks acquire the organism from the blood of an infected host and transmit the disease when they infest a new host. However, *Coxiella* is probably more commonly acquired by inhaling dust contaminated with the organism.

Q fever is a zoonosis and causes fever and sometimes endocarditis in man, although the disease may be asymptomatic. In small ruminants, infection is often inapparent although large numbers of the organism may be excreted in the fetal membranes, birth fluids, faeces, and milk at and after parturition. In intensive lambing and kidding systems this can lead to a heavily infected environment and has caused epidemics in man.

C. burnetii has been implicated as a cause of infectious abortion in small ruminants. Polydorou (1981b) described the occurrence of Q fever in Cyprus and reported that it was first diagnosed there as the cause of abortion in sheep and goats in 1971. Between December 1974 and June 1975, 78 British soldiers stationed in Cyprus were found to be infected with Q fever. This outbreak coincided with an epizootic of abortions in sheep and goats in the same area that was attributed to Q fever.

Ovine enzootic abortion (OEA)

OEA, caused by *Chlamydia psittaci* (*ovis*) has become increasingly important in Europe during the past 10 years and is the most commonly diagnosed cause of ovine abortion in the UK (Wilsmore and Dawson 1986). OEA was diagnosed in goats in Cyprus in 1959 (Polydorou 1981a) and is now emerging as a cause of perinatal loss in southern Europe and Africa, for example, in Chad (Lefevre et al. 1979) and South Africa (Schutte and Pienaar 1977). Recently, the causal organism has spread from infected sheep to pregnant women and caused abortion (Buxton 1986).

C. psittaci (*ovis*) can affect goats but has been more commonly described in sheep. Typically, it causes abortion in the last 3 weeks of pregnancy, premature birth, stillbirth, or the birth of weak, full-term lambs or kids. It does not appear to be a cause of barrenness or early embryonic death.

While an aborted or stillborn fetus usually appears macroscopically normal, the fetal membranes are purulent and thickened, affected cotyledons are necrotic, and intercotyledonary areas appear leathery. In cases of abortion, the whole of the fetal membrane may be affected while in full-term lambs and kids only part of the membranes may be affected and, when the area affected is small, the lamb or kid may appear to be normal.

In smears made from material taken from affected fetal membranes, stained by the modified Ziehl-Neelsen technique, and examined under the light microscope ($\times 1000$), many infective particles, the so-called elementary bodies, can usually be seen. An alternative method of examination is to stain with 1% methylene blue and use dark ground microscopy. This is more sensitive, but can be less specific. Using both staining methods, care must be taken to differentiate between *C. psittaci* and *Coxiella burnetii* which looks similar.

C. psittaci (*ovis*) is an intracellular bacterium with a predilection for the chorionic epithelial cells of the small ruminant fetal placenta. It has a unique growth cycle consisting of a fragile reticulate body which is capable of multiplying within the host cell but cannot survive outside it, and the elementary body, derived from a generation of reticulate bodies, which cannot multiply but is released from ruptured host cells and is infectious. The organism can be cultured in McCoy cell tissue cultures treated by irradiation or with chemicals such as cycloheximide. The chlamydiae are then centrifuged onto McCoy cell monolayers. The technique is the definitive method of diagnosis of OEA and the best method of isolating the organism. Formerly, this was done in embryonated hens' eggs, a technique still used for growing the organism for vaccine production.

Although the organism is sensitive to ultra-violet light and desiccation, it can survive in dark, damp places for many days. The products of an infected parturition are highly contagious so transmission normally occurs during lambing or kidding. The organism can also be excreted in the faeces or transmitted by the venereal route but neither are important routes of transmission. It can be inferred, therefore, that when lambing/kidding conditions are crowded, particularly indoors, transmission of the disease is more likely.

The shortest period between infection and abortion is 6 weeks, but most sheep become infected at lambing and if they are going to abort they will not do so until the following lambing season. Infection and abortion only occur in the same pregnancy when the lambing season is prolonged, allowing aborting ewes to infect sheep that are still in the first half of pregnancy. The incubation period can be much shorter in goats and therefore infection and abortion in the same pregnancy may be more common than in sheep.

Serological responses to infection with *C. psittaci* (*ovis*) can be monitored using the complement fixation test (CFT) or the enzyme linked immunosorbent assay (ELISA). In an intensive lambing environment where animals are aborting, all in-contact animals seroconvert transiently. After 4–6 weeks, detectable antibodies fall to pre-infection levels so, between lambing seasons, latently infected animals cannot be detected by serological tests. A proportion of the affected animals will eliminate the infection between pregnancies, while the remainder will develop clinical OEA at the next pregnancy and will seroconvert once more. This time, anti-chlamydia antibody levels will remain high. Although all infected animals develop a humoral response at infection, these antibodies do not provide protection.

When OEA is enzootic, mostly younger animals are affected, including sheep lambing for the first time. These animals have been infected in their own perinatal period, either at birth or from a contaminated environment. However, most cases of OEA usually occur during the second pregnancy. The lack of abortions in older animals indicates that animals that recover develop a solid immunity. Our experiments confirm this and show that sheep previously suffering from clinical OEA have good fertility and do not excrete chlamydiae at a subsequent parturition.

Control. Vaccines against OEA have been available for over 25 years. They are usually made from organisms which have been grown in embryonated hens' eggs, killed, and then suspended in an oil adjuvant. During the past 10 years, these vaccines have appeared to be less effective and it has been suggested that antigenically different strains of *C. psittaci* (*ovis*) have emerged. Our current research indicates that modern isolates are more virulent than the organism first identified by Stamp et al. (1950). However, the original isolate is still protective if sufficient antigen is incorporated in each dose of vaccine to overcome the increased virulence of the organism and the increased challenge encountered in modern intensive lambing and kidding environments. While vaccination can control the clinical signs of OEA, it does not prevent the excretion of chlamydiae at parturition.

The administration of long-acting preparations of oxytetracycline to pregnant sheep during an outbreak of OEA has been shown to be effective in reducing clinical OEA but, as with vaccination, treatment does not prevent the excretion of chlamydiae at parturition (Aitken et al. 1982).

The isolation of aborting animals, the cleansing and disinfection of lambing and kidding pens between occupants, the liberal use of clean bedding, and the removal and destruction by burial or burning of all fetal membranes and any aborted or stillborn fetuses are routine procedures that, when adopted, will considerably reduce the number of cases of OEA.

International movement of small ruminants. The common policy of importing exotic sheep and goats for cross-mating to improve production of native breeds can introduce OEA to areas where it has not previously existed. Therefore, such introductions should be made with caution and only where necessary. If possible, importation of genetic material should be confined to semen and embryos. This will help to avoid the importation of a whole range of exotic diseases of which OEA is only one.

Where exotic adult breeding stock is imported it should come from flocks which have been declared free of OEA by serological tests of a significant proportion of the whole flock. Blood samples for these tests are best obtained when the flock of origin is lambing or kidding.

Mastitis

Mastitis is an infectious disease of lactating animals, characterised in the peracute and acute forms by severe, usually unilateral, necrotising inflammation of the mammary gland with a systemic reaction and, in some cases, death. Peracute and acute forms include gangrenous mastitis whereas the chronic form, which generally follows the acute disease, may only be detected by careful examination of the udder. Mastitis also occurs in a subclinical form which is detected by bacteriological and cellular examination of the milk. Acute mastitis may cause permanent damage to udder tissue and it is an important reason for culling.

Gangrenous mastitis is said to be the most common form of the disease in milking animals, particularly in Mediterranean countries. It is not confined to young dams nor to breeds with high milk production.

The importance of mastitis

Mammary diseases are generally considered to contribute to perinatal mortality and reduce weaning weight. Mastitis appears to be the most serious mammary disease, especially in countries where animals are intensively managed for milk production and where hygiene is poor during milking.

Mastitis occurs in both range and farm flocks or herds and causes significant financial loss in terms of reduced milk production, inferior milk quality and discarded milk, suboptimal performance and increased mortality of offspring, higher veterinary and replacement costs, loss of function of affected glands, and sometimes death.

In small ruminants mastitis is caused by a wide variety of organisms. The principle aetiological agents are staphylococci (*Staphylococcus aureus* and coagulase negative staphylococci), *Pasteurella mastitidis* (*P. haemolytica*), streptococci (*Streptococcus agalactia, Str. uberis, Str. zooepidemicus*), mycoplasmata (*Mycoplasma agalactia, M. mycoides* subsp. *mycoides, M. capricolum*), and coliforms (*Escherichia coli, Klebsiella pneumoniae*).

Staph. aureus is traditionally assumed to be the only pathogen of importance in ovine mastitis, but our surveys have shown that *P. haemolytica* is the major cause of acute mastitis, especially in flocks kept for meat production.

The information currently available on the epidemiology and pathogenesis of mastitis is limited. There are also gaps in our knowledge of the properties of the causative agents, host susceptibility, and predisposing causes. Many factors related to udder health need to be elucidated.

Reliable information on the incidence of mastitis within large sheep and goat populations is not available, but the disease is widespread. The literature indicates that the various pathogens capable of causing mastitis are likely to vary between geographical areas (El-Massannat 1978).

Possible sources of infection have not been fully investigated. It may be that the main sources are the nasopharynx of the sucking neonate, milkers' hands, milking machines, and an environment contaminated by faeces and discharges from diseased lambs, kids, and their dams.

Mastitis occurs sporadically in animals kept under different systems of husbandry, varying from open mountain pasture to enclosed barns. Many outbreaks occur in sheep and goats managed extensively.

Control

General guidelines should be established for controlling mastitis, regardless of specific control measures for one causative agent. Control of only one agent is not likely to be successful in controlling mastitis because of the wide variety of aetiological agents. For example, in bovine mastitis there is a view that if one type of organism is removed from susceptible animals, it will be replaced by another.

Instead, efforts should be concentrated on determining the predisposing factors involved in the pathogenesis of mastitis and finding ways of reducing their occurrence. Perhaps the most challenging problem is determining which factors predispose animals to mastitis. Several factors have been suggested, including breed and parity of the animal, the presence of teat lesions i.e., abrasions or contagious pustular dermatitis, vigorous and indiscriminate sucking, chilling of the udder by excessive fleece removal, soiling of the udder, and arthropod vectors. Determining the role of these or other factors is necessary before rational preventive measures can be suggested.

Control is a major issue, from both an economic and a public health viewpoint as subclinical mastitis can reduce milk production and quality and a number of the causal organisms are of public health significance e.g., enterotoxin-producing staphylococci. But control in small ruminants has not attracted much attention from research workers. However, there are a few general measures for controlling this disease. Affected animals should be segregated and treated early and all injured teats or udders treated. Animals with severe mastitis should be culled to avoid contamination of the environment. Indeed, culling is often an essential part of a control programme. Pasture should be frequently changed by moving animals to a new place every night. New bedding should be provided frequently and the ground where animals are kept should be disinfected to help prevent contamination of teats. Finally, insecticides should be used to control flies.

These measures are intended to reduce the spread of infections, rather than eliminate those already existing. If infections are reduced to a low level by other means, such as culling and therapy, hygienic routines must still be practised. Other measures include ensuring offspring are well fed and watered to prevent udder damage, using intramammary preparations in slow-release bases at the end of lactation, and practising immunoprophylaxis. Vaccination has so far proved to be of limited value in controlling mastitis. Many reports from different countries give details of immunization but, despite numerous experiments and field trials on a variety of vaccines and regimens, the immunological status of the udder has not been significantly boosted. In the most successful cases, only limited protection has been demonstrated in vaccinated animals and a reduction in the severity of clinical mastitis was the most frequently reported advantage. Although there is doubt about the efficacy of vaccines against mastitis, they are commercially available in many countries.

Treatment

Mastitis is generally considered to be incurable. Treatment is not easy under range conditions because early detection is difficult and the disease develops and progresses rapidly.

It seems that treatment for mastitis is likely to be of limited use. The only advantage may be that the animal's life may be saved as in most cases the damage to the parenchyma of the mammary gland is irreversible. Research is needed to assess the effectiveness of various forms of therapy.

References

Aitken, I.D., Robinson, G.W. and Anderson, I.E. 1982. Long acting oxytetracycline in the treatment of enzootic abortion of ewes. Veterinary Record 111: 446.

Alton, G.G. 1987. Control of *Brucella mellitensis* infection in sheep and goats–a review. Tropical Animal Health and Production 19: 65–74.

Buxton, D. 1986. Potential danger to pregnant women of *Chlamydia psittaci* from sheep. Veterinary Record 118: 510–511.

El-Masannat, E.T. 1987. A study of ovine mastitis with special reference to mastitis caused by *Pasteurella haemolytica*. PhD thesis. University of London, UK.

Lefevre, P.C., Baketana, K. and Bertaudiere, L. 1979. (An outbreak of abortion due to *Chlamydia ovis* in goats in Chad.) In French. Revue d'Elevage et de Medecine Veterinaire des Pays Tropicaux 32: 33–35.

Pegram, R.G., Roeder, P.L. and Scott, J.M. 1979. Two new serotypes of *Pasteurella haemolytica*. Research in Veterinary Science 22: 130–131.

Polydorou, K. 1981a. The control of enzootic abortion of sheep and goats in Cyprus. British Veterinary Journal 137: 411–415.

Polydorou, K. 1981b. Q fever in Cyprus: a short review. British Veterinary Journal 137: 470–477.

Rajan, A., Maryamma, K.I. and Krishnan Nair, M. 1976. Mortality in goats – a study based on post mortem observations. Kerala Journal of Veterinary Science 7: 79–83.

Schutte, A.P. and Pienaar, J.G. 1977. Chlamydiosis in sheep and cattle in South Africa. Journal of the South African Veterinary Association 48: 261–265.

Stamp, J.T., McEwen, A.D., Watt, J.A.A. and Nisbet, D.I. 1950. Enzootic abortion in ewes. 1. Transmission of the disease. Veterinary Record 62: 251–254.

Wilsmore, A.J. 1981. Field observations on the epidemiology of enzootic abortion in a commercial flock. Sheep Veterinary Society Proceedings 5: 48–52.

Wilsmore, A.J., Cain, B.C., Dawson, M. and Venables, C. 1986. Skin sensitivity tests in naturally infected and vaccinated sheep. Pages 13–16 in Agriculture. Chlamydial Diseases of Ruminants (Aitken, I.D., ed.). Publications of the European Communities, Luxembourg.

Wilsmore, A.J. and Dawson, M. 1986. Chlamydial diseases of ruminants in Britain. Pages 107–111 in Agriculture. Chlamydial Diseases of Ruminants (Aitken, I.D., ed.). Publications of the European Communities, Luxembourg.

E.F. Thomson and F.S. Thomson (eds), Increasing Small Ruminant Productivity in Semi-arid Areas
© *1988 ICARDA . ISBN 978-94-010-7086-7*

The Economic Significance and Control of Small Ruminant Viruses in North Africa and West Asia

R.P. Kitching

Introduction

I would like to be able to answer the question that the title of the paper poses, particularly as it relates to the economic importance of viral diseases of small ruminants in the countries of North Africa and West Asia, but there have been no properly conducted assessments of the economic importance of healthy small ruminants. Without doubt they are important to the small farmer whose total wealth may be represented by the size of his sheep and goat flock. Diseases such as sheep and goat pox (capripox) and peste des petits ruminants (PPR) do cause major losses, but as the incidence, prevalence, and mortality rates for these diseases have not been properly investigated and the total small ruminant population is frequently unknown, economic evaluations are at best meaningless and at worst totally misleading. For a variety of reasons, cattle and their diseases have attracted much of the research effort, but recently more attention has been given to small ruminants which, in my opinion, are of far greater importance than cattle in many of the poorer communities (Fig. 1).

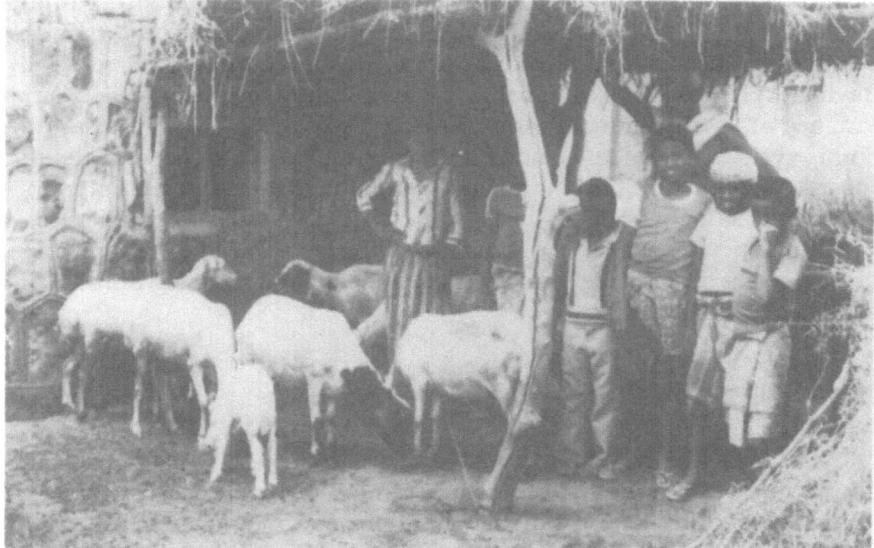

Fig. 1. Small ruminants are of considerable economic importance to village farmers.

Table 1. Major viral diseases of small ruminants in North Africa and West Asia.

Virus Family	Disease
Poxviridae	Capripox
	Contagious pustular dermatitis
Picornaviridae	Foot-and-mouth disease
Togaviridae	Border disease
Bunyaviridae	Rift Valley fever
Reoviridae	Bluetongue
Paramyxoviridae	Peste des petits ruminants
	Rinderpest
Rhabdoviridae	Rabies
Retroviridae	Maedi-visna
	Arthritis-encephalitis

Table 1 lists the major viral diseases of sheep and goats present in North Africa and West Asia. They represent a permanent threat to animals already suffering a variety of chronic parasitic diseases and nutritional deficiencies and a constraint to any attempt to upgrade indigenous stock or introduce more productive exotic animals and more intensive husbandry methods. An important criticism of much research, including my own, is that diseases are studied in isolation without considering the effect of a combination of diseases on a flock; diseases which singly may have relatively minor economic consequences, but together can be extremely serious. For example, foot-and-mouth disease is usually a mild disease in adult sheep and goats, but the damage it causes to the buccal mucosa could facilitate the spread of capripox.

Having explained why I am unable to give absolute figures on the economic importance of small ruminant viral diseases, I will briefly review what information is available. The deficiencies that will be apparent may persuade those responsible for research funding to encourage investigations which attempt to explain what actually happens in the field. Agricultural biotechnology is an extremely powerful science, but it must be directed to solving real problems, which can cost a subsistence farmer his livelihood and ultimately even his life.

Sheep and goat pox

In 1982 the Overseas Development Administration of the British government financed a project to examine the natural history of sheep and goat pox with the intention of formulating rational programmes to control the disease. At that time, the malignant pox diseases of sheep and goats were classified as sheep pox, goat pox, sheep and goat pox, and goat dermatitis, and the viruses

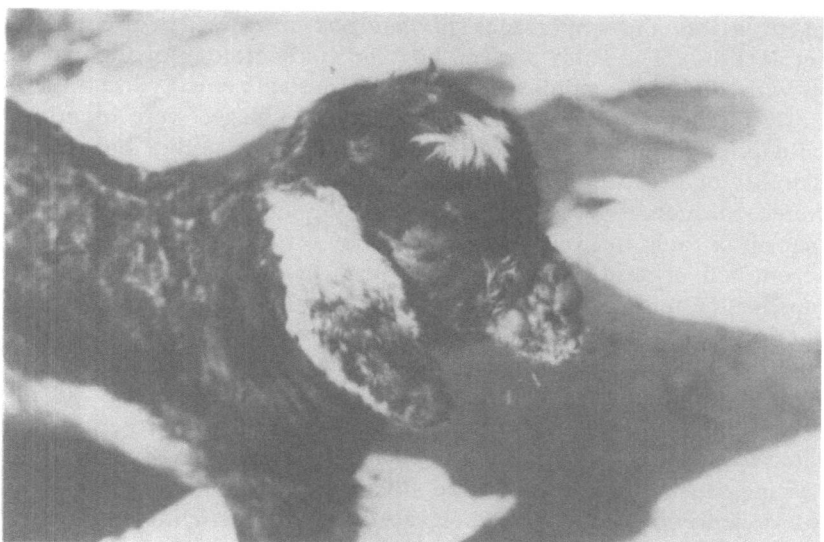

Fig. 2. Capripox in the Sultanate of Oman.

that caused them were similarly separately classified. At the Institute for Animal Disease Research at Pirbright (formerly the Animal Virus Research Institute), we collected isolates of pox virus from Sudan, Nigeria, Kenya, Yemen Arab Republic, Sultanate of Oman, Turkey, Pakistan, India, Bangladesh, and China to represent strains from the region in which the diseases are enzootic. We found that the strains were not host specific, and although many strains were more pathogenic in either sheep or goats, all the strains could infect both species. The pathology of the diseases they produced was indistinguishable, as were the serology and morphology of the viruses (Kitching and Taylor 1985; Kitching and Smale 1986). It was only possible to separate the strains by treating their DNA with restriction endonucleases and comparing the patterns produced by the separated fragments on agarose gel (Black et al. 1986). Even then it was found that all shared a genome sequence homology of greater than 95%. In addition, animals that had recovered from infection from one isolate, however mild the disease, were totally resistant to challenge with any of the other isolates, regardless of the geographical origin of the initial and challenge isolates. These findings led to the concept that all malignant pox diseases of sheep and goats are caused by strains of a single species of capripoxvirus, and the diseases they cause are now referred to as capripox (Fig. 2). A single vaccine has subsequently been developed for use in sheep and goats throughout the capripox enzootic area (Kitching, Hammond and Taylor 1987).

In association with the British veterinary team in the Yemen Arab Republic and the veterinary authorities in the Sultanate of Oman investigations were undertaken to assess the importance of capripox in these two countries (Kitching et al. 1986). The study showed how the epidemiology of the disease could vary with different population densities. In the Yemen, disease was predominantly restricted to young animals, although villages were identified from which capripox had been absent for 4 or more years, either because of poor accessibility or because of isolation due to surrounding dry areas. When disease entered, all animals were susceptible and the mortality could be high. In Oman capripox came in cycles, with periods of very low incidence. When the disease entered, it spread rapidly, aided by a good road system which allowed transport of animals incubating capripox to all parts of the country. A similar situation has recently been seen in Bangladesh where capripox has been absent for a considerable time (Kitching, McGrane et al. 1987). The disease spread slowly at first and then erupted as a major epizootic, causing high mortality. Even in India, where capripox is enzootic, a virulent strain closely related to the strain now present in Bangladesh has been spreading for the past 3 years, causing high mortality in all age groups.

Capripox is clearly of economic importance but, without reliable statistics, any estimates of financial losses would be only guesses. Sufficient information is probably available to formulate a model and extrapolate the economic consequences, but at present there is no way of testing whether the model is a true reflection of what is actually happening in the field. However, advantage could be taken of studies on human disease. For example, Carrasco and Lardinois (1987) analysed the costs and benefits of vaccination programmes for diseases of known attack rates affecting human populations at different levels of risk. When this is applied to vaccination against capripox, the benefits appear to be exceptionally favourable (Kitching and Pearson, unpublished). The problem, of course, is getting sufficient vaccine for the population at risk.

Contagious pustular dermatitis (orf)

A second important pox virus infection of small ruminants is contagious pustular dermatitis or orf. Although it is prevalent throughout the world, the low level of research funding that the disease attracts would suggest that it is of little economic importance. It is my opinion that orf is of considerable significance, if only because it affects almost 100% of all sheep and goats. Therefore, while an individual animal may suffer only a mild infection which has only a slight effect on its performance, when this effect is multiplied by the total sheep and goat population, the losses must be enormous. Some animals suffer more than just a mild disease and secondary bacterial or viral infections or fly strike can lead to death. In Sicily, where the sheep and goats are hand milked, orf lesions on the udder are widespread and animals are predisposed to secondary mastitis, which seriously reduces production (Kitching, unpublished). A similar situation probably exists in North Africa and West Asia.

Simple hygienic measures could reduce this problem, although it is difficult to change long established practices. The orf vaccine is a poorly attenuated field strain, it is difficult to apply, and its only advantage is that it allows the stockowner to decide at which time of year his animals will become infected. Once started, orf vaccination must be continued as the vaccine strain itself will become established in the flock and will infect the young lambs if the ewes do not have their own immunity boosted by vaccination prior to lambing. An additional complication is the existence of sheep and goats persistently infected with orf virus. These animals are difficult to identify and provide a persistent source of infection to susceptible young stock and humans.

Peste des petits ruminants and rinderpest

Peste des petits ruminants (PPR) is another viral disease of small ruminants causing major losses, against which there is a very efficient vaccine. The epidemiology of PPR differs from capripox in that it spreads much more quickly and requires a larger animal population to maintain itself. The disease thus tends to appear in rapidly spreading epizootics affecting all age groups and causing high mortality. In association with other diseases such as capripox, mortality can approach 100%. However, not much is known about the natural history of this disease and attempts are being made at Pirbright to characterise the strains and identify the relationship between PPR and rinderpest using modern biochemical techniques. In India where rinderpest is enzootic, it is said that small ruminants are affected by rinderpest and not PPR. They are reservoirs of the disease, which periodically spreads to the cattle population. Scott (1985) quotes Crawford (1947) as suggesting that rinderpest became a problem in small ruminants in India following the introduction of the goat-adapted strain of rinderpest vaccine. Certainly there are now strains of morbillivirus (PPR and rinderpest) in India which are pathogenic for sheep, goats, and cattle. In Africa there is serological evidence that rinderpest infects small ruminants, but that serious disease is caused only by strains of PPR.

Like capripox, PPR and rinderpest are clearly of economic importance, particularly as they relate to disease in cattle, but it would be futile to guess their financial cost. Taylor (1984) emphasized how much was still unclear about the epidemiology of PPR and that what was required was basic information about its incidence and seasonal patterns. There are many reports of epizootics with mortality rates of up to 82% in areas previously clear of disease (Appel et al. 1981), but results of serological surveys to define areas of enzootic PPR are scarce.

The vaccine routinely used in Africa and West Asia to protect sheep and goats against PPR is Plowright's attenuated rinderpest vaccine. This provides heterologous immunity against PPR for at least a year (Taylor 1979), although it is unlikely that the vaccine is as efficient in small ruminants as it is in protecting cattle against rinderpest. Work continues on the development of an attenuated PPR vaccine.

Foot-and-mouth disease

Foot-and-mouth disease (FMD) in cattle is of major economic importance, but its significance in small ruminants has received relatively little attention. In 1986, of a total 98 positive samples received by the World Reference Laboratory at Pirbright for FMD, four were from sheep or goats. This reflects the less obvious clinical signs of the disease more than the incidence of FMD in sheep and goats. Nevertheless, FMD virus can kill lambs and goat kids by destroying the cells of the developing heart muscle and can cause agalactia in lactating goats. In a day, an infected adult sheep can excrete up to $10^{5.6}$ tissue culture infective doses $(TCID_{50})$ of FMD virus in particles in its breath. Inhalation of 10 $TCID_{50}$ is sufficient to infect a sheep and 25 $TCID_{50}$ are sufficient to infect a cow (Donaldson 1986). In order to survive optimally, airborne FMD virus requires a relative humidity of at least 60%, a condition not frequently observed in arid regions except perhaps at night. However, the freedom given to sheep and goats to forage for food frequently brings them into close proximity to cattle. In the few studies undertaken, it has not been shown that small ruminants are significant vectors of FMD in Africa and Asia. Anderson et al. (1976) considered that they were not important in the dissemination of FMD in Kenya, but there is circumstantial evidence that small ruminants can maintain FMD in countries which attempt to control the disease solely by vaccinating cattle. Again, this is an area where more research is required. The role that FMD could play in predisposing infected animals to other viral infections, such as pox, by damaging the integrity of the skin and mucous membranes, should be examined.

Bluetongue

The distribution of bluetongue is defined by the distribution of its main vectors, certain tropical and subtropical species of midges of the genus *Culicoides*, in particular *C. imicola*, *C. variipennis*, and *C. brevitarsis*. They are distributed roughly between latitudes 40°N and 35°S. Within this area there is serological evidence that bluetongue virus, consisting of at least 24 serological types, circulates usually unobserved. The virus affects sheep, goats, and cattle but disease is commonly only seen in the fine wool and mutton breeds of sheep (Taylor 1986). Indigenous animals rarely show clinical signs of blue-tongue, but when exotic breeds of sheep, particularly Merinos, are introduced disease can cause severe losses. Bluetongue is most frequently seen on the borders of the enzootic area when weather conditions are favourable to the spread of the vector or when unseasonal winds carrying infected *Culicoides* beyond their normal boundaries allow virus to enter new areas. Under these conditions, explosive epizootics can occur with major losses. For example, in 1956 approximately 180000 sheep died of bluetongue disease in southern Spain and Portugal (Taylor 1986) and more recently major epizootics have occurred in Cyprus and Turkey.

In 1977 an outbreak of bluetongue caused by serotype 4 was identified in western Turkey which persisted until 1979 (Taylor et al. 1985). By examining serum samples from representative groups of animals in Turkey, Syria, and Jordan, Taylor et al. (1985) were able to develop a picture of the distribution of bluetongue virus types throughout the eastern Mediterranean basin. However, it is evident that this picture was only of a moment in time, and that the prevalent serotypes and their distribution vary considerably from year to year.

The serotypes of bluetongue virus are separated and classified using the virus neutralisation test. However, recent work at Pirbright questions the epidemiological significance of this classification (Mertens 1986). The genome of bluetongue virus consists of 10 segments of double-stranded RNA. The capsid proteins which characterise the virus antigenically are coded by segments numbered two and five, the remaining eight segments code for the core proteins and other non-structural proteins and play no part in defining the antigenic identity of the different serotypes. Mertens (1986) has shown a higher degree of sequence homology between different serotypes from geographically close areas than between isolates classified as the same serotype from geographically distant regions. For instance, serotypes 1 and 20 from Australia have a greater sequence homology with each other than with African serotypes, and conversely the African and Cypriot isolates, serotypes 1, 3, and 4, have considerable sequence homology. An American isolate of serotype 10 has sufficient sequence homology with the African serotypes to suggest that it may have originated in Africa. Such studies are extremely useful in indicating the evolution of bluetongue virus and emphasize the danger of making conclusions on serological evidence alone. An additional complication is the ability of different serotypes to produce hybrids when coinfecting single cells, so that the daughter viruses may contain segments derived from each of the parents. It is not clear whether this occurs in the field. In areas such as Sudan where animals may be infected with any or all of up to 16 serotypes, the opportunity for mixed infections is obvious, and the potential must exist for new strains to develop by this mechanism.

The need to control bluetongue is confined to those situations in which clinically susceptible sheep are exposed to virus. This is true throughout North Africa and West Asia. In most of this area, attempts to control the vector would be fruitless and vaccination is the only recourse. On the borders of the enzootic area, bluetongue may be present some years and absent in others. Even within the enzootic area bluetongue is very dynamic, with one or more serotypes being present one year and other serotypes the following year. It has been assumed that it is necessary to vaccinate against each of the prevalent serotypes, so in South Africa sheep are vaccinated annually against 15 serotypes, usually by three vaccinations each containing five serotypes. Using live vaccines, Jeggo (1986) has shown that simultaneous vaccination with three serotypes resulted in the replication of only two of the three component vaccines. However, he also showed that vaccination with one serotype, followed 1 month later by vaccination with a second serotype produced immunity not only to these two serotypes but also a heterologous immunity to a third serotype. Nevertheless, there is still a need to be able to identify the predominant serotypes in an area and it should be emphasized that vaccination with a live preparation is not without risk, particularly to pregnant animals. Further studies on immunity to bluetongue are needed, and there is considerable scope to improve vaccination protocols, particularly in areas such as Turkey that only periodically suffer outbreaks of clinical bluetongue.

Maedi-visna and arthritis-encephalitis

In the European sheep and goat herd the diseases caused by lentiviruses, maedi-visna in sheep and arthritis-encephalitis in goats, are of increasing importance. These diseases are undoubtedly present in North Africa and West Asia and the regular imports of exotic sheep and goats present a constant potential source of infection. The lentiviruses incorporate themselves as proviral DNA into the genome of the host cell. When activated, these acquired genes produce infectious viral RNA which then codes for the viral proteins and the disease process can begin. Classically, maedi is the pneumonic manifestation of the disease and visna the central nervous expression, but signs of mastitis and arthritis can also be evident. A closely related lentivirus causes arthritis and encephalitis in goats.

These diseases are referred to as slow virus infections, as the incubation period is very long and recognisable clinical signs are rarely observed before the infected animal is 3 years old. However, by this time the disease process is usually well advanced. Concurrent infection with the virus of pulmonary adenomatosis predisposes sheep to the more rapid development of maedi (Dawson 1987).

Maedi-visna is transmitted by milk from an infected ewe to her lamb or by the respiratory route amongst housed sheep. The virus is restricted to monocytes which form only a very small percentage of the total leucocyte population. Experimental evidence (Dawson 1987) suggests that it is very unlikely that the disease can be spread by contaminated syringe needles during routine flock treatment or vaccinations.

There are no reports indicating that lentiviruses are of economic importance among the small ruminant populations in Africa and West Asia. This may be due to a low prevalence, the short average life span of most of the potential victims, or that the diseases are submerged in the prevailing level of ill health amongst flocks and have not yet been recognised. Simple tests exist for identifying seropositive animals and attempts should be made to at least investigate the prevalence of lentivirus disease. There are no vaccines and the only effective control is the slaughter of all seropositive animals.

Border disease

Border disease in sheep is caused by a pestivirus closely related to, if not indistinguishable from, bovine diarrhoea virus. It is characterised by persistently infected animals which are themselves frequently poor growers but more importantly can introduce infection into previously uninfected flocks. The infertility, abortions, and birth of abnormal lambs associated with border disease may remain unrecognised in animals already suffering from low fertility due to the nutritional deficiencies and more obvious infections prevalent in the region that are characterised by abortion. There are no vaccines against border disease; the only effective control is to identify and slaughter persistently infected animals. However, identification can be extremely difficult without a laboratory capable of maintaining pestivirus-free cell lines.

Pestiviruses are notorious for contaminating tissue cultures, as they are frequently introduced with the bovine serum used in cell culture growth media. When these cells are used to produce live vaccines for ruminants, the results can be catastrophic. All live vaccines should be tested for pestivirus, but I suspect this is not always properly carried out.

Rabies

Sheep and goats, like all other mammals, are susceptible to rabies. Rabies is enzootic in most of North Africa and West Asia although strenuous attempts are being made by many countries to control it. Rabies cannot be considered of economic importance in ruminants in this region but it is of obvious public health importance. The incidence of rabies amongst sheep and goats reflects the success of campaigns to control the disease amongst its main vectors in the region, domestic and feral dogs and cats, and wolves. The need to vaccinate ruminants against rabies would be an admission that rabies control was ineffective.

Rift Valley fever

Another important zoonosis which periodically spreads into North Africa is Rift Valley fever. This is a mosquito-borne disease usually restricted to South, Central, and East Africa and which, like bluetongue, can cause epizootics in previously free areas depending on climatic conditions. Rift Valley fever causes major losses among lambs as well as focal hepatitis in older sheep. In humans it can cause dengue-like symptoms and recently it caused many human fatalities in Egypt (Meegan et al. 1979). Control is by vaccination with a live vaccine but it is not recommended in pregnant sheep. However, in non-enzootic regions it is difficult to predict the onset of a new epizootic and animals are not generally vaccinated until the disease has broken out.

Recombinant DNA and viral disease control

Recombinant DNA technology is advancing rapidly. Initially, research concentrated on the comparatively simple genomes of viruses and bacteria, and recombinant vaccines have already been developed. Genes encoding the important antigenic determinants of rabies, vesicular stomatitis, and hepatitis viruses have been inserted into the genome of vaccinia virus. These vaccines have the advantage of being live without causing the diseases which they are intended to prevent. At Pirbright we are working to produce a recombinant capripox vaccine by inserting genes from PPR virus. Such a vaccine would have the advantage that small ruminants would be protected against two important diseases following a single vaccination. The genome of capripox is sufficiently large to contain genes from more than one other virus and it is possible that ruminants could be protected against a range of other viral diseases in one vaccination.

The genome of mammals is considerably more complex, but important genes have been identified which are responsible for hormone production. In terms of disease resistance, it is apparent that animals living in areas in which certain viral diseases are enzootic have a degree of natural resistance to these diseases. At present, the only way to transfer these resistance factors to higher yielding exotic animals is by long-term interbreeding programmes. If it were possible to transfer the genes or groups of genes responsible for disease resistance to the embryo of another animal, considerable time could be saved. Already there is the technology for embryo transfer so engineered embryos could be quickly introduced.

Discussion

In describing the viral diseases of small ruminants I have, in most cases, considered control only in terms of vaccination. Such control usually acknowledges that the disease is enzootic. However, vaccination is only the first stage in reducing the level of disease, before other more stringent control measures can be applied. Import restrictions, quarantine, movement restrictions, and ultimately slaughter are all effective in maintaining a low level of disease incidence. However, throughout North Africa and West Asia, where the movement of nomadic people with their animals is common, these additional measures are difficult to enforce and cannot realistically be considered as a replacement for continued vaccination. In addition, disease surveillance is frequently inadequate and viral disease can spread rapidly in fully susceptible, non-vaccinated populations.

It is difficult to be optimistic about the present situation concerning the viral diseases in North Africa and West Asia. Basic information about their epidemiology is lacking and disease surveillance and control policies are inadequate. The vast sums of money required to establish the infrastructure that conventional thinking would suggest are necessary are unlikely to be forthcoming. An alternative, considerably cheaper approach that could bypass the traditional methods of disease control may be to concentrate on the development of a completely new concept. By identifying the genes which have been acquired over generations and which allow the indigenous animals to survive in the harsh environment of the Middle East, and placing them directly into the genome of highly productive animals, years of selective breeding could be saved. Advances in biotechnology conjure a vision of genetically engineered animals which resist disease and thereby produce more meat and milk.

Considerable advances will probably be made in the coming decades, but there will be many failures and there are many potential dangers. Nevertheless, there is the prospect that new technology can be applied on a large scale to improve the productive potential of agriculture in developing countries. Inevitably, much of the research will be carried out in Europe and North America, but with such a goal there is some justification in concentrating funding in a few centres of excellence, instead of dispersing what money is available in laudable disease control programmes which are inevitably doomed to failure. While I acknowledge that such a view might sound selfish and almost heretical, there are too many examples to support the argument. I have outlined the vast gaps in our knowledge of very fundamental aspects of important viral diseases. These gaps must be filled, not only to formulate rational control programmes but also to identify the problems which the biotechnologist is being asked to solve. Increased cooperation is needed between epidemiologists, agriculturalists, biochemists, and most important, governments and international funding organisations.

References

Anderson, E.C., Doughty, W.J. and Anderson, J. 1976. The role of sheep and goats in the epizootiology of foot-and-mouth disease in Kenya. Journal of Hygiene, Cambridge 76: 395–402.

Appel, M.J.G., Gibbs, E.P.J., Martin, S.J., Ter Meulen, V., Rima, B.K., Stephenson, J.R. and Taylor, W.P. 1981. Morbillivirus diseases of animals and man. Pages 235–297 in Comparative Diagnosis of Viral Diseases. Volume IV. (Kurstak, E. and Kurstak, C., eds).

Black, D.N., Hammond, J.M. and Kitching, R.P. 1986. Genomic relationship between capripoxviruses. Virus Research 5: 277–292.

Carrasco, J.L. and Lardinois, R. 1987. Formula for calculating vaccine profitability. Vaccine 5: 123–127.

Crawford, M. 1947. The immunology and epidemiology of some virus diseases. Veterinary Record 59: 537–540.

Dawson, M. 1987. Pathogenesis of maedi-visna. Veterinary Record 120: 451–454.

Donaldson, A.I. 1986. Aerobiology of foot-and-mouth disease (FMD): an outline and recent advances. Revue Scientifique et Technique Office International des Epizootics 5: 315–321.

Jeggo, M.H. 1986. A review of the immune response to bluetongue virus. Revue Scientifique et Technique Office International des Epizootics 5: 357–362.

Kitching, R.P. and Smale, C. 1986. Comparison of the external dimensions of capripoxvirus isolate. Research in Veterinary Science 41: 425–427.

Kitching, R.P. and Taylor, W.P. 1985. Clinical and antigenic relationship between isolates of sheep and goat pox viruses. Tropical Animal Health and Production 17: 64–74.

Kitching, R.P., Hammond, J.M. and Taylor, W.P. 1987. A single vaccine for the control of capripox infection in sheep and goats. Research in Veterinary Science 42: 53–60.

Kitching, R.P., McGrane, J.J. and Taylor, W.P. 1986. Capripox in the Yemen Arab Republic and the Sultanate of Oman. Tropical Animal Health and Production 18: 115–122.

Kitching, R.P., McGrane, J.J., Hammond, J.M., Miah, A.H., Mustapha, A.H.M. and Majumder, J.R. 1987. Capripox in Bangladesh. Tropical Animal Health and Production. In press.

Meegan, J.M., Hoogstraal, H. and Moussa, M.I. 1979. An epizootic of Rift Valley fever in Egypt in 1977. Veterinary Record 105: 124–125.

Mertens, P.P.C. 1986. The genome segments of bluetongue virus: the proteins they encode and the relationship between different isolates by cross-hybridisation. Revue Scientifique et Technique Office International des Epizootics 5: 333–349.

Scott, G.R. 1985. Rinderpest in the 1980's. Progress in Veterinary Microbiology and Immunology 1: 145–174. Karger, Basel.

Taylor, W.P. 1979. Protection of goats against peste des petits ruminants. Research in Veterinary Science 27: 321–324.

Taylor, W.P. 1984. The distribution and epidemiology of peste des petits ruminants. Preventive Veterinary Medicine 2: 157–166.

Taylor, W.P. 1986. The epidemiology of bluetongue. Revue Scientifique et Technique Office International des Epizootics 5: 351–356.

Taylor, W.P., Sellers, R.F., Gumm, I.O., Herniman, K.A.Z. and Owen, L. 1985. Bluetongue epidemiology in the Middle East. Pages 527–530 in Progress in Clinical and Biological Research. Vol. 178. Bluetongue and Related Orbiviruses. Alan R. Liss Inc., New York, USA.

E.F. Thomson and F.S. Thomson (eds), Increasing Small Ruminant Productivity in Semi-arid Areas
© 1988 ICARDA. ISBN 978-94-010-7086-7

Controlling Livestock Diseases in the Tropics by Breeding: A Perspective

O.B. Kasali, B.C. Njau and T. Bekele

Introduction

Of the 30 million km^2 of the African continent, 15 million km^2 have good quality and plentiful water supplies and are thus well suited for livestock production. In almost half of this area, however, livestock rearing is severely limited by tsetse-transmitted animal trypanosomiasis, a chronic parasitic disease usually fatal in susceptible species (Finelle 1983). If trypanosomiasis could be controlled, a large part of this region could be immediately used for livestock or mixed agriculture. With an increasing human population in the region, there is mounting pressure for increased food production on tsetse-free pastures and farmland. But many of these tsetse-free areas are in the drier regions of Africa where the local ecology is too fragile to support continuous heavy use. Problems associated with overgrazing in these areas further emphasize the need to bring into full production the more favourable agricultural areas currently under-utilized due to trypanosomiasis (Trail 1987).

The production of small ruminants in the tropics is largely constrained by gastrointestinal parasites. These parasites are a potential cause of reduced production (Allonby and Urquhart 1975), which has very important economic implications (Akerejola et al. 1979). Although many species of parasites are involved, only a few are of major economic importance due to their greater pathogenicity and relative abundance, e.g., *Haemonchus contortus, Trichostrongylus colubriformis, Oesophagostomum columbianum*, and *Ostertagia* spp. The importance of the major parasites also varies with climate due to differences between species in the effects of climate on transmission dynamics (Schillhorn Van Veen 1978; Michel 1982; Vercruysse 1983; 1985).

Trypanosomiasis

Current efforts to control African animal trypanosomiasis are aimed at the vector and chemotherapy. Efforts to control the disease are hampered by the high cost and complex logistics required, the lack of a field vaccine, and the small numbers of trypanotolerant livestock available. Thus, producers must depend on chemotherapy, chemoprophylaxis, vector control, and vaccine development, all of which have severe limitations (Murray 1982).

Small populations of humpless, *Bos taurus* cattle, dwarf sheep, and goats possessing some degree of resistance to trypanosomiasis are found in West and Central Africa. This trypanotolerance is generally attributed to the N'Dama and West African Shorthorn cattle, Djallonke sheep, and Dwarf West African goats. The humped *Bos indicus* cattle which are prevalent today are generally susceptible to trypanosomiasis, although some may exhibit a degree of trypanotolerance (Trail 1987).

A survey of trypanotolerant livestock in West and Central Africa (ILCA 1979) indicated that trypanotolerant breeds of cattle were at least as productive as other indigenous African breeds in areas with no or low tsetse challenge and, in areas where tsetse challenge was substantial, only the trypanotolerant breeds could survive. However, it was clearly illustrated that as tsetse challenge increased, the productivity of trypanotolerant livestock diminished.

The N'Dama breeding programme

Results from the first 2 years of the ILCA/ILRAD Trypanosomiasis Network suggest an important variation between and within cattle breeds for measures of trypanotolerance. Other studies in cattle and mice, involving tolerant and susceptible strains, all indicate a polygenic basis for trypanotolerance control. This polygenic variation could be used in two ways; using the proven selection techniques of quantitative genetics, which first require the definition of an easily and cheaply measured selection criterion, or through the identification of genetic markers.

The Network is starting to evaluate suitable criteria for the trypanotolerant trait using information from relevant sites. At the same time, the genetic and phenotypic variation and co-variation among performance traits and the trypanotolerant trait are being determined. It should then be possible to devise optimal programmes for breeding improved trypanotolerant N'Dama cattle using proven selection techniques.

Evidence from the Network suggests that packed cell volume (PCV) might be a suitable measure of trypanotolerance. The repeatability of PCV level of around 0.32 indicates that it may have a sufficiently high heritability to be useful in selection programmes.

Studies are being carried out where single-sire matings are possible which give paternal half-sib groups. This allows the most accurate determination of heritabilities and genetic correlations between the trypanotolerance trait and the other health and production traits.

The major histocompatibility complex (MHC) has been linked to susceptibility to two important cattle diseases, mastitis and enzootic bovine leucosis (ILRAD 1987). Therefore, research is being conducted at ILRAD on the basic structure of the bovine MHC and functional aspects of MHC in the immunoresponse in African animal trypanosomiasis and East Coast fever. Cattle are being studied to determine total genetic identity, MHC identity, partial

MHC identity, MHC homozygous animals inheriting identical MHC genes from both parents, and haematopoietic chimaric twins which have blood cells of two different gene types. These factors can be determined with a conventional breeding programme, using bulls and cows selected on the basis of MHC type. However, it is possible to produce multiple offspring from a single mating pair using embryo transfer techniques. This considerably increases the likelihood of obtaining the required genotypes in a shorter period of time (ILRAD 1987).

Gastrointestinal parasites

Current control of parasitic diseases focuses on reducing the contamination of pastures with the ova and developing larvae in faecal droppings of animals. This has been achieved mainly with anthelmintic treatment and controlled grazing. Tactical or strategic treatment with anthelmintics contributes little to the control of helminthiasis in Africa. This is due to the high cost of chemotherapeutic agents, the widespread use of communal pastures, and the difficulty of forecasting and monitoring the weather. Also, the frequent use of drugs leads to resistance, which is an important problem in the successful control of parasites.

Controlled grazing helps to prevent heavy infection or reinfection (Michel 1982) and is practiced by rotational and/or alternative grazing by different species of animals. However, this is not feasible in certain areas of Africa where nomadic pastoralists are constantly moving. Even the settled agropastoralists who practice mixed farming must constantly decide whether to allot separate plots of land to agriculture or livestock.

Vaccination against endoparasites has not been successful, except against lungworms under certain conditions. An attempt to immunize sheep with the irradiated larvae of *H. contortus* did not produce good results (Sivanathan et al. 1984) and young lambs, unlike adults, cannot be immunized against *H. contortus* infection using irradiated larvae because they are immunologically immature (Urquhart 1980). A major handicap in the development of vaccines against gastrointestinal nematodes is the poor immunological response of the hosts, especially the young ones, to parasites such as *H. contortus* and other trichostrongyles (Soulsby 1985). Furthermore, the lack of systemic host responses to gastrointestinal parasites, and the quantitative aspects of parasitism have substantially limited the development of vaccines.

Host-parasite interactions have tended toward equilibrium between the parasites and their hosts. This has helped the mechanisms of hypobiosis, self cure, genetic resilience, and genetic resistance to evolve in *H. contortus* infection. The first two are advantageous to the parasite in that they allow it to avoid adverse environmental conditions and/or replace aged forms with a more vigorous young generation (Urquhart et al. 1987).

There is a great deal of variation between animals in susceptibility to helminthiasis, much of it apparently genetic. This finding has stimulated interest in the possibility of selecting breeds or strains of ruminants, especially sheep, which are genetically resistant to parasitic worms (Dineen 1985; Soulsby 1985). The genetic variation of host responsiveness to helminths appears early in the life of outbred animal populations (Windon et al. 1980) and may be marked with increased responsiveness as the host ages (Le Jambre 1978). Hence, genetic variation between animals should be determined before the majority have become responsive (Soulsby 1985).

Genetic resistance to economically important helminths such as *H. contortus* has been reported in some breeds of sheep and goats in Africa (Preston and Allonby 1978). The genotype of the host influences the immune response to helminth infections, particularly the chronic forms, and consequently the overall outcome of the infection (Soulsby 1985).

In the past, it was necessary to infect hosts with nematodes to determine genotype variation (Windon et al. 1984). Sheep haemoglobin types have been used but at present, there is no evidence of a genetic correlation between them and resistance (Le Jambre 1978). An association has recently been observed between ovine lymphocyte antigen Sydney (SYI) (thought to be part of the sheep major histocompatibility complex (MHC)) and the immune response against *Trichostrongylus colubriformis* infection (Outteridge et al. 1985). This would allow direct identification and hence selection for resistance without requiring infection. The antigen, the genetic marker for this immune response, was present at high frequency (72.2%) on the lymphocytes of responder rams and at a lower frequency (21.9%) on the cells of lower responder rams, while for ewes the frequencies were 65.7 and 33.5%, respectively. Riffkin and Dobson (1979) and Luffau et al. (1986) identified sheep with genetic resistance to parasitic infections using the SYI antigen. Dineen and Wagland (1982) indicated that although heritability of resistance to parasites is high, the long generation interval of the host would slow progress in selecting for this parameter.

Conclusion

Animal production using genetically resistant germplasm can be cost effective in Africa where traditional animal management predominates. However, initiation of a selective breeding programme for such resistance is hampered by a lack of basic data on the genetic variation of the diseases involved, identification of relevant genes, and the desired level of breeding compatible with productivity.

A breeding program to produce livestock with improved disease resistance could play a particularly important and valuable role in the control of livestock diseases because useful genes, once established in target populations, do not require sophisticated management or other disease control measures to continue functioning. Once genes with the potential to improve disease resistance are identified, they could be rapidly introduced into livestock populations using artificial insemination and embryo transfer techniques. In the future, the development of technologies for transferring single genes or groups of genes directly into embryos at an early stage of development might be expected to increase the pace of genetic improvement in livestock.

References

Akerejola, O.O., Schillhorn Van Veen, T.W. and Njoku, C.O. 1979. Ovine and caprine diseases in Nigeria: a review of economic losses. Bulletin of Animal Health and Production in Africa 27: 65–70.

Allonby, E.W. and Urquhart, G.M. 1975. The epidemiology and pathogenic significance of haemonchosis in a Merino flock in East Africa. Veterinary Parasitology 1: 129–143.

Armour, J. 1980. The epidemiology of helminth disease in farm animals. Veterinary Parasitology 6: 7–46.

Armour, J. and Gettinby, G. 1983. A critical review of the evaluation of production effects of helminth disease and mismanagement of livestock production. Pages 164–172 in the Third International Symposium on Veterinary Epidemiology and Economics, Arlington, Virginia, USA, 6–10 Sept 1984. Veterinary Medicine Publishing Company, Kansas, USA.

Barger, I.A. 1982. Helminth parasites and animal production. Pages 133–155 in Biology and Control of Endoparasites (Symons, L.E.A., Donald, A.D. and Dineen, J.K., eds). Academic Press, Sydney, Australia.

Dineen, J.K. 1984. Immunological control of helminthiasis by genetic manipulation of host and parasite. Pages 1–9 in Proceedings of a workshop on Immunogenetic Approaches to the Control of Endoparasites with Particular Reference to Parasites in Sheep, University of Sydney, 22–23 Oct 1983 (Dineen, J.K. and Outteridge, P.M., eds). Division of Animal Health, Commonwealth Scientific and Industrial Research Organization, Australia.

Dineen, J.K. and Wagland, B.M. 1982. Immunoregulation of parasites in natural host-parasite systems with special reference to the gastrointestinal nematodes of sheep. Pages 297–329 in Biology and Control of Endoparasites. McMaster Laboratory 50th Anniversary Symposium on Parasitology, University of Sydney, 5–6 Nov 1981 (Symons, L.E.A., Donald, A.D. and Dineen, J.K., eds). Academic Press, Sydney, Australia.

Finelle, P. 1983. African animal trypanosomiasis. Pages 1–23 in FAO Animal Production and Health Paper No. 37. FAO, Rome, Italy.

ILCA (International Livestock Centre for Africa). 1979. Typanotolerant Livestock in West and Central Africa. Vol I. General Study. Monograph No. 2. ILCA, Addis Ababa, Ethiopia. 148 p.

ILRAD Reports. 1987. Towards improved disease resistance. The bovine major histocompatibility complex. Nairobi (Kenya), Vol. 5, No. 3.

Le Jambre, L.F. 1978. Host genetic factors in helminth control. Pages 137–141 in The Epidemiology and Control of Gastrointestinal Parasites of Sheep in Australia (Donald, A.D., Southcott, W.H. and Dineen, J.K., eds). Academic Press, Sydney, Australia.

Luffau, G., Nguyen, T.C., Cullen, P., Vu Tien Khang, J. and Ricordeau, G. 1986. Genetic resistance to *Haemonchus contortus* in Romanov sheep. Pages 683–689 in Proceedings of the Third World Congress on Genetics Applied to Livestock Production. XI. Genetics of Reproduction, Lactation, Growth, Adaptation, Disease, and Parasite Resistance. 16–22 July 1986, Lincoln, Nebraska, USA. Groupe Lab. Path. Animale, INRA, France (Abstract No. 307 (1987)). Veterinary Bulletin 57: 50.

Michel, J.F. 1982. Some thoughts on the control of parasitic gastroenteritis. Pages 113 – 131 in Biology and Control of Endoparasites (Symons, L.E.A., Donald, A.D. and Dineen, J.K., eds). Academic Press, Sydney, Australia.

Murray, M., Morrison, W.I. and Whitelaw, D.D. 1982. Host susceptibility to African trypano-somiasis: trypanotolerance. Pages 1–68 in Advances in Parasitology. Vol. 21 (Baker, J.R. and Muller, R., eds). Academic Press, London and New York.   ,

Outteridge, P.M., Windon, W.I. and Dineen, J.K. 1985. An association between a lymphocyte antigen in sheep and the response to vaccination against the parasite *Trichostrongylus colubri-formis*. International Journal for Parasitology 15: 121–127.

Preston, J.M. and Allonby, E.W. 1978. The influence of breed on the susceptibility of sheep and goats to a single experimental infection with *Haemonchus contortus*. Veterinary Record 103: 509–512.

Riffkin, G.G. and Dobson, C. 1979. Predicting resistance of sheep to *Haemonchus contortus* infections. Veterinary Parasitology 5: 365–378.

Schillhorn Van Veen, T.W. 1978. Haemonchosis in sheep during the dry season in the Nigerian Savanna. Veterinary Record 102: 364–365.

Sivanathan, S., Duncan, J.L. and Urquhart, G.M. 1984. Some factors influencing the immuniza-tion of sheep with irradiated *Haemonchus contortus* larvae. Veterinary Parasitology 16: 313–323.

Soulsby, E.J.L. 1985. Advances in veterinary parasitology, animal health and productivity. Pages 211–221 in Proceedings of an International Symposium, 26 June–2 July 1985, Cambridge, UK.

Trail, J.C.M. 1987. The African Trypanotolerance Livestock Network. Paper presented at the International Trypanotolerance Centre. Inauguration Conference, Banjul, Gambia.

Urquhart, G.M. 1980. Application of immunity in the control of parasitic disease. Veterinary Parasitology 6: 217–239.

Urquhart, G.M., Armour, J., Duncan, J.L., Dunn, A.M. and Jennings, F.W. 1987. Veterinary Parasitology. Longman Scientific and Technical, Essex, UK. 286 p.

Vercruysse, J. 1983. A survey of seasonal changes in nematodes faecal egg count levels of sheep and goats in Senegal. Veterinary Parasitology 13: 239–244.

Vercruysse, J. 1985. The seasonal prevalence of inhibited development of *Haemonchus contortus* in sheep in Senegal. Veterinary Parasitology 17: 159–163.

Windon, R.G., Dineen, J.K., Cregg, P., Griffiths, D.A. and Donald, A.D. 1984. The role of thresholds in the response of lambs to vaccination with irradiated *Trichostrongylus colubrifor-mis* larvae. International Journal for Parasitology 14: 423–428.

Windon, R.G., Dineen, J.K. and Kelly, J.D. 1980. The segregation of lambs into "responders" and "non-responders" response to vaccination with irradiated *Trichostrongylus colubriformis* larvae before weaning. International Journal for Parasitology 10: 65–73.

E.F. Thomson and F.S. Thomson (eds), Increasing Small Ruminant Productivity in Semi-arid Areas
© 1988 ICARDA . ISBN 978-94-010-7086-7

Impact on Productivity and Epidemiology of Gastrointestinal and Lungworm Parasites in Sheep in Morocco

A. Dakkak and H. Ouhelli

Introduction

There are at least 15 million sheep in Morocco and they occupy an important place in the agricultural economy. They produce a significant quantity of protein, amounting to 78750 t of lamb or about 32% of the total meat consumption. They also produce wool estimated at 9 million shearings per year.

Only sheep can utilize the vast pastural zones in Morocco which cover more than 25 million ha (Michel and Ruelan 1967). Sheep rearing is quite extensive over nearly the whole area and so the animals are exposed to numerous infectious and parasitic diseases. Of the latter, the gastrointestinal and lung helminths have the greater economic significance, according to our observations and those of the regional services involved in sheep production and health. The information cited above has provided the impetus to establish a research program on the epidemiology of these infections. Such a program is necessary for the development of rational treatment and prevention schemes.

Effects of helminthiasis on productivity

Gastrointestinal helminths

Marinov and Fassi-Fehri (1974) have compared the growth of lambs from ewes dewormed monthly with thiabendazole (50 mg/kg liveweight) for 8 months with the growth of lambs from ewes which were not dewormed but managed under identical conditions. Liveweight gains and carcass efficiency at slaughter of lambs from treated ewes were 17.5 and 2.5% greater, respectively, than those of lambs from untreated ewes. Also, treated ewes produced more milk than untreated ewes.

In the same study, liveweight gains of lambs treated monthly with thiabendazole (50 mg/kg liveweight) from weaning to 3 months were compared with liveweight gains of untreated lambs of the same age and in the same environment. Weight gains in treated lambs were 11.9% greater than those in untreated lambs.

Table 1. Effects of three treatments with morantel tartrate in June, November, and February on ewe and lamb mortality and lambing rate of ewes.

	Ewe mortality (%)	Lamb mortality (%)	Perinatal mortality (%)	Lambing rate (%)
Untreated (n = 132)	5.5	18.7	16.2	74.7
Treated (n = 125)	3.4	9.3	6.4	80.1
Difference (%)	2.1	9.4	9.8	5.5

Source: Fikri (1980); Pandey et al. (1984).

In a more recent study Dakkak et al. (1979a) compared liveweight gains of fattening lambs treated with morantel tartrate (8 mg/kg liveweight) every 3 weeks for 2 months prior to slaughter with those of untreated lambs of the same age, under the same conditions, and over the same period. At slaughter, treated lambs had gained 2.6 kg per animal more than untreated lambs.

Marinov and Fassi-Fehri (1974) also reported that in ewes treated with thiabendazole (50 mg/kg liveweight) 2 months before breeding and monthly during gestation, lambing rate and wool production were 7.0 and 15.6% greater, respectively, than in identical control ewes.

The effects of three strategic treatments against gastrointestinal parasites in June, November, and February on the survival and productivity of ewes have recently been studied by Fikri (1980) and Pandey et al. (1984). The results are shown in Table 1. The animals from the control flock received no anthelmintic treatment during the year and grazed the same pastures under the same management as those ewes treated three times with morantel tartrate (8 mg/kg liveweight). These studies demonstrated that three strategically-timed treatments against gastrointestinal helminths reduced the mortality rate of ewes and lambs, lowered perinatal mortality, and increased lambing rate.

Lungworms

In an experimental design identical to that just quoted, Fikri (1980) and Pandey et al. (1981) treated ewes with fenbendazole instead of morantel tartrate. By using a drug active against lung and gastrointestinal parasites the role of lungworms in mortality and reducing ewe productivity could be studied. Table 2 shows the effect of treatment against both types of parasite. At a dosage of 10 mg/kg liveweight, fenbendazole removed 95% of the lung population of protostrongylid worms and 100% of that of *Dictyocaulus filaria* (Dakkak et al. 1979b). The mortality and reduction in productivity attributable to the protostrongylids can be estimated by calculating the differences between the totals obtained after each type of treatment (Table 3).

Table 2. Effects of three treatments with fenbendazole in June, November, and February on ewe and lamb mortality and lambing rate of ewes.

	Ewe mortality (%)	Lamb mortality (%)	Perinatal mortality (%)	Lambing rate (%)
Untreated (n = 132)	5.5	18.4	16.2	74.7
Treated (n = 128)	1.9	4.9	2.1	84.6
Difference (%)	3.6	13.8	14.0	9.9

Source: Fikri (1980); Pandey et al. (1984).

Table 3. Estimates of the effects of protostrongylids on the mortality and production of ewes.

Anthelmintic	Ewe mortality (%)	Lamb mortality (%)	Perinatal mortality (%)	Lambing rate (%)
Morantel tartrate (n = 132)	3.4	9.3	6.4	80.1
Fenbendazole (n = 128)	1.9	4.9	2.1	84.6
Difference (%)	1.6	4.4	4.3	4.4

Source: Fikri (1980); Pandey et al. (1984).

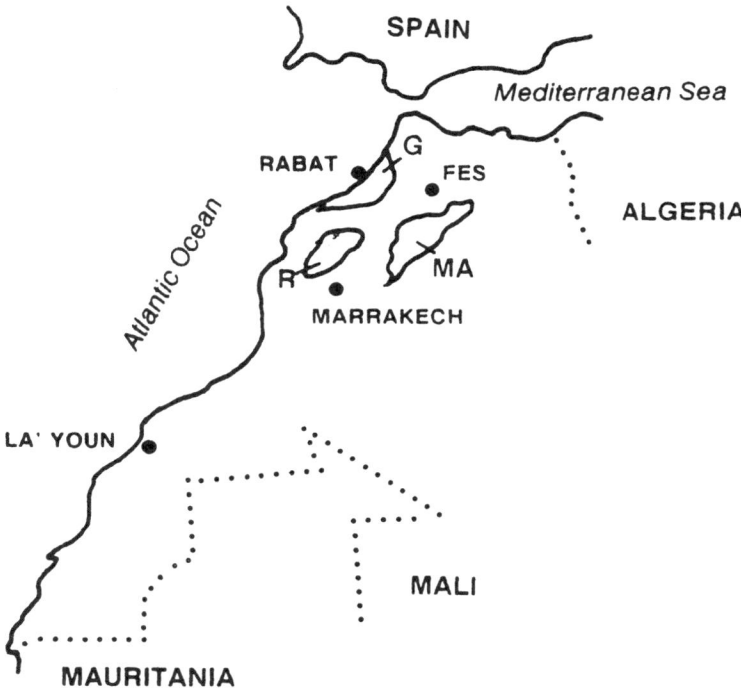

Fig. 1. Sheep rearing regions in which the studies were conducted: Middle Atlas (MA), Gharb (G), and Rhamna (R).

Epidemiology of gastrointestinal and lungworm infections

The epidemiology of sheep parasites in general and gastrointestinal and lung helminthiases in particular have been studied to determine the annual pasture contamination and degree of infection of the animals. Fig. 1 shows the three sheep rearing regions where the studies were conducted. Each of the three regions has a unique climate. In the Middle Atlas mountain range the climate is semi-arid with a cold winter, in the Gharb plain it is humid with a warm winter, while in the Rhamna plain it is arid with a mild winter. The total sheep population in the three regions is approximately 7.8 million or 52% of the total sheep in Morocco.

Methods

Pasture contamination was ascertained by monthly determination of the gastrointestinal helminth egg count per gram of faeces (EPG) and the number of lungworm larvae shed per gram of faeces (LPG) and of infective larvae of gastrointestinal worms per gram of herbage. The prevalence of molluscan intermediate hosts for trematodes (primarily *Fasciola hepatica*) and proto-strongylids on pasture and the rate and degree of infection of the molluscs by these parasites were also determined monthly.

The degree of infection of sheep was determined monthly with six animals (three ewes and three lambs) taken from a flock of untreated "tracer" animals. These sheep were slaughtered and all the parasites collected from the gastrointestinal tract, lungs, liver, and head.

Results and discussion

Detailed results for gastrointestinal parasites (Cabaret and Dakkak 1978; Cabaret and Ouhelli 1978; Ouhelli et al. 1980; 1981; Pandey et al. 1980; Dakkak et al. 1982) and for lungworms (Cabaret and Dakkak 1979a; 1979b; Cabaret et al. 1978; 1980a; 1980b; 1980c; Dakkak and Cabaret 1984) have been published and will only be summarized here.

Climate. The influence of climate on the development of parasitism in general and of gastrointestinal and lungworm parasitism in particular is very important. To alleviate the effects of climatic variations, both within and between years, epidemiological research should be conducted over at least 3–4 years. The results reported here are averages over 2 years for each of the regions.

Helminth fauna. Tables 4 and 5 present the different species of helminths of the gastrointestinal tract and lungs which have been identified in the three regions.

Table 4. Species and frequency [1] of helminth parasites in the gastrointestinal tract of sheep.

Parasite species	Region		
	Middle Atlas	Gharb	Rhamna
Abomasum			
Ostertagia circumcincta	+ + +	+ + +	+ + +
O. trifurcata	+	+	+
O. lyrata	+	+	−
O. ostertagi	−	+	−
O. pinnata	+	−	−
Marshallagia marshalli	+ +	+	+
Haemonchus contortus	+	+	+
H. longistipes	−	+	−
Trichostrongylus axei	+ + +	+ + +	+ + +
T. vitrinus	+ +	+	+
T. andreievi	+	+	−
Camelostrongylus mentulatus	+	+	−
Small intestine			
T. axei	+	+	+
T. colubriformis	+ +	+	+
T. vitrinus	+	+ +	+
T. probolurus	+	+	−
T. andreievi	+	+	−
Cooperia oncophora	+	+	+
Cooperia spp.	+	+	+
Nematodirus filicollis	+ +	+ + +	+ + +
N. spathiger	−	+	−
Large intestine			
Chabertina ovina	+	+	+
Bunostomum trigonocephalum	+	+	+
Oesophagostomum venulosum	+	+	+
O. columbianum	+	+	+
Trichuris ovis	+	+	+

[1] Occurrence: − = never; + = infrequent; + + = frequent; + + + = very frequent.

Table 5. Species and frequency [1] of helminth parasites in the lungs of sheep in three regions in Morocco.

Parasite species	Region		
	Middle Atlas	Gharb	Rhamna
Dictyocaulus filaria	+ +	+ +	+
Protostrongylus rufescens	+	+ +	+ + +
Muellerius capillaris	+ + +	+ + +	+ + +
Cystocaulus ocreatus	+	+	+ +
Neostrongylus linearis	+ + +	+ + +	+ +

[1] Occurrence: − = never; + = infrequent; + + = frequent; + + + = very frequent.

Gastrointestinal strongyles. Seasonal and regional variations in the shedding of eggs and pasture contamination by infective larvae of gastrointestinal helminths are presented in Fig. 2. In general, the shedding of eggs reaches higher levels in

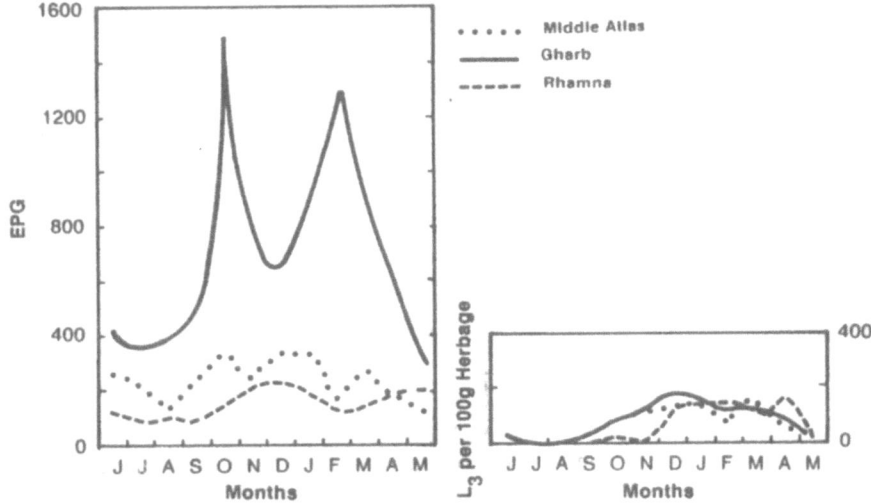

Fig. 2. Seasonal changes in the faecal output of gastrointestinal nematode eggs per gram (EPG) of faeces and the density of infective larvae (L_3) on herbage in Rhamna, Gharb, and Middle Atlas.

fall, during winter, and at the beginning of spring than at the end of spring and in the summer in the three regions. In these cool and moist periods, conditions are most favorable for the development and survival of free-living stages of the parasites. This explains the high density of infective larvae on pasture herbage, which puts the sheep at a high risk of infection.

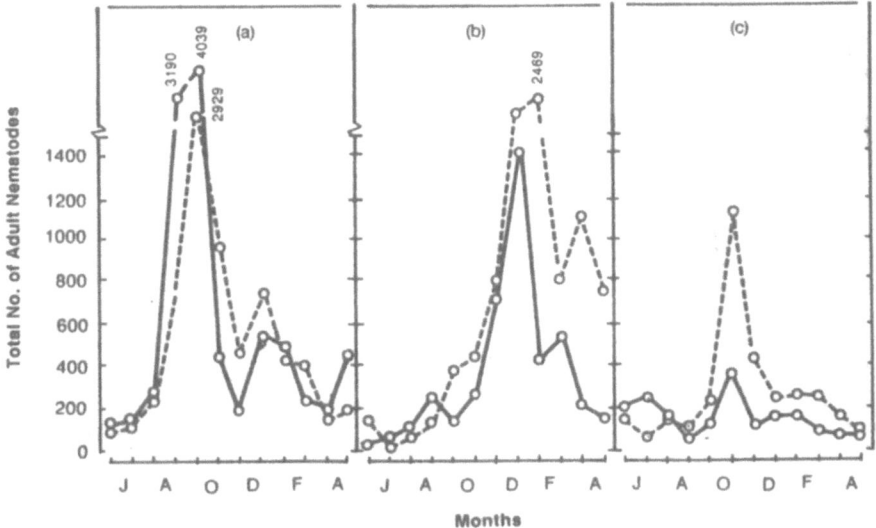

Fig. 3. Seasonal changes in the number of adult nematodes in the abomasum (– – –) and small intestine (———) of sheep in the Middle Atlas (a), Gharb (b), and Rhamna (c) regions.

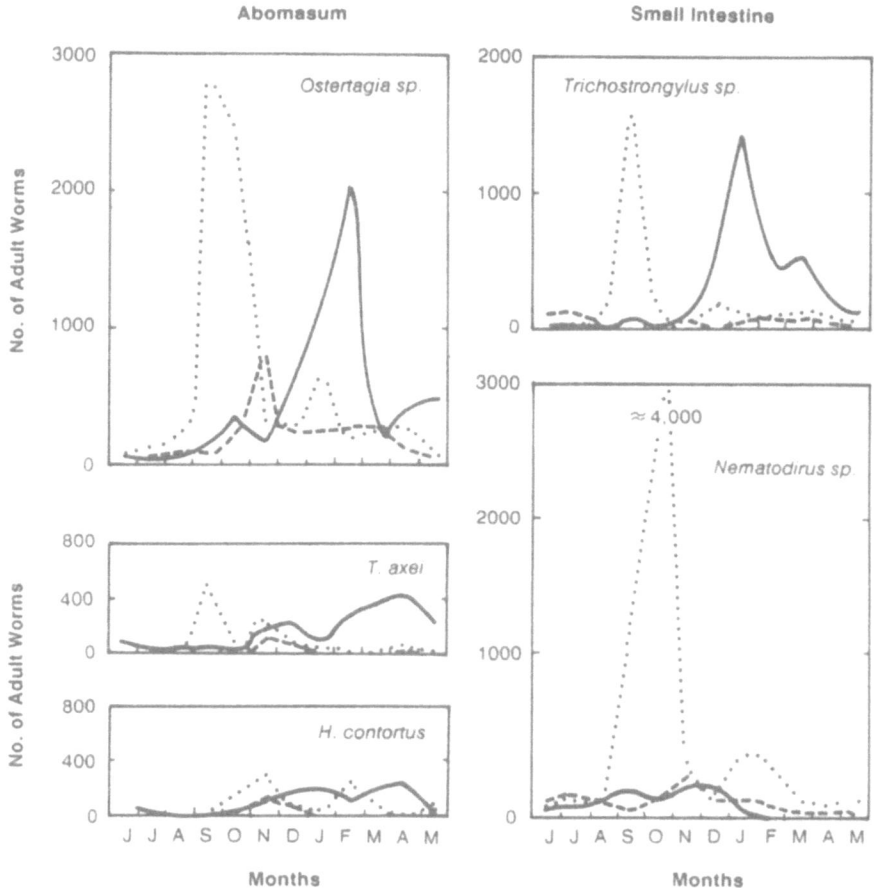

Fig. 4. Seasonal changes in the population of abomasal and small intestinal adult nematodes in the Middle Atlas ($\cdots$), Gharb (————), and Rhamna (– – –) regions. Other species are not shown as numbers were < 20 every month.

Fig. 3 shows the seasonal changes in the number of adult abomasal and small intestinal parasites in sheep in the three regions. The period of greatest infection occurs during fall, winter, and spring in the Middle Atlas, the second half of fall, winter and spring in Gharb, and the second half of fall and in early winter in Rhamna.

The primary abomasal parasites in the three regions are species of *Ostertagia*, *Trichostrongylus*, and *Haemonchus* (Fig. 4) while in the small intestine, they are predominantly *Trichostrongylus* and *Nematodirus* species.

The intermediate hosts of lungworms. The seasonal and regional variation in the density, the rate and degree of infection of molluscs, and the proportion of infective larvae harbored by them are shown in Fig. 5. First-stage larvae of protostrongylid species can only become infective third-stage larvae in ter-

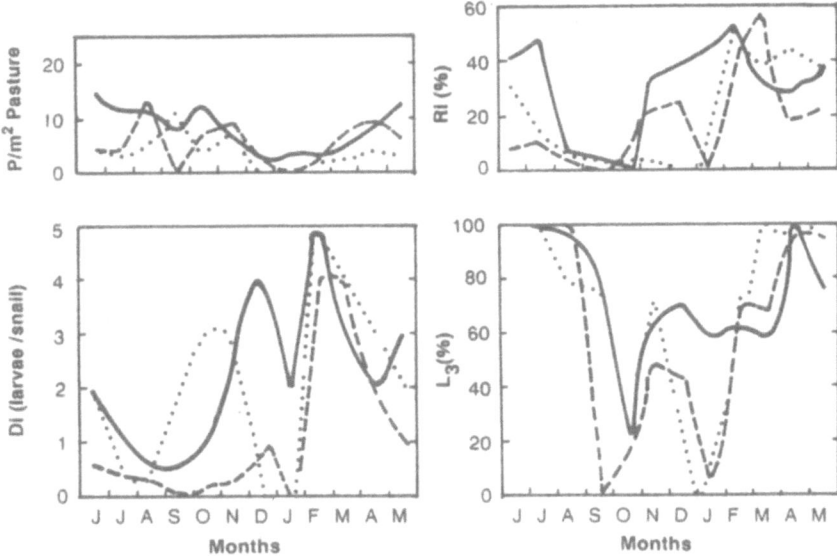

Fig. 5. Seasonal changes in the population (P) of snails, the rate (Ri) and degree (Di) of infection of snails by the larvae of the protostrongylids, and the percentage L$_3$ of the total larvae infecting snails in the Middle Atlas (· · ·), Gharb (————), and Rhamna (– – –) regions.

restrial molluscs. Thus the biology and ecology of the intermediate hosts, as well as their rate and degree of infection with the parasites, must be studied so that the epidemiology of protostrongylid species can be understood (Cabaret 1981).

The same genera and species of molluscs have been identified in the three regions and include *Euparypha pisana, Otala lactea, Helicella marioni, H. conspurcata, Cochlicella conoidea, C. ventricosa, C. acuta, Cochliocopa lubrica, Rumina decollata, Limax maximus*, and *Milax gagates*. The species which are most prevalent are, in decreasing order of frequency, *C. acuta, C. ventricosa, H. virgata, O. lactea, E. pisana*, and *L. maximus* in the Middle Atlas; *H. virgata, E. pisana, O. lactea, C. acuta*, and *L. maximus* in Gharb; and *O. lactea, H. virgata, C. acuta*, and *C. ventricosa* in Rhamna.

For the three regions the ecological niches of the different species of snail have been identified. *C. conoidea, C. ventricosa, H. conspurcata*, and *L. maximus* occur on rangelands with dense and regular vegetation, *E. pisana, H. virgata, O. lactea, C. acuta*, and *L. maximus* occur on scrub brush land of *Chaemerops humilus* and *Asparagus albus*, while *C. ventricosa, H. virgata*, and *L. maximus* are found in forest pastures. *M. gagates* is found near small streams and temporary stagnant pools, *C. lubrica* under stones, and *H. turcia* around limestone-bearing rocks.

Receptivity of the different species of molluscs to infection with protostrongylid larvae is, in decreasing order, *M. gagates, O. lactea, E. pisana, Cochliella* spp., *Helicella* spp., *L. maximus*, and *C. acuta*.

The appearance of molluscs on pasture varies between seasons. The majority of Helicidae species collect in clusters high upon vegetation that survives the dry season (mid-June to mid-September). The groups separate in fall with the arrival of the rains. This period coincides with the beginning of the reproductive period for the snails and it is characterized by disbursement over wide areas.

The molluscs generally start to lay eggs 15 days after the first rain and laying continues until the beginning of December. This is followed by a period of high mortality and predation by birds and rodents can result in a decrease in snail numbers of up to 95% during winter.

The fall period in each cycle is most important because the snails are older and therefore more susceptible to infection (Cabaret et al. 1980a) and after a dry summer, rainfall in this period stimulates the snails to become active (Dakkak and Cabaret 1984). The resumption of sexual reproduction results in a wide distribution of the snails, thus increasing the opportunity of infection by larvae (Cabaret et al. 1980b).

The periods of maximum infection in snails with infective larvae (L_3) occur in March–April and June–July in the Middle Atlas region, in April and from June–August in Gharb, and in April and from June–August in Rhamna (Fig. 5).

Lungworms. The seasonal and regional variation in faecal output of first-stage larvae of *D. filaria* and protostrongylid species and of adult worms in the lung are shown in Figs 6 and 7, respectively. For *D. filaria*, free-living larvae are particularly sensitive to temperature extremes and dryness or excessive rainfall (Rose 1955; 1965) and under such conditions the risk of larval development and transmission to sheep is low. High risk periods occur in September–October in the Middle Atlas region for spring lambs and in March–April for winter lambs, in October–November in Gharb for spring lambs and in April for winter lambs, and in November–December in Rhamna for spring lambs and March–April for winter lambs.

For the protostrongylid lungworms, the period of high risk of infection of

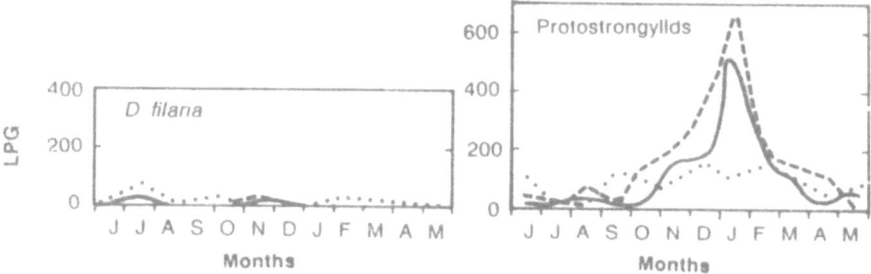

Fig. 6. Seasonal changes in the faecal output of first stage larvae of *D. filaria* and protostrongylids per gram of faeces (LPG) in the Middle Atlas ($\cdots$), Gharb (———), and Rhamna (– – –) regions.

252

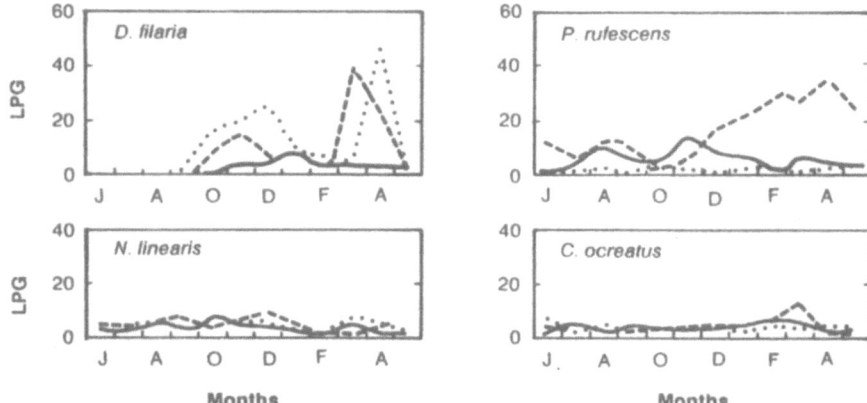

Fig. 7. Seasonal changes in the faecal output of several species of lungworm first stage larvae per gram (LPG) of faeces in the Middle Atlas ($\cdots$), Gharb (———), and Rhamna (– – –) regions. *M. capillaris* not shown as LPG always < 2.

sheep is from February–May and September–October in the Middle Atlas, February–May and November–December in Gharb, and February–May and November–December in Rhamna (Fig. 5). The period of highest numbers of molluscs is from October–March in the three regions (Fig. 6).

Only a small part of the total population of *Muellerius capillaris* and *Neostrongylus linearis* can be harvested using the techniques for recovering protostrongylid larvae from the lungs because these worms are located in very small nodules which they stimulate in the lung tissue. This is a common

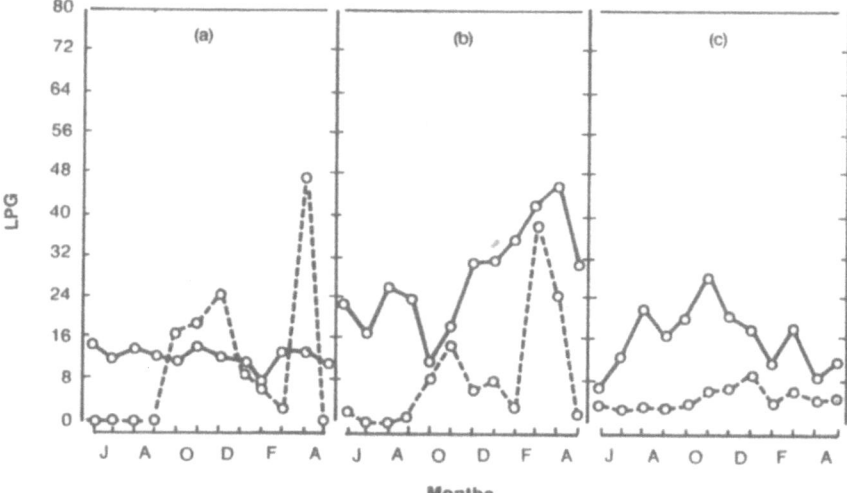

Fig. 8. Seasonal changes in the number of adult *D. filaria* (– – –) and protostrongylids (———) in the Middle Atlas (a), Gharb (b), and Rhamna (c) regions.

problem in studying protostrongylid diseases (Rose 1958; Kassai 1962; Jubb and Kennedy 1970; Dakkak et al. 1979b; 1986). Therefore, the numbers of protostrongylid parasites represented in Fig. 7 do not adequately reflect the true level of infection by each protostrongylid species. Thus the total number of these lungworms (Fig. 8) is apparently stable at a low level in the Middle Atlas region where *Protostrongylus rufescens* is not abundant (Alahkam 1977; Ait Taleb 1987). In other regions where *P. rufescens* is more abundant (Bahaida 1978; Dakkak et al. 1979b; 1986; Ait Taleb 1987) total population numbers follow those of *P. rufescens*, which is more easily recovered from the small bronchii and bronchioles of the lung. Sheep are subjected to the highest levels of protostrongylid infection throughout the year in the Middle Atlas, October–November and March–April in the Gharb, and August–March in the Rhamna (Fig. 7).

Acknowledgement

Parts of the results quoted in this paper have been extracted from regular reports of the EPOM project (contract No. TSD 214-MA (MR)) between the Hassan II Agronomy and Veterinary Institute and the Commission of European Communities, Section for Science, Research and Development (DG XII). We extend our thanks to them for the generous financial aid which permitted the studies in the three regions.

References

Ait Taleb, A. 1987. Epidemiologie des parasitoses ovines au Moyen Atlas (Timahdit-El Hajeb) et au Rhamna. These Doctorat Veterinaire. Institute Agronomique et Veterinaire Hassan II, Rabat, Morocco. 202 p.

Alahkam, L. 1977. Contribution a l'etude parasitologique, epidemiologique et lesionnelle des broncho-pneumonies vermineuses du mouton dans la region de Tadla. These Doctorat Veterinaire. Institute Agronomique et Veterinaire Hassan II, Rabat, Morocco. 137 p.

Bahaida, B. 1978. Contribution a l'etude des Protostrongylidoses du mouton. Production des larves L_1, et leur devenir chez les mollusques terrestres hotes intermediaires. These Doctorat Veterinaire. Institute Agronomique et Veterinaire Hassan II, Rabat, Morocco. 173 p.

Cabaret, J. 1981. Receptivite des mollusques terrestres de la region de Rabat a l'infestation par les Protostrongyloses dans les conditions experimentales et naturelles. These Doctorat es Sciences. Universite Pierre et Marie Curie, Paris, France. 214 p.

Cabaret, J. and Dakkak, A. 1978. Les nematodes parasites de la caillette du mouton au Maroc. Premiers resultats. Maroc Veterinaire 1: 5–7.

Cabaret, J. and Dakkak, A. 1979a. Infestation experimentale de *Cochlicella ventricosa* (Draparnaud, 1801) par des larves L_1 de Protostrongylides. Annales de Parasitologie, Paris 54: 57–64.

Cabaret, J. and Dakkak, A. 1979b. La survie des adultes de *Euparipha pisana* (Muller, 1774) dans la region de Rabat (Maroc). Interet pour le comprehension de l'epidemiologie des Proto-strongylidoses des petits ruminants. Colloque International d'Heliculture-Auzeville, 14–16 September. France.

Cabaret, J. and Ouhelli, H. 1978. Etude d'une population de nematodes parasites du tube digestif des ovins dans la regions de Moulay-Bouazza (Moyen Atlas, Maroc). Revue de Medecine Veterinaire 129: 603–610.

Cabaret, J., Dakkak, A. and Alahkam, L. 1978. Considerations sur l'elimination des larves L$_1$ de Protostrongylides dans les feces des ovins; nature de la distribution, influence de l'age de l'animal et des traitements anthelminthiques. Annals de la Societe Belge de Medecine Tropicale 58: 309–314.

Cabaret, J., Dakkak, A. and Bahaida, B. 1980a. Etude de l'infestation des mollusques terrestres de le region de Rabat (Maroc) par les larves de Protostrongylides dans les conditions naturelles. Revue d'Elevage et de Medecine Veterinaire 33: 159–165.

Cabaret, J., Dakkak, A. and Bahaida, B. 1980b. Facteurs de risques de l'infestation des ovins par les Protostrongylides. Bulletin de l'Office International des Epizootic 92: 1351–1356.

Cabaret, J. Dakka, A. and Bahaida, B. 1980c. On some factors influencing the output of the larvae of Protostrongylids of sheep in natural infections. The Veterinary Quarterly 2: 115–120.

Dakkak, A. and Cabaret, J. 1984. Des mollusques terrestres hotes intermediaires des Protostrongylides dans les paturages de la region de Rabat. Actes de l'Institut Agronomique et Veterinaire Hassan II 4: 41–46.

Dakkak, A., Cabaret, J. and Ouhelli, H. 1979a. Interets zootechnique et epidemiologique des traitements anthelminthiques des agneaux de boucherie par le tartrate de morantel dans les conditions de l'elevage marocain. Maroc Veterinaire 2: 3–11.

Dakkak, A., Cabaret, J. and Ouhelli, H. 1979b. Efficacite comparee du fenbendazole et du tetramisole sur les helminthes parasites du mouton au Maroc. I. Protostrongylides et Dictyocaulus filaria. Recueil de Medecine Veterinaire 155: 785–793.

Dakkak, A., Chaer, M. and Pandey, V.S. 1982. Etude du developpement et de la survie des formes libres d'Ostertagia circumcincta sur les paturages de la region de Rabat. IIe Congres Scientifique de l'Union des Biologistes Arabes, March, Fes, Morocco. Arab Biologists Union.

Dakkak, A., Robin, B. and Kachani, Malika. 1986. Efficacite de l'Ivermectine dans le traitement des bronchopneumonies vermineuses des strongyloses digestives et de l'oestrose du mouton. Revue de Medecine Veterinaire 137: 781–787.

Fikri, A. 1980. Traitement strategique des brebis par deux types d'anthelminthiques: interets zootechnique et parasitaire. These Doctorat Veterinaire. Institute Agronomique et Veterinaire Hassan II, Rabat, Morocco. 92 p.

Jubb, K.V.F., Kennedy, P.C. 1970. Pathology of Domestic Animals. Academic Press, New York and London. 237 p.

Kassai, T. 1962. Reproductive life span of Cystocaulus, Muellerius and Neostrongylus species in the lungs of sheep. Maguar Allatorvosok Lapja 17: 262–264.

Marinov, A. and Fassi-Fehri, M. 1974. Lutte contre les strongyloses des ovins avec le thiabendazole. Etude de rentabilite dans les conditions maghrebines. Recueil de Medecine Veterinaire 150: 135–144.

Michel, C. and Ruelan, A. 1967. L'agriculture et les forets au Maroc. Pages 103–140 in Les Cahiers de la Recherche Agronomique, Institute National de la Recherche Agronomique (ed.).

Ouhelli, H., Benzaouia, T., Pandey, V.S. and Dakkak, A. 1980. Application de la methode des "animaux traceurs" a l'etude de l'epidemiologie de certaines parasitoses du mouton. Bulletin de l' Office International des Epizootics 92: 1343–1344.

Ouhelli, H., Benzaouia, T., Pandey, V.S. and Dakkak, A. 1981. Etude epidemiologique de certaines parasitoses du mouton au Maroc atlantique par utilisation de la methode des "animaux traceurs". Revue d'Elevage et de Medecine Veterinaire des Pays Tropicaux 34: 319–324.

Pandey, V.S., Cabaret, J. and Dakkak, A. 1981. Effect of treating ewes with fenbendazole during pregnancy and lactation in a mediterranean climate. Veterinary Record 109: 15.

Pandey, V.S., Cabaret, J. and Fikri, A. 1984. The effect of strategic anthelmintic treatment on the breeding performance and survival of ewes naturally infected with gastro-intestinal strongyles and Protostrongylids. Annals de Recherches Veterinaire 15: 491–496.

Pandey, V.S., Cabaret, J., Ouhelli, H. and Dakkak, A. 1980. Etude des nematodes parasites du tube digestif des ovins adultes dans deux regions du Maroc. Bulletin de l'Office International des Epizootics 92: 1345–1349.

Rose, J.H. 1955. Observation on the free-living larvae of the lungworm *Dictyocaulus filaria*. Journal of Comparative Pathology and Therapeutics 65: 370–381.

Rose, J.H. 1958. Site of development of the lungworm *Muellerius capillaris* in experimentally infected lambs. Journal of Comparative Pathology and Therapeutics 68: 359–362.

Rose, J.H. 1965. Some observations on the transmission of lungworm infection in a flock of sheep at pasture. Research in Veterinary Science 6: 189–195.

E.F. Thomson and F.S. Thomson (eds), Increasing Small Ruminant Productivity in Semi-arid Areas
© *1988 ICARDA . ISBN 978-94-010-7086-7*

Resistance of Sheep and Goats to Helminth Infections: A Genetic Basis

L. Gruner and J. Cabaret

Introduction

The increasing appearance of nematode strains resistant to anthelmintics has revived interest in the search for alternative control methods. Local epidemiological studies are a necessary preliminary to any control program and they should identify which are the most important parasites, the periods of high risk of infection, and highly contaminated pastures. Integrated control programs may then be designed to include consideration of the choice of anthelmintic in relation to target parasite, periods of treatment, and pasture management. Where farmers rely solely on anthelmintics and *Haemonchus contortus* is prevalent, the emergence of resistance increases rapidly, as has occurred in Australia and New Zealand. Integrated control might reduce the number of anthelmintic drenchings required and thus reduce the probability of resistance. Vaccination has proved to be effective against *Dictyocaulus viviparus* in calves but much work remains to be done before vaccines will be available for other parasitic nematodes (Urquhart 1988).

Susceptibility and resilience to helminth infection vary between breeds or individuals and are affected by nutritional, physiological, and genetic factors. In the past 10 years there has been increasing interest in genetic factors (Le Jambre 1978; Dargie 1982; Albers and Gray 1987; Courtney 1986; Gray 1987). In this paper we will assess the contribution of animal selection to developing resistance, discuss the value of screening methods for resistance in small ruminants, and estimate the interest in selection programs.

Selection of sheep resistant to *Haemonchus contortus*: the Australian example revisited

H. contortus is one of the most common parasitic helminths in sheep and is widespread in Australia. Le Jambre et al. (1978) investigated the genetic variation within Australian Merinos artificially infected with *H. contortus* and estimated the heritability of resistance (h^2) to be 0.28 with a standard error of 0.15.

A large program was initiated at Armidale in 1982 in which 20 unrelated rams were randomly mated to 25 ewes and the offspring evaluated in a field test system. Half the lambs born were infected with a single dose of 11000 infective larvae and the other half were used as controls. Egg counts and packed cell volume (PCV) were recorded at 4 and 5 weeks after infection. The infected lambs were then treated with anthelmintics and after a 4-week period of recovery, the control lambs were treated and the previously infected group used as controls (Albers et al. 1984). To date, 157 rams and 1583 offspring have been used in the study (Albers and Gray 1987; Gray 1987).

Resistance, defined as the ability to suppress establishment and/or subsequent development of worm infection, was measured directly from faecal egg counts or indirectly using PCV depletion. A similar heritability value of 0.29 (standard error, 0.12) was recorded for both these parameters.

From an economic point of view, resistance is the ability of infected sheep to maintain existing levels of production. This has been termed resilience by Australian researchers and it had a heritability of 0.18 (standard error, 0.10). Resistance and resilience were positively correlated so selection for resistance will induce better resilience and a higher level of production.

From these results, a heritability value of 0.3 for resistance to *H. contortus* seems realistic although a coefficient of variation of 40% within a flock might be expected. A selection intensity of 5% for males and 30% for females is reasonable. Flock resistance would then increase on average by 6% every year and egg output would be reduced by 50% in three generations. A more realistic scheme of selection would be to increase resistance at approximately 1% per year. These data were obtained for wool and meat production systems but should be reconsidered if milk or cheese production are the economic goals.

An important question is whether resistance to helminths is dependent on a major resistance gene or is under the control of several genes. If control depends on a major gene, a decrease in egg output of over 50% per year might be expected on farms where homozygous resistant rams are used. Conversely, if resistance to helminth infection is polygenic, the expected progress is slow and an increase in resistance of 30% in 12 years is likely. The existence of a major resistance gene has still not been confirmed and this information is necessary before any large-scale selection program is designed.

Criteria for genetic selection for resistance

A universal criterion for determining resistance to helminths has yet to be found but in experimental infections, worm burdens, sex-ratio, length of worms, and number of eggs *in utero* are of interest as these parameters may underline some specific mechanism of resistance. In young kids infected with *Teladorsagia circumcincta*, the only significant difference was in the fecundity of females expressed as eggs per female worm (Richard and Cabaret 1986).

Usually, faecal egg counts are used to measure resistance but other parameters can be used. For example, Courtney et al. (1986) used the periparturient rise in egg count to measure resistance. Antibody response and indirect indicators of anaemia (for *H. contortus*) can also be used. Windon and Dineen

(1984) vaccinated sheep with irradiated larvae of *Trichostrongylus colubriformis* and showed that the response differs between low and high responder lambs and has a heritability of 0.41 (standard error, 0.19). Riffkin and Yong (1984) used purified nematode antigen and then recorded the response in treated sheep. While these methods are interesting they are of limited use in selection programs.

What we need are genetic markers of susceptibility to helminths. In sheep, haemoglobin type is correlated to resistance to *H.contortus* infection (Evans et al. 1963). This finding has been reported in different regions and for different breeds of sheep (Jilek and Bradley 1969; Allonby and Urquhart 1976; Altaif and Dargie 1978; Preston and Allonby 1979). Sheep with AA haemoglobin type were more resistant than those with AB or BB type. However, this marker was not related to resistance in the Romanov breed in France (Luffau et al. 1986) or in Australian Merinos (Albers and Gray 1987) so it is of limited value. Outteridge et al. (1985) have shown an association between resistance to *T. colubriformis* and major histocompatibility gene complex (MHC), while one of the three experimented ovine lymphocyte antigens (OLA) appeared to be an interesting predictive marker worthy of further investigation.

The role of breed in resistance

Australian selection programs use intra-breed selection. Breed is an important factor in resistance and according to Gray and Raadsma (1986), crossbreds had similar resistance but greater resilience to helminth infections than purebreds. The susceptibility of several breeds of sheep to natural or experimental infection is shown in Table 1 which illustrates that in general *H. contortus* has been used most often to infect sheep and little information is available for other nematodes. The criterion of resistance has been the output of nematode eggs in faeces and further studies are required on true infection i.e., number of worms or intensity of lesions. Natural infections usually occurred in ewes while experimental infections occurred in lambs so the two sets of information are difficult to compare. Further studies are required on the mechanisms of resistance to infection and reinfection and, as resistance has been extensively studied in sheep, more studies are needed on goats in view of their importance in the economy of developing countries. Most studies have been made on infection by strongyles in the gastrointestinal (GI) tract and these should be extended to other helminth infections e.g., protostrongylids, *Moniezia*, and flukes.

Specificity of resistance to helminths

Most experimental studies have dealt with resistance to one particular nematode but we should consider whether to create lines of sheep resistant to one species or to a wider group such as a genus, family, or order.

Windon and Dineen (1984) have studied several GI strongyles belonging to the family Trichostrongylidae. They showed that following vaccination against *T. colubriformis*, high responder lambs were more resistant than low responder lambs to challenge with *T. rugatus* and *Teladorsagia circumcincta*. There was no difference between high and low responders to challenge with *H. contortus* and while lambs were partly protected against the target parasite and several other taxonomically related nematodes, there was no protection against another of the same family.

Table 1. Fluctuations in resistance to natural (N) or experimental (E) infection with gastrointestinal and pulmonary strongyles in various breeds of sheep and goats.

Hosts and helminths	Type of infection	Criteria of resistance [1]	Breeds arranged in decreasing order of resistance	References
SHEEP				
H. contortus	N	epg, PCV	Florida native Rambouillet	Jilek and Bradley (1969)
idem	E	epg, no. of worms	idem idem	Radhakrishnan et al. (1972)
idem	E	idem idem	idem idem	Bradley et al. (1973)
idem	E	idem idem	idem idem	Knight et al. (1973)
idem	E	epg, no. of worms, albumin, catabolism	Scottish Blackface/ Finn Dorset	Altaif and Dargie (1978)
idem	N	epg, no. of worms	Red Masai Merino Corriedale Hampshire	Preston and Allonby (1978)
idem	E	epg, no. of worms, survival of sheep	idem idem idem idem	Preston and Allonby (1979)
idem	E	epg, no. of worms, PCV	Merino Awassi	Al-Khshali and Altaif (1979)
idem	E	idem idem	St Croix, 3/4 St Croix Florida native Barbados, domestic lambs	Courtney et al. (1985)
Ostertagia circumcincta	N	epg	Romney marsh, 3 other breeds	Stewart et al. (1973)
Ostertagia spp.	N	epg, no. of worms	Targhee, 3 other breeds	Scrivner (1964)
Trichostrongylus axei	E	no. of worms, bodyweight	Dorset, Scottish blackface	Ross (1970)

Table 1 (continued).

Hosts and helminths	Type of infection	Criteria of resistance [1]	Breeds arranged in decreasing order of resistance	References
Nematodirus and others (*Ostertagia*)	N	epg	Crossbred of Dorsethorn, 2 Merino strains Corriedale	Piper et al. (1978)
Mixed (*H. contortus*)	N	epg	Dorset Blackbelly /4 other pure or crossbreeds	Yazwinski et al. (1979)
Mixed	N	epg	Finn and Romney. Columbia/Dorset and North Country Cheviot. Suffolk	Norman and Hohenboken (1979)
Mixed	N	epg (peri-parturient rise)	Florida native, Barbados Blackbelly and St Croix/ Rambouillet, Finn Dorset. Rambouillet	Courtney et al. (1984; 1986)
Mixed	N,E	epg, no. of worms	Lacaune/ Ramanov	Gruner et al. (1986)
Mixed	N	epg, no. of worms, bodyweight	3/4 Ost-Friesian .1/4 Corriedale /Corriedale (resilience)	Suarez (1985)
Mixed lungworms	N	lungs lesions	Sardi = Timahdit	Alahkam (1977)
Mixed lungworms	N	lungs lesions no. of worms	Suffolk/ Hampshire/ Texel	Benakhla (1982)
Mixed gastrointestinal, lungworms	N	epg (lgp)	Merino of Arles /Merino. Romanov /Romanov	Gruner et al. (1987)
GOATS				
H. contortus	E	epg, no. of worms	Saanen /East African /Galla	Preston and Allonby (1978)
Mixed gastrointestinal, *Muellerius*		epg, lpg	Alpine /Saanen	Cabaret and Anjorand (1984)

[1] epg = eggs per gram of faeces; lpg = larvae per gram of faeces; PCV = packed cell volume.

In field conditions, polyparasitism occurs and we are interested to know how resistance to one group of parasites interacts with resistance to another group. For this reason, we have studied the epidemiology of helminthiasis in

Table 2. Comparison of natural infection of Merino of Arles, Romanov, and their crosses (Rom. Mer) in southern France.

Intensity of infection	Helminth species
Merino < Rom.Mer < Romanov	Trichostrongyles (all spp.)
	Teladorsagia circumcincta and
	Trichostrongylus vitrinus
	Chabertia ovina
	Nematodirus spp.
	Dictyocaulus filaria
	Moniezia sp.
Merino = Rom.Mer = Romanov	*Dicrocoelium lanceolatum*
Merino > Rom.Mer > Romanov	*Neostrongylus linearis*
	Fasciola hepatica

sheep and adaptability of prolific Romanov sheep in the south of France for the past 10 years (Gruner and Cabaret 1985). Heavy, mixed infections of nematodes, trematodes, and cestodes were observed in experimental flocks grazing irrigated pastures. In December 1985 and 1986, three groups of sheep were compared, Merino of Arles, Romanov, and their crosses. The period of lambing and the availability of mountain pastures in summer were important environmental factors affecting infection.

Adjusted helminth egg and larval counts and larval diagnoses on coprocultures are presented in Table 2. There were differences in infection in the three groups with Merino of Arles being less infected by trichostrongylids than Romanov, but more infected by *Fasciola* and protostrongylids. The host-parasite relationship is complex and resistance may differ greatly from one breed to another.

Conclusions: limits for a selection program

Selection programs are run for several years and it is necessary to compare the cost with the expected benefits. It is promising that selection for resistance and resilience to parasites does not adversely affect selection for increased production. Indeed, selecting for resistance will positively influence production. Two particular problems remain unsolved and may be important in the adoption of such selection programs. Firstly, we do not yet have genetic markers that permit selection at an early age. Secondly, resistance tends to be restricted to a few target parasites and for practical purposes several lines of resistant sheep are required. Even though these problems remain unsolved, the most susceptible animals should be removed from flocks. The suggestion that contaminative individuals are few and remain contaminative for the rest of their lives should be examined.

References

Alakham, L. 1977. Contribution a l'etude pathologique, epidemiologique et lesionnelle des bronchopneumonies vermineuses du mouton dans la region de Talda. These de Doctorat Veterinaire, Institut Agronomique et Veterinaire Hassan II. Rabat, Morocco. 99 p.

Albers, G.A.A., Burgess, S.E., Adams, D.B., Barker, J.S.F., Le Jambre, L.F. and Piper, L.R. 1984. Breeding *Haemonchus contortus* resistant sheep. Problems and prospects. Pages 41–51 in Immunogenetic Approaches to the Control of Endoparasites (Dineen, J.K. and Outteridge, P.M., eds). Division of Animal Health, CSIRO, Melbourne, Australia.

Albers, G.A.A. and Gray, G.D. 1987. Breeding for worm resistance: a perspective. International Journal for Parasitology 17: 559–565.

Al-Khshali, M.N. and Altaif, K.I. 1979. The response of Awassi and Merino sheep to primary infection with *Haemonchus contortus*. Tropical Animal Health and Production 11: 164–170.

Allonby, E.W. and Urquhart, G.M. 1976. A possible relationship between haemonchosis and haemoglobin polymorphism in Merino sheep in Kenya. Research in Veterinary Science 20: 212–214.

Altaif, K.I. and Dargie, J.D. 1978. Genetic resistance to helminths. The influence of breed and haemoglobin type on the response of sheep to primary infections with *Haemonchus contortus*. Parasitology 77: 161–175.

Bradley, R.E., Radhakrishnan, C.V., Patil-Kulkarni, V.C. and Loggins, P.E. 1973. Responses of Florida Native and Rambouillet lambs exposed to one or two oral doses of *Haemonchus contortus*. American Journal of Veterinary Research 34: 729–735.

Benakhla, A. 1982. Les pneumonies vermineuses ovines: frequence, lesions, traitement. Memoire Magister en Science Veterinaire, Faculte de Medecine Veterinaire de Liege, Belgium. 61 p.

Cabaret, J. and Anjorand, N. 1984. Comparaison de l'infestation naturelle par les strongyles et *Moniezia* sp. chez les races caprines Alpine et Saanen. Bulletin de la Societe francaise de Parasitologie 2: 49–52.

Courtney, C.H. 1986. Host genetic factors in helminth control in sheep. Veterinary Clinics of North America, Food and Animal Practice 2: 433–438.

Courtney, C.H., Gessner, R., Sholz, S.R. and Loggins, P.E. 1986. The periparturient rise in fecal egg counts in three strains of Florida Native ewes and its value in predicting resistance of lambs to *Haemonchus contortus*. International Journal for Parasitology 16: 185–189.

Courtney, C.H., Parker, C.F., McClure, K.E. and Herd, R.P. 1984. A comparison of the periparturient rise in fecal egg counts of exotic and domestic ewes. International Journal for Parasitology 14: 377–381.

Courtney, C.H., Parker, C.F., McClure, K.E. and Herd, R.P. 1985. Resistance of exotic and domestic lambs to experimental infection with *Haemonchus contortus*. International Journal for Parasitology 15: 101–109.

Dargie, J.D. 1982. The influence of genetic factors on the resistance of ruminants to gastro-intestinal nematode and Trypanosome infections. Pages 17–51 in Animal Models in Parasitology (Owen, D.G., ed.). McMillan Press Ltd., London, UK.

Evans, J.V., Blunt, M.H. and Southcott, W.H. 1963. The effects of infection with *Haemonchus contortus* on the sodium and potassium concentrations in the erythrocytes and plasma in sheep of different haemoglobin types. Australian Journal of Agricultural Research 4: 549–558.

Gray, G.D. 1987. Genetic resistance to haemonchosis in sheep. Parasitology Today 3: 253–255.

Gray, G.D. and Raadsma, H.W. 1986. Resilience to *Haemonchus contortus* infection in lambs crossbred between Merino strains and bloodlines. Pages 691–696 in Proceedings of the Third World Congress on Genetics Applied to Livestock Production, 16–22 July 1986, Lincoln Nebraska, USA. University of Nebraska, USA.

Gruner, L. and Cabaret, J. 1985. Utilisation des parcours mediterraneens et parasitisme interne des ovins. Pages 307–335 in Exploitation des milieux difficiles par les ovins et les caprins. 10em Journees de la Recherche Ovine et Caprine. INRA-ITOVIC, ITOVIC-SPEOC, Paris, France.

Gruner, L., Cabaret, J., Sauve, C. and Pailhories, R. 1986. Comparative susceptibility of Romanov and Lacaune sheep to gastrointestinal nematodes and small lungworms. Veterinary Parasitology 19: 85–93.

Gruner, L., Cabaret, J., Bouix, J. and Molenat, G. 1987. Comparative susceptibility of Merinos and Romanov sheep to different helminth parasites. Page 57 in Proceedings of 12th Conference of the World Association for the Advancement of Veterinary Parasitology, 12–15 July 1987, Montreal, Canada. McGill University, Montreal, Canada.

Jilek, A.F. and Bradley, R.E. 1969. Haemoglobin types and resistance to *Haemonchus contortus* in sheep. American Journal of Veterinary Research 30: 1778–1779.

Knight, R.A., Vegors, H.H. and Glimp, H.A. 1973. Effects of breed and date of birth of lambs to gastro-intestinal nematode infections. American Journal of Veterinary Research 34: 323–327.

Le Jambre, L.F. 1978. Host genetic factors in helminth control. Pages 137–141 in The Epidemiology and Control of Gastro-intestinal Parasites of Sheep (Donald, A.D., Southcott, W.H. and Dineen, J.K., eds). Division of Animal Health, CSIRO, Melbourne, Australia.

Luffau, G., N'Guyen, T.C., Cullen, P., Vu Tien Khang, J., Bouix, J. and Ricordeau, G. 1986. Genetic resistance to *Haemonchus contortus* in Romanov sheep. Pages 683–689 in Proceedings of the Third World Congress on Genetics Applied to Livestock Production, 16–22 July 1986, Lincoln Nebraska, USA. Univeristy of Nebraska, USA.

Norman, L.M. and Hohenboken, W. 1979. Genetic and environmental effects on internal parasites, foot soundness and attrition in crossbred ewes. Journal of Animal Science 48: 1329–1336.

Outteridge, P.M., Windon, R.W. and Dineen, J.K. 1985. An association between a lymphocyte antigen in sheep and the response to vaccination against the parasite *Trichostrongylus colubriformis*. International Journal for Parasitology 15: 121–127.

Piper, L.R., Le Jambre, L.F., Southcott, W.H. and Chang, T.S. 1978. Natural worm burdens in Dorset horn, Merino and Corriedale weaners and their crosses. Proceedings of the Australian Society of Animal Production 12: 276.

Preston, J.M. and Allonby, E.W. 1978. The influence of breed on the susceptibility of sheep and goats to a single experimental infection with *Haemonchus contortus*. Veterinary Record 103: 509–512.

Preston, J.M. and Allonby, E.W. 1979. The influence of breed on the susceptibility of sheep to *Haemonchus contortus* infection in Kenya. Research in Veterinary Science 26: 134–139.

Radhakrishnan, C.V., Bradley, R.E. and Loggins, P.E. 1972. Host responses of worm-free Florida Native and Rambouillet lambs experimentally infected with *Haemonchus contortus*. American Journal of Veterinary Research 33: 817–833.

Richard, S. and Cabaret, J. 1986. Caracteristiques de la reponse de jeunes chevreaux a une primo-infestation par le nematode *Teladorsagia circumcincta*. Bulletin de la Societe francaise de Parasitologie 4: 245–246.

Riffkin, G.G. and Yong, W.K. 1984. Recognition of sheep which have innate resistance to trichostrongylid nematode parasites. Pages 30–38 in Immunogenetic Approaches to the Control of Endoparasites (Dineen, J.K. and Outteridge, F.M., eds). Division of Animal Health, CSIRO, Melbourne, Australia.

Ross, J.G. 1970. Genetic differences in the susceptibility of sheep to infection with *Trichostrongylus axei*: a comparison of Scottish Blackface and Dorset breeds. Research in Veterinary Science 11: 465–468.

Scrivner, L.H. 1964. Breed resistance to ostertagiosis in sheep. Journal of the American Veterinary Medical Association 144: 883–887.

Stewart, M.A., Miller, R.F. and Douglas, J.R. 1937. Resistance of sheep of different breeds to infestation by *Ostertagia circumcincta*. Journal of Agricultural Research 55: 923–930.

Suarez, V.H. 1985. Comparacion del effecto de la parasitosis gastrointestinales sobre razas ovinas, 3/4 Ost. Friesian × 1/4 Corriedale y Corriedale en la region semiarida pampeana. Veterinaria Argentina 2: 554–561.

Urquhart, G.M. 1988. The potential use of vaccines or genetically resistant animals in the control of helminthiasis. In Proceedings of a Workshop on Increasing Small Ruminant Productivity in

Semi-Arid Areas, 30 Nov–3 Dec 1987, ICARDA, Aleppo, Syria, (Thomson, E.F. and Thomson, F.S., eds). Kluwer Academic Publishers, Dordrecht, The Netherlands.

Windon, R.G. and Dineen, J.K. 1984. Parasitological and immunological competence of lambs selected for high and low responsiveness to vaccination with irradiated *Trichostrongylus colubriformis*. Pages 13–28 in Immunogenetic Approaches in the Control of Endoparasites (Dineen, J.K. and Outterridge, P.M., eds). Division of Animal Health, CSIRO, Melbourne, Australia.

Yazwinski, T.A., Goode, L., Moncol, D.J., Morgan, G.W. and Linnerud, A.C. 1979. Parasitic resistance in straightbred and crossbred Barbados Blackbelly sheep. Journal of Animal Science 49: 919–926.

E.F. Thomson and F.S. Thomson (eds), Increasing Small Ruminant Productivity in Semi-arid Areas
© 1988 ICARDA . ISBN 978-94-010-7086-7

The Potential Use of Vaccines or Genetically Resistant Animals in the Control of Helminthiasis

G.M. Urquhart

Introduction

In a paper I gave recently on the control of helminthiasis in the tropics, I tried to emphasize that a viable sheep or cattle enterprise depended, among other things, on the control of gastrointestinal nematodes (Urquhart 1987). For example, in Australia there is a highly profitable wool industry based on some 150 million Merinos which earn about 1800 million USD in exports. However, the cost of controlling parasitic worms, in terms of anthelmintics alone and excluding labour, is around 40 million USD. Nevertheless, the control of gastrointestinal worms is essential if farmers' profit margin is to be sustained. Sheep or cattle husbandry which ignores the control of these diseases is almost inevitably doomed to failure.

Nematode control using anthelmintics

My remit is to discuss the relative merits of artificial immunization and genetic selection as potential methods of controlling gastrointestinal nematodes but this implies that something is wrong with our current control techniques. By control techniques I mean attempts to prevent disease and not merely the treatment of clinically affected animals, which is of very limited value.

Basically, control depends on anthelmintic drugs given in one of two ways (Urquhart et al. 1987). In the first, the worms are killed in the host before they have time to develop to sexual maturity. This prevents contamination of the pasture with worm eggs and so limits further challenge with infective larvae. A less effective method is to allow a very modest infection of adult worms to develop, killing these with an anthelmintic, and then immediately moving the stock to fresh and rested pastures.

During the past few years, a modification of the first technique has been developed using long-acting devices (LADS) or boluses which, given orally, remain in the reticulum or rumen. These operate either by continuously leaking small quantities of drug which kill the infective larvae as they enter the abomasum or, alternatively, as a series of four or five pulsed releases of therapeutic doses of drug about every 3 weeks i.e., before the worms become adult. These are not yet available for sheep, but are likely to become so in the near future.

Although all of these techniques are highly effective there are several problems, both real and potential, which I will briefly discuss.

The cost of anthelmintics and labour

Anthelmintic treatment absorbs a significant amount of potential profit and while the use of long-acting devices is less labour intensive, they tend to be expensive.

Drug-resistance

This is now a significant problem (Waller 1987), especially in areas of Australia, Africa, and South America where the blood-sucking nematode *Haemonchus contortus* is found. Apparently this has arisen because of the necessity for repeated and frequent treatments. In Australia, the benzimidazoles or levamisole may need to be given on eight occasions at intervals of 3–4 weeks to prevent the development of adult worms and about 50% of sheep are now thought to be infected with strains of *Haemonchus* resistant to one or other of these drugs. The onset of the problem was probably accelerated by the use of minimally effective doses of anthelmintics.

Failure to develop immunity

In the UK there is some evidence (Urquhart et al. 1987) that calves and lambs reared with effective anthelmintic treatment during their first year of life may fail to develop a high degree of acquired immunity and are therefore susceptible to helminthiasis in their second year or later.

Drug residues

Problems with drug residues have not figured greatly in anthelmintic literature although long-acting anthelmintics may change this. For example, Wall and Strong (1987) reported that cattle dung pats apparently failed to degrade normally due to the absence of dung beetles caused by the insecticidal effect of ivermectin excreted in the faeces. In Australia and South Africa, a new anthelmintic, closantel, is currently being used to control *Haemonchus*, as a single dose gives 6–8 weeks protection against reinfection, presumably because drug residues in the plasma continue to exert an anthelmintic effect. While this may be suitable for wool sheep its use in lambs destined for meat production requires attention to drug withdrawal periods.

Vaccines

It would certainly be advantageous if vaccines were available which would give prolonged periods of protection or, alternatively, sheep breeds were available which were naturally resistant to helminth diseases.

There is only one vaccine commercially available, that against *Dictyocaulus viviparus*, the bovine lungworm (ABPI 1987). Calves are vaccinated orally at 2 months or older with 1000 x-irradiated larvae on two occassions with an interval of 1 month between doses. Since dairy calves in northern Europe are normally reared indoors for the first few months vaccination is conveniently carried out during this time and, 1 month after the second dose, calves are immune and can go to grass.

The efficacy of this vaccine in the field is unquestionable. Breakdowns are few and are often due to other causes such as failure to vaccinate the second crop of younger calves which go to grass for the first time in mid-summer. It is not 100% effective against challenge and a small number of worms may become established in the lungs of vaccinated calves, but this is rarely associated with clinical signs. The few larvae which are passed in the faeces of such calves and overwinter successfully on pasture boost the immunity of previously vaccinated cattle. This means, however, that pastures remain contaminated and so each calf crop must be vaccinated annually.

It is an expensive vaccine to produce and the short shelf-life (28 days) necessitates an efficient postal service and refrigeration if not used immediately. It is also specific as it only protects against *Dictyocaulus*, and so farmers must continue to use anthelmintic to control gastrointestinal worms.

Following the success of this vaccine, efforts were made to develop one of a similar type against *Haemonchus*, undoubtedly the most serious helminth disease of sheep in tropical and subtropical areas (Urquhart 1980). Initially, experiments were conducted with sheep over 7 months old and vaccination resulted in a high degree of immunity and a 98% reduction in worm burdens. Since haemonchosis also affects young lambs, subsequent experiments were conducted with 2–5 month old lambs. The lambs, aged up to 3 months old at vaccination, had no immunity whatsoever and the 5 month old lambs were protected only slightly (Urquhart 1980).

A series of subsequent investigations has shown that sheep aged up to 7 months and calves, up to perhaps 12 months, are generally immunologically unresponsive to infection (or vaccination) with gastrointestinal nematodes. Since calves and lambs can be immunized successfully with bacterial and viral vaccines long before these ages and since the lungworm vaccine works perfectly well in calves of a few weeks old, the defect is presumably associated with delayed maturation of the immune response in the gut. So far, the precise cause of this defect is unknown and it suggests that any future vaccines will have to solve, or at least circumvent, this problem.

In the long run, vaccines against common helminth diseases such as ostertagiasis and haemonchosis will become available as a by-product of the current explosion of knowledge in molecular biology and immunology (Murray 1987) but this is likely to take several decades. Presumably these will be small sub-unit vaccines produced by either recombinant DNA technology or chemical synthesis and they will probably require suitable adjuvants to potentiate their immunogenicity. Alternatively, the antigen may be expressed in the host by genetically engineered viruses which could provide a more vigorous and sustained stimulation of the immune system. The possible use of anti-idiotype antibodies (i.e., an antibody against the antigen-combining site of a helminth antibody which mimics the structure of the helminth antigen) is particularly interesting since neonatal mice that are unresponsive to vaccination with *E. coli* K13 polysaccharide can be successfully protected with anti-idiotype vaccine which mimics the polysaccharide (Stein and Soderstrom 1984). This finding may be useful in overcoming immunological unresponsiveness to helminth vaccines in young ruminants.

Unfortunately, the mechanisms underlying the immune response against gastrointestinal helminths are still being unravelled and the respective roles of antibody and a wide range of cell-mediated responses are still undetermined. However, such information may not be an essential prerequisite to vaccine development since there are probably several complementary but independent mechanisms and artificial stimulation of one of these might be sufficient to produce satisfactory immunity.

Vaccines are likely to be highly specific and therefore of greatest value where a single infection predominates. This is certainly the case with ostertagiasis in most of the temperate world and with haemonchosis in tropical zones. However, there are areas where helminthiasis is caused by several genera of worms and where a single vaccine would be less effective. Also, because of the economic significance of subclinical helminthiasis in cattle and sheep (Coop 1982) any vaccine would have to be highly efficient in protecting against infection as opposed to merely preventing clinical signs.

Genetic resistance to helminthiasis

Most of the work on developing animals genetically resistant to helminthiasis has been done in Australia where helminthiasis and drug-resistance are always potential threats to wool production. Since sheep may be infected with *Haemonchus, Trichostrongylus*, and *Ostertagia*, genetically resistant sheep should preferably be resistant to all these species. However, to date, work has concentrated largely on *Haemonchus*, the greatest problem. Also, because of the specialised nature of the industry i.e., Merino wool production, the emphasis is on the selection of individuals rather than breeds, and so progress is inevitably slow.

Evidence of genetic resistance (Gray 1987) has been based on the numbers of worms in sheep at necropsy, the faecal egg output (EPG), and anaemia as measured by the packed red cell volume (PCV). Using single-sire mating of 157 rams with randomly selected ewes, 1583 lambs were studied. After artificial infection with *Haemonchus* at 5–18 months old, resistance to haemonchosis was moderately heritable as judged by differences in EPG and PCV i.e., of the order of 0.3. Although this may not appear to be highly significant, similar heritabilities were found for weaning weight and fleece weight for which selection has been highly successful. Assuming a heritability of 0.3, variation of resistance within a flock of 40%, and a selection intensity of 5% in males and 30% in females, the Australian workers have calculated that resistance traits in a flock would increase by 6% each year. Selection experiments under natural infection have been in progress since 1978 and indicate a similar trend.

These studies have shown that in uninfected resistant and susceptible sheep there is no difference in liveweight gain or wool growth, indicating that breeding for resistance to *Haemonchus* does not reduce productivity. On the other hand, if subjected to infection, resistant sheep will produce more meat and wool than susceptible sheep.

One of the problems of such studies is their extrapolation to the field where laboratory parameters cannot be used. To overcome this, Gray (1987) suggested that it may be adequate to simply select individual, highly productive sheep using liveweight gains at the beginning and end of a period of exposure to natural infection. While this is perhaps a useful technique under light or modest challenge, it is unlikely that a farmer would be willing to allow the productivity of a proportion of his flock to decline over an entire grazing season without resort to anthelmintic treatment.

The constraint to the development of worm-resistant sheep, i.e., it depends on the selection of individual animals, is largely removed if one can find an entire breed which is resistant and which has already evolved, at least to some degree, for meat production.

It seems that this may be the case with the Red Masai sheep in East Africa. Preston and Allonby (1979) describe the relative *Haemonchus* resistance of six breeds of sheep grazed over a period of 2 years and subjected to natural challenge. The Red Masai were by far the most resistant to infection as judged by faecal egg counts, flock mortality, and worm counts at necropsy. The resistance appeared to be genetic in origin rather than attributable to previously acquired immunity.

The Masai sheep have evolved for centuries in an area of endemic haemonchosis in a system of seminomadic husbandry in which anthelmintic therapy has played little or no part. It is not a commercially developed breed but there is little doubt that it could be improved by selection. For those parts of the developing world where, despite the threat of haemonchosis, commercial sheep husbandry is being developed and especially where veterinary surveillance is inadequate the possibility of developing *Haemonchus*-resistant breeds of economic worth presents a fascinating challenge and one of great potential.

Conclusions

It will be several decades before acceptable helminth vaccines are available for commercial use but, as pointed out by Murray (1987), "the development of molecular vaccines against parasites is now an inevitable process and the growing accumulation of basic facts about these organisms indicates that there are no major technical obstacles which cannot be overcome". Until these vaccines are developed, applied research will probably concentrate on the use of effective long-acting anthelmintic devices during the first year of grazing. These will be so designed that they will also allow the acquisition of a degree of immunity, preferably towards the end of the grazing season as the animals become immunologically responsive. This immunity will then give protection in later years without the necessity of repeated anthelmintic treatment. Unfortunately, haemonchosis is likely to prove an exception to this approach since Merino sheep at least seem to acquire little immunity even with repeated exposure.

The imponderables with this approach are the development of drug-resistant strains of parasites, public attitudes to possible tissue residues of drugs, and most recently, concern about the environmental effects of anthelmintics excreted in the faeces. However, veterinary parasitologists are aware of these problems and they are unlikely to be insuperable.

The possibility of developing cattle or sheep genetically resistant to helminth infections is still in its infancy both technically and philosophically but it has great potential. Perhaps the greatest stimulus to this approach will be the development of helminth vaccines since there is some evidence that resistance might be restricted to animals with certain MHC haplotypes i.e., the set of alleles on a single chromosome, collectively termed the Major Histocompatibility Complex, which controls immune response (see Murray 1987). However, the immediate prospects are infinitely greater if one can show that a specific breed, rather than an individual, is highly resistant. Evidence of such a trait clearly exists in Ndama cattle against trypanosomiasis (Murray et al. 1984) and in Red Masai sheep against haemonchosis. Perhaps it is time that more attention was given to the qualities of indigenous breeds in developing countries.

References

ABPI (Association of British Pharmaceutical Industry). 1987. Compendium of Data Sheets 1987/88. Datapham Publications, Whitehall, London, UK. 347 p.

Coop, R.L. 1982. The impact of subclinical parasitism in ruminants. Pages 439–450 in Parasites–Their World and Ours (Mettrick, D.F. and Resser, S.S., eds). Elsevier Biomedical Press, Amsterdam, The Netherlands.

Gray, G.D. 1987. Genetic resistance to haemonchosis in sheep. Parasitology Today 3: 253–255.

Murray, P.K. 1987. Prospects for molecular vaccines in veterinary parasitology. Veterinary Parasitology 25: 121–133.

Murray, M., Trail, J.C.M., Davis, C.E. and Black, S.J. 1984. Genetic resistance to African trypanosomiasis. Journal of Infectious Diseases 149: 311–319.

Preston, J.M. and Allonby, E.W. 1979. The influence of breed on the susceptibility of sheep to *Haemonchus contortus* infection in Kenya. Research in Veterinary Science 26: 134–139.

Stein, K.E. and Soderstrom, T. 1984. Neonatal administration of idiotype or anti-idiotypic primes for protection against *Escherichia coli* K13 infection in mice. Journal of Experimental Medicine 160: 1001–1011.

Urquhart, G.M. 1980. Application of immunity in the control of parasitic disease. Veterinary Parasitology 6: 217–239.

Urquhart, G.M. 1987. Seminar on Animal Health in the Tropics. To be published in the Newsletter of Tropical Agricultural Association, ODA, London, UK.

Urquhart, G.M., Armour, J., Duncan, J.L., Dunn, A.M. and Jennings, F.W. 1987. Veterinary Parasitology. Longman Scientific and Technical, Essex, UK. 286 p.

Wall, R. and Strong, L. 1987. Environmental consequences of treating cattle with the antiparasitic drug ivermectin. Nature 327: 418–421.

Waller, P.J. 1987. Anthelmintic resistance and the future for roundworm control. Veterinary Parasitology 25: 177–191.

E.F. Thomson and F.S. Thomson (eds), Increasing Small Ruminant Productivity in Semi-arid Areas
© *1988 ICARDA . ISBN 978-94-010-7086-7*

Mechanisms of Immunity to Gastrointestinal Nematodes of Sheep

W.D. Smith

Introduction

There is unequivocal evidence that sheep can acquire immunity to gastrointestinal nematodes. In Western Europe, for example, while clinical parasitic gastroenteritis is common in lambs during their first grazing season, disease outbreaks are unusual in subsequent years. It has been shown experimentally with three different species of nematode that substantial immunity to incoming larvae develops after about 2 months in continuously infected lambs (Barger, Le Jambre, Georgi and Davis 1985; Fig. 1).

Despite this, there are no vaccines for controlling gastrointestinal nematodes in sheep and little or no immunity has been stimulated experimentally by parenteral injection of either live worms or extracts of dead ones (reviewed by Lloyd 1981). Partial success has been achieved experimentally with vaccines consisting of irradiation attenuated larvae similar to Dictol, the commercially available cattle lungworm vaccine. But this method is, at most, only partially effective in growing lambs (Urquhart, Jarrett, Jennings, McIntyre and Mulligan 1966; Dineen, Gregg and Lascelles 1978), which need to be protected

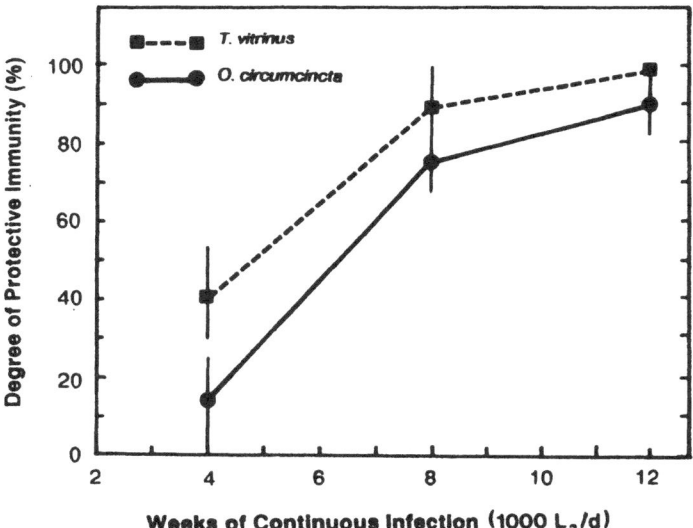

Fig. 1. Development of immunity to incoming larvae in continuously infected lambs. (Vertical bars show standard error of means (SEM)).

most. Also, this approach does not appear to work with certain important species e.g., *Ostertagia circumcincta* (Smith, Jackson and Jackson 1982).

Because of these difficulties, our approach has been to attempt to understand the mechanisms involved in naturally acquired immunity in the hope that such information will eventually lead to a rational approach to vaccination. Consequently, this paper is biased towards progress achieved at our institute in this field in the past few years. Several more general reviews of immunity to gastrointestinal parasites have been published recently (Miller 1984; Barger 1987; Miller 1987; Wakelin 1987).

Biology of *Ostertagia circumcincta*

Most of our research on immunity to the gastrointestinal nematodes of sheep has been conducted with *O. circumcincta*, the most important species in the United Kingdom and other temperate parts of the world including, I suspect, the semi-arid regions of North Africa and West Asia.

The normal life cycle of *Ostertagia* is simple. Infective larvae on grass are ingested by the sheep, exsheath in the rumen, and pass into the abomasum where they invade the gastric glands. There, they develop and grow rapidly, emerging about 7–10 days after infection and causing much damage to the mucosa (Fig. 2). The rest of their life is spent mainly on the surface of the mucosa and, by about 18 days after infection, the now mature females lay eggs which pass out in the faeces to the pasture where they hatch and develop into infective larvae, thus completing the cycle.

Ostertagia can arrest its development in the gastric glands at the early fourth stage when the worms are 1–1.5 mm long. Such larvae can remain

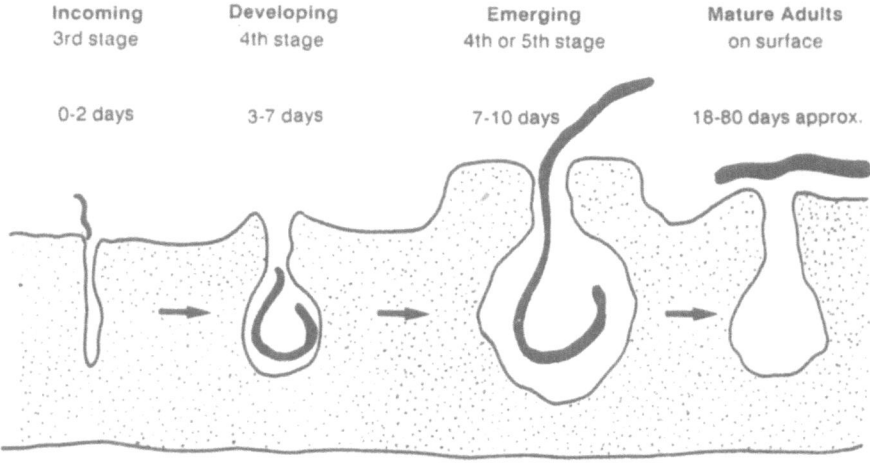

Incoming 3rd stage	Developing 4th stage	Emerging 4th or 5th stage	Mature Adults on surface
0-2 days	3-7 days	7-10 days	18-80 days approx.

Worms can be arrested in their development at the early 4th stage

Fig. 2. The parasitic phase of *O. circumcincta* in the mucosa of the abomasum.

dormant for weeks or months before resuming development in the normal way. Arrested development can occur either if the sheep is immune or if the infective larvae on the pasture have experienced certain climatic conditions e.g., autumn weather in Western Europe.

In naive animals, worms from a single infection can persist in the abomasum for 3 months or more, while in sheep which have previously been infected with the parasite, challenge infections are expelled more rapidly and the rate of growth of the worms is reduced or arrested. Thus, protective immunity to a challenge infection can be quantified by comparing both the number and the length of parasites recovered from immune and control sheep.

Chronic cannulation of the gastric lymph duct: a method for measuring local immune responses to *Ostertagia*

Since *Ostertagia* is confined to the surface of the abomasum and its mucosa, we have concentrated on the local immunological response and have attempted to assess the function of various components of the response in relation to protective immunity. Several aspects of the response have been followed by monitoring day-to-day changes in the composition of the gastric lymph of immune and susceptible sheep challenged with the parasite. The composition of the plasma in the gastric lymph reflects that of the interstitial fluid of the abomasal mucosa and aspects of the local cellular response can easily be studied by following changes in the flow and composition of the lymphocytes which are present in it (Fig. 3).

The lymphatic drainage of the ovine stomachs is anatomically separate from that of the intestine. We usually cannulate the common gastric lymph

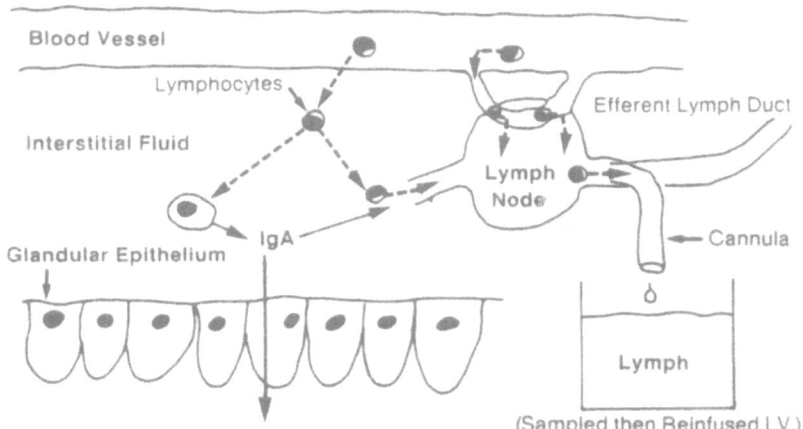

Fig. 3. A simplified view of abomasal lymph formation. Cannulation of the gastric lymph duct allows serial measurement of locally produced proteins and the traffic of lymphocytes via the draining node.

278

Table 1. Worm data from previously infected [1] and control sheep 10 days after challenge with 50000 *Ostertagia*.

Group	Mean worm count	Mean % of worms arrested in their development
Previously infected	2500	97
Control	23000	<1

[1] 2000 larvae per day, 5 days a week for 2 months, followed by anthelmintic.

duct which contains lymph efferent from all four stomachs (Nickel, Schummer and Sieferle 1976). Lymph flow is usually 10–30 ml/h with a lymphocyte output of about 5×10^8 cells/h. In our experiments we routinely subsample the collected lymph once a day and reinfuse the remainder (more than 95% of the collection) intravenously (Smith et al. 1983b).

Responses in the gastric lymph of sheep infected with **50000** *Ostertagia* **larvae**

The only consistent finding in worm-free sheep has been a lymphoblast response which began some 8 days after infection and was maintained for at least 3 weeks (Smith et al. 1983b). Sheep previously infected with 2000 larvae per day for 2 months and which were immune to the challenge infection (Table 1) showed a vigorous secondary immune response in the lymph. The response consisted of an immediate-type hypersensitivity reaction followed by

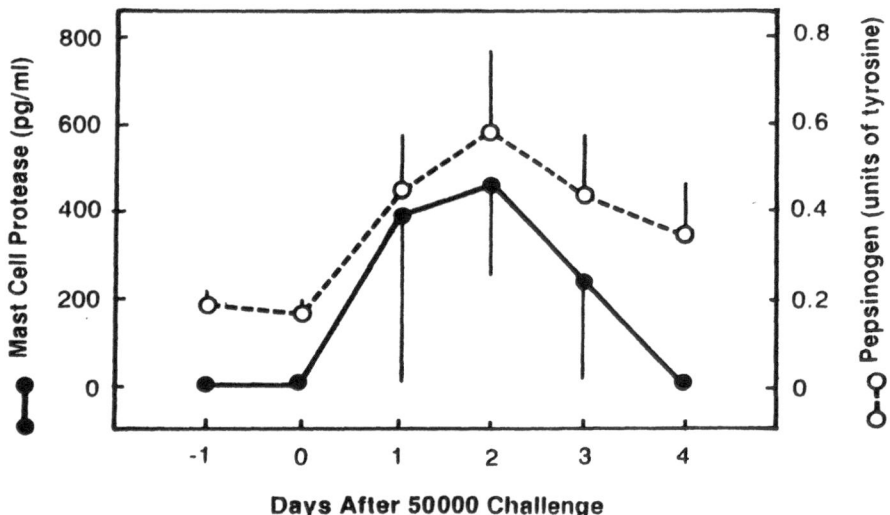

Days After 50000 Challenge

Fig. 4. Changes in the concentrations of pepsinogen and mast-cell protease in the gastric lymph of previously infected sheep after challenge with 50000 L_3 *O. circumcincta*. (Vertical bars show SEM).

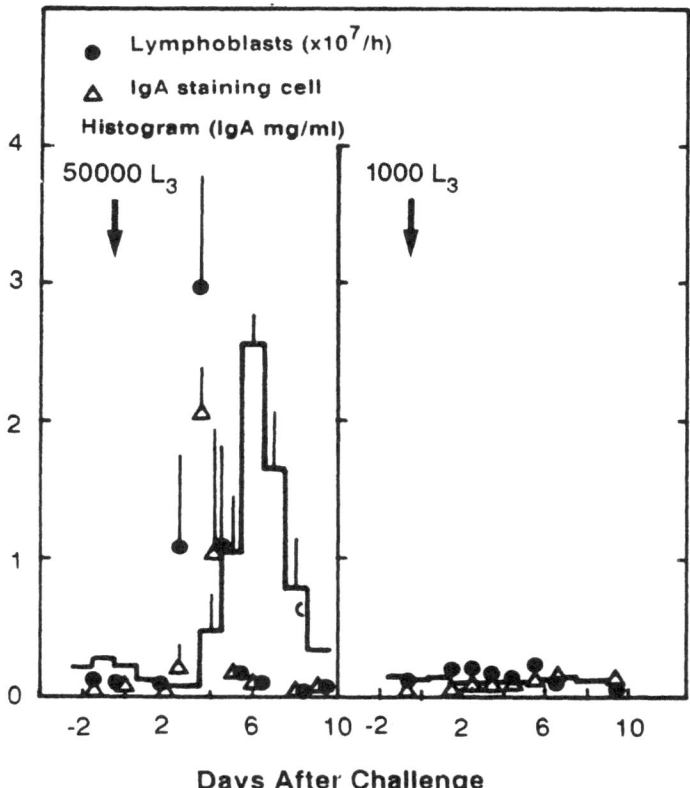

Fig. 5. Changes in the output of lymphoblasts and IgA staining cells and in IgA concentrations in the gastric lymph of previously infected sheep after challenge with either 50000 or 1000 L_3 *O. circumcincta*. (Vertical bars show SEM).

a cellular response which in turn was followed by large increases in total and specific anti-worm IgA (Figs 4 and 5).

The immediate-type hypersensitive reaction

This was detected 24–72 h after challenge by increases in the concentrations of mast cell protease and pepsinogen in the gastric lymph (Fig. 4; Huntley, Gibson, Brown, Smith, Jackson and Miller 1987). There are large numbers of mast cells and globule leucocytes in the gastric mucosa of immune sheep and these cells are probably coated with parasite-specific reaginic antibodies including IgE, although there is no direct evidence for this yet. On exposure to parasite antigens, these sensitised mast cells degranulate releasing their products, which include the protease, into the interstitial fluid and hence the lymph. The function, if any, of this protease is not yet known but it is a useful marker of ovine mast cell degranulation. A range of other components, including histamine and possibly leucotrienes, are also released from the sensitised mast cells. Histamine and other vasoactive amines are thought to increase the permeability of the mucosal epithelium allowing plasma proteins and antibodies to pass into the mucous layer (Yakoob, Holmes and Armour 1983). The same process allows back flow of secreted pepsinogen into the lamina propria, which accounts for the temporary rise in pepsinogen in the lymph and blood of immune sheep after challenge (Fig. 4; Yakoob et al. 1983).

The leucotrienes, formerly known collectively as the slow reacting substance of anaphylaxis, are another type of inflammatory mediator thought to be released when mast cells degranulate. Douch, Harrison, Buchanan and Greer (1983) showed that intestinal mucosal scrapings from sheep previously infected with *Trichostrongylus colubriformis* contained substances which inhibited the migration of the parasite *in vitro* and had biochemical properties similar to the slow reacting substance of anaphylaxis. Douch has subsequently shown that the purified leucotriene C4 appears to have a direct paralysing action on both larvae and adults of several ovine nematodes *in vitro*. Our own results indicate that the concentrations of the leucotrienes B4, C4, and D4 are not increased in mucosal extracts of sheep immune to either *T. vitrinus* or *O. circumcincta* compared to worm-free controls (Moqbel, MacDonald, Miller, Jackson and Smith, unpublished). Clearly, this requires further investigation.

The cellular response

This reaches a peak 3 days after challenge and is composed of a large transient increase in the output of lymphoblastic and IgA containing cells in the lymph (Fig. 5). In several species, including sheep, these cells tend to selectively migrate back to the gut (Hall, Hopkins and Orlans 1977). We have shown in adoptive immunization experiments with genetically identical sheep that partial immunity to *Ostertagia* and *Haemonchus* can be transferred from immune to susceptible animals by such cells (Smith, Jackson, Jackson, Williams, Willadsen and Fehilly 1986; Smith, Jackson, Jackson, Williams, Willadsen and Fehilly; 1984). This has provided direct evidence that at least those aspects of the local immune response we have been measuring can be important.

It is not clear how these cells mediate protection. An indirect mechanism seems much more plausible than a direct cytotoxic one. It has been shown that IgA immunity is transferred by the cells, although whether this immunoglobin was actually involved in the effector mechanism is by no means clear (Smith et al. 1984; 1986).

The antibody response

Large temporary increases in the concentration of lymph antibodies, peaking around 6 days after challenge, have been consistently recorded in immune sheep (Fig. 5). Those of the IgA isotype are almost certainly produced in the abomasal mucosa rather than the gastric nodes which contain relatively few IgA plasma cells. But their role in relation to protective immunity to *Ostertagia* is by no means clear. Attempts to transfer protection against gastrointestinal nematodes by intravenous infusion of large quantities of immune lymph plasma have been unsuccessful (Adams, Merritt and Cripps 1980; Smith and Graham, unpublished). This does not rule out a role for antibody because the concentrations of antibody in the mucosa of the recipients of such lymph are much lower than those in immune sheep after challenge.

There is a close negative correlation between the size of the gastric lymph IgA response of a sheep and the length of its worms (Smith, Jackson, Jackson and Williams 1985). It may be that IgA antibodies retard the development of *Ostertagia*, perhaps by interfering with the worms' ability to feed.

Some factors affecting the local immune response of previously infected sheep

Size and frequency of challenge dose

We found in our gastric lymph/*Ostertagia* system that if the challenge was reduced from a single dose of 50000 to 1000 larvae then no response could be detected in the lymph (Fig. 5) and functional immunity, in terms of both relative numbers and state of development of the challenge worms, was reduced (Smith, Jackson, Jackson, Williams and Miller 1984).

In further experiments we challenged sheep with 2000 larvae per day, a dose rate likely to be encountered on moderately contaminated pasture. The sheep were highly immune to this type of challenge and only a few inhibited parasites were found at slaughter. The continuous challenge stimulated only transient increases in lymphoblast and IgA containing cell output in the lymph whereas IgA and pepsinogen concentrations remained elevated throughout the experiment. Temporary interruption of the challenge in a second group of previously infected sheep showed that elevated IgA and pepsinogen values were maintained only if larval intake was continuous (Smith, Jackson, Graham, Jackson and Williams 1987).

Age of the sheep

The above experiments were all conducted on mature sheep aged 10 months or more, but lambs are more susceptible than adult sheep to experimental infection with gastrointestinal nematodes. For example, most lambs aged 6 months or less which have been immunized with either normal *H. contortus* or irradiated *H. contortus* or *T. colubriformis* are not resistant to homologous challenge with normal larvae, whereas the same immunizing procedure pro-

Table 2. Worm data from 4.5 and 10 month old lambs with identical previous experience of *Ostertagia* after challenge with 50000 larvae.

Age of lambs (months)	Mean % protection[1]	Mean % arrested
4.5	27	14
10	76	97

[1] $\% \text{ Protection} = 100 \times \left(1 - \dfrac{\text{Worm count of previously infected group}}{\text{Worm count of age matched controls}}\right)$

duces a consistently high degree of protection in older sheep (Manton, Peacock, Poynter, Silverman and Terry 1962; Urquhart et al. 1966; Dineen et al. 1978). The reason for this age-related unresponsiveness is unknown and is difficult to understand because neonatal and even foetal lambs are capable of mounting protective immune responses against various bacterial and viral infections (Soulsby 1981). It may be necessary to understand the basis of this unresponsiveness in order to develop successful immunization strategies for lambs.

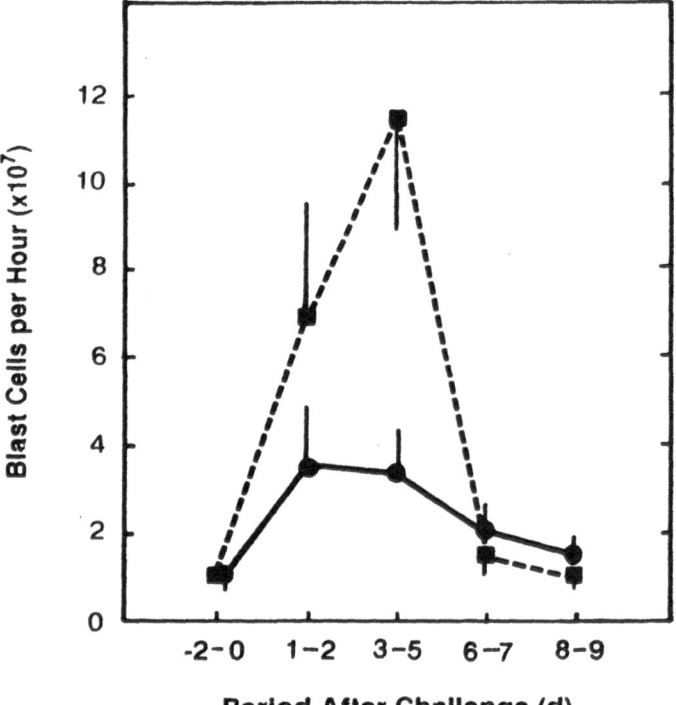

Period After Challenge (d)

Fig. 6. Comparison of the output of lymphoblasts in the gastric lymph of 10 and 4.5 month old lambs (dotted and solid line, respectively) after challenge with 50000 L$_3$ *O. circumcincta*. (Vertical bars show SEM).

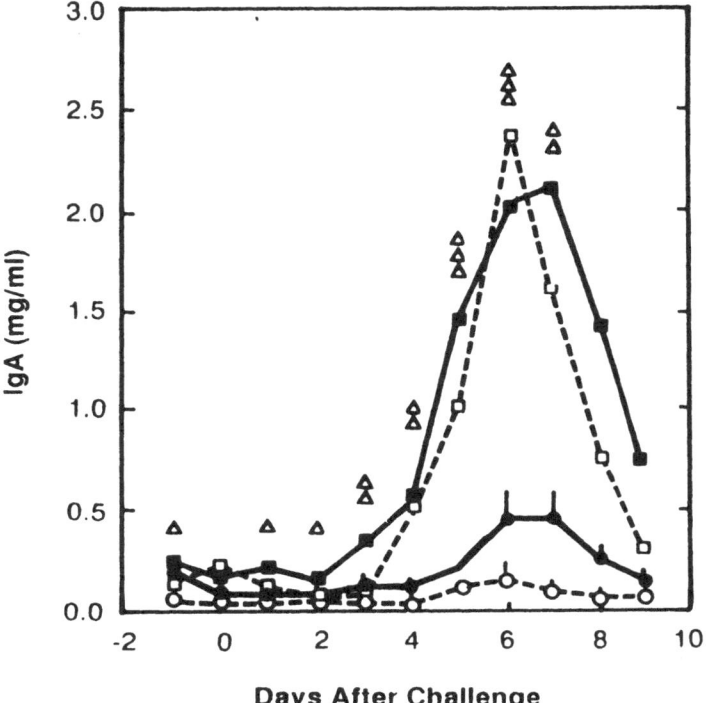

Fig. 7. Comparison of the lymph IgA responses of 10 and 4.5 month old previously infected lambs following challenge with 50000 L₃ *O. circumcincta*. Squares and circles represent data from experiments with 10 and 4.5 month old sheep, respectively. Open and solid symbols show two different experiments. (Vertical bars show SEM and △ equals p < 0.05, △△ equals p < 0.02 and △△△ equals p < 0.01).

We compared the local immune responses of 4.5 and 10 month old previously infected lambs to a single challenge with 50000 larvae in two experiments with each age group (Smith et al. 1984). The younger animals were more susceptible than the older sheep to the challenge infection (Table 2) and both cellular and IgA components were significantly less well developed in the younger lambs (Figs 6 and 7).

The basis for this age difference is obscure. It is unlikely that it was merely due to the suppressive effect of maternal antibody in the younger lambs because Dineen, Gregg and Lascelles (1978) found that previously infected colostrum-deprived lambs were no more immune to challenge with *T. colubriformis* than colostrum-fed lambs.

Genotype of the sheep

We have not yet examined the effect of the genetics of the sheep in our *Ostertagia* immunity system. However, it is well recognised in some countries that indigenous sheep are much more resistant to *Haemonchus* than imported breeds (Preston and Allonby 1979; Courtney, Parker, McLure and Herd 1985). Several Australian groups have demonstrated that resistance to gastrointestinal nematodes is heritable in Merinos (Albers and Gray 1987) and one report indicates that, with *T. colubriformis* at least, this trait is associated with a particular lymphocyte surface antigen (Outteridge, Windon and Dineen 1985).

Plane of nutrition

The effect of diet on the immune response to *Ostertagia* has not yet been examined in our system. Others have clearly shown that lambs on a high plane of nutrition and vaccinated with an irradiated vaccine of *T. colubriformis* were better protected against challenge than similar lambs fed a low protein diet (Wagland, Steel, Windon and Dineen 1984). Clearly, this could be important in dry areas where animals are likely to be undernourished at certain times of the year.

Conclusion

The mechanism by which sheep acquire immunity to gastrointestinal nematodes is undoubtedly complex and despite considerable advances in our knowledge over the past 2 decades, the process is not yet understood. In immune sheep, worm exclusion or expulsion is probably brought about by a combination of immunologically specific (e.g., parasite specific T cells and antibodies) and non-specific components (e.g., mucus and inflammatory mediators) interacting in concert. This response is influenced by the age and genotype of the sheep as well as by its nutritional and hormonal status.

Very little is known about the antigens of the nematodes, and obviously it will be particularly important to identify and characterise those antigens which stimulate protective immune responses. The application of recombinant DNA and ovine monoclonal antibody techniques to this subject will undoubtedly advance our knowledge and perhaps eventually lead to a worm vaccine.

References

Adams, D.B., Merritt, G.C. and Cripps, A.W. 1980. Intestinal lymph and the local antibody response to infection by *Trichostrongylus colubriformis* in sheep. Australian Journal of Experimental Biology and Medical Science 58: 167–177.

Albers, G.A.A. and Gray, G.D. 1987. Breeding for worm resistance: a perspective. International Journal for Parasitology 17: 559–566.

Barger, I.A. 1987. Population regulation in trichostrongylids of ruminants. International Journal for Parasitology 17: 531–540.

Barger, I.A., Le Jambre, L.F., Gerogi, J.R. and Davies, H.I. 1985. Regulation of *Haemonchus contortus* populations in sheep exposed to continuous infection. International Journal for Parasitology 15: 529–533.

Courtney, C.H., Parker, C.F., McClure, K.E. and Herd, R.P. 1985. Resistance of exotic and domestic lambs to experimental infection with *Haemonchus contortus*. International Journal for Parasitology 15: 101–109.

Dineen, J.K., Gregg, P. and Lascelles, A.K. 1978. The response of lambs to vaccination at weaning with irradiated *Trichostrongylus colubriformis* larvae: segregation into "responders" and "non-responders". International Journal for Parasitology 8: 59–66.

Douch, P.G.C., Harrison, G.B.L., Buchanan, L.L. and Greer, K.S. 1983. *In vitro* bioassay of sheep gastrointestinal mucus for nematode paralysing activity mediated by a substance with some properties characteristic of SRS-A. International Journal for Parasitology 13: 207–212.

Hall, J.G., Hopkins, J. and Orlans, E. 1977. Studies on lymphocytes in sheep. III Destination of lymph-borne immunoblasts in relation to their tissues of origin. European Journal of Immunology 7: 30–37.

Huntley, J.F., Gibson, S., Brown, D., Smith, W.D., Jackson, F. and Miller, H.R.P. 1987. Systemic release of a mast cell proteinase following nematode infections in sheep. Parasite Immunology. In press.

Lloyd, S. 1981. Progress in immunization against parasitic helminths. Parasitology 83: 225–242.

Manton, V.J.A., Peacock, R., Poynter, D., Silverman, P.H. and Terry, R.J. 1962. The influence of age and naturally acquired resistance to *Haemonchus contortus*. Research in Veterinary Science 3: 308–314.

Miller, H.R.P. 1984. The protective mucosal response against gastrointestinal nematodes in ruminants and laboratory animals. Veterinary Immunology 6: 167–259.

Miller, H.R.P. 1987. Gastrointestinal mucus, a medium for survival and for elimination of parasitic nematodes and protozoa. 94: 77–100.

Outteridge, P.M., Windon, R.W. and Dineen, J.K. 1985. An association between a lymphocyte antigen in sheep and the response to vaccination against the parasite *Trichostrongylus colubriformis*. International Journal for Parasitology 15: 121–127.

Preston, J.M. and Allonby, E.W. 1979. The influence of breed on susceptibility of sheep to *Haemonchus contortus* in Kenya. Research in Veterinary Science 26: 134–139.

Smith, W.D., Jackson, E. and Jackson, F. 1982. Attempts to immunize sheep against *Ostertagia circumcincta* with irradiated larvae. Research in Veterinary Science 32: 101–105.

Smith, W.D., Jackson, F., Jackson, E. and Williams, J.T. 1983a. Studies on the local immune response of the lactating ewe infected with *Ostertagia circumcincta*. Journal of Comparative Pathology 93: 295–305.

Smith, W.D., Jackson, F., Jackson, E. and Williams, J. 1983b. Local immunity and *Ostertagia circumcincta*; changes in the gastric lymph of sheep after a primary infection. Journal of Comparative Pathology 93: 471–478.

Smith, W.D., Jackson, F., Jackson, E., Williams, J. and Miller, H.R.P. 1984. Manifestations of resistance to ovine ostertagiasis associated with immunological response in the gastric lymph. Journal of Comparative Pathology 94: 591–601.

Smith, W.D., Jackson, F., Jackson, E. and Williams, J. 1984. Age immunity to *Ostertagia circumcincta*: comparison of the local immune responses of 4 and 10 month old lambs. Journal of Comparative Pathology 94: 591–601.

Smith, W.D., Jackson, F., Jackson, E., Williams, J., Willadsen, S.M. and Fehilly, C.B. 1984. Resistance to *Haemonchus contortus* transferred between genetically histocompatible sheep by immune lymphocytes. Research in Veterinary Science 37: 199–204.

Smith, W.D., Jackson, F., Jackson, E., Williams, J., Willadsen, S.M. and Fehilly, C.B. 1986. Transfer of immunity to *Ostertagia circumcincta* and IgA memory between identical sheep by lymphocytes collected from gastric lymph. Research in Veterinary Science 41: 300–306.

Smith, W.D., Jackson, F., Graham, R., Jackson, E. and Williams, J. 1987. Mucosal IgA production and lymph cell traffic following prolonged low level infections of *Ostertagia circumcincta* in sheep. Research in Veterinary Science. In press.

Soulsby, E.J.L. 1981. Immunological unresponsiveness of the neonatal ruminant to gastrointestinal helminths. Isotopes and Radiation in Parasitology IV. International Atomic Energy Agency, Vienna, Austria.

Urquhart, G.M., Jarrett, W.F.H., Jennings, F.N., MacIntyre, W.I.M. and Mulligan, W. 1966. Immunity to *Haemonchus contortus* infection. Relationship between age and successful vaccination with irradiated larvae. American Journal of Veterinary Research 27: 1645–1648.

Wakelin, D. 1987. The role of the immune response in helminth population regulation. International Journal for Parasitology 17: 549–558.

Wagland, B.M., Steel, J.W., Windon, R.G. and Queen, J.K. 1984. The response of lambs to vaccination and challenge with *Trichostrongylus colubriformis*: effect of plane of nutrition on, and the inter-relationship between, immunological responsiveness and resistance. International Journal for Parasitology 14: 39–44.

Yakoob, A., Holmes, P.H. and Armour, J. 1983. Pathophysiology of gastrointestinal trichostrongyles in sheep. Plasma losses and changes in plasma pepsinogen levels associated with parasite challenge of immune animals. Research in Veterinary Science 34: 305–309.

E.F. Thomson and F.S. Thomson (eds), Increasing Small Ruminant Productivity in Semi-arid Areas
© 1988 ICARDA . ISBN 978-94-010-7086-7

Workshop Recommendations for Research at ICARDA

The recommendations of the three working groups are presented under three headings, in order of priority for ICARDA: ruminant nutrition, small ruminant genetics, and animal health.

Ruminant nutrition

Crop residues: the priorities were considered to be:
- completion of research on degradability and intake of cereal straws;
- development of methodologies to assist cereal breeders screen large numbers of genotypes;
- use of new techniques (e.g., infrared spectroscopy) to include measurement of fibre and lignin; and
- investigation of the effect of straw protein and mineral contents on voluntary intake.

Annual medics: the work on medics to replace fallows was considered to have enormous implications for the region, and, although not in the terms of reference, the Workshop urged ICARDA to focus on management methods.

Feed resource / genotype interactions: the Workshop considered this to be a complex area and urged preliminary work on 'improved' and 'unimproved' genotypes including
- voluntary intake potential of the different genotypes;
- rate of flow of different feedstuffs through the digestive tract of improved and unimproved genotypes; and
- selection of highly productive animals to relate performance with feed intake.

Supplementary feeding: strategies to improve the utilization of stubbles, rangelands, and native pastures need to be developed. Recommendations included
- considering the role of urea and sulphur molasses blocks to improve utilization of low-protein feeds;
- developing methods of administering anthelmintics, trace elements and vitamins through blocks; and
- determining the optimum strategy for feeding other supplements such as bran and barley grain.

Palatability of forage legumes: research is needed to study anti-quality factors, especially in forage peas, but also in other forage legumes where appropriate.

Grazing behaviour: this is important in mixed flocks of sheep and goats and the Workshop thought there was a need to:
– determine the actual nutrients consumed by cannulated sheep and goats in various grazing situations and
– define the optimum ratio of sheep and goats for weed control in pastures, most efficient utilization of pastures, and maximum farm profitability.

Adaptation to the environment: Awassi sheep are adapted to an environment with a fluctuating nutrient supply. Research was recommended to:
– determine how best to utilize body-fat reserves;
– relate use of fat reserves to time of lambing;
– relate fat utilization with protein intake and the role of undegraded dietary protein; and
– determine how to reduce rumen degradability of locally available sources of protein.

Water metabolism: the effect of saline water on production, and the reasons for different performance between genotypes and species drinking saline water need to be determined to formulate the best strategies for livestock production where supplies of fresh water are limited.

Small ruminant genetics

Efficiency of feed utilization: research should include:
– comparison of the efficiency of different sheep genotypes in utilizing straw, other crop by-products, pastures, and forages and
– determination of the best way of managing improved sheep genotypes in extensive and intensive farming systems.

Development of methodologies to evaluate improved livestock: objectives should be to:
– develop methods of screening populations for specific characters (e.g., milk production, disease resistance);
– analyse genotype × environment interactions, especially in relation to existing stocking rate experiments;
– determine the effect of breeding season on reproduction and other traits; and
– compare improved and unimproved genotypes in farm flocks, including the effect of releasing 'improved sires' on flock productivity.

Survey of sheep and goat breeds: information should be collected and collated on the existing genetic wealth of sheep and goats and its utilization in livestock-producing farming systems.

Evaluation of breeding objectives: research should be carried out in relation to existing farming systems and the economic situation of farmers. It should include:
- assessment of the Awassi in more frequent breeding systems;
- economic assessment (including allowance for the provision of adequate feed) of increasing the twinning rate of Awassi sheep;
- evaluation of the significance of improving wool quality and quantity; and
- assistance in the formation of networks to develop and evaluate national breeding schemes.

Animal health

Parasitology: the present studies at ICARDA headquarters and on farmers' fields should be broadened to obtain a more general picture of disease constraints facing existing and improved feeding systems.

Disease control: many of the technologies to control diseases which are appropriate in the developed world may not be appropriate in developing countries. It was recommended that:
- social and economic constraints to utilization of modern disease control techniques be determined;
- on-farm research to develop appropriate technologies be commenced with an initial emphasis on control of external and internal parasites; and
- the role of genetic control of diseases should be investigated.

Flock management: concern was expressed that the health of ICARDA's own flock may be at risk. It was emphasized that ICARDA's priority is rightly the provision of improved feeding systems, and to ensure that livestock play their proper part in such research ICARDA should:
- include a comprehensive flock health program in its management strategy;
- quarantine new sheep and goat introductions until vaccinations take effect;
- maintain enzootic stability against endemic diseases by continued contact with local sheep through grazing of the same pastures in succession, while at the same time avoiding direct contact; and
- develop an ability to diagnose and treat diseases as they occur.

The workshop participants recognised that ICARDA would need additional resources to conduct most of this research on small ruminant nutrition, genotype evaluation, and health. Participants from several institutions expressed willingness to collaborate with ICARDA, either as consultants or as co-supervisors of post-graduate students who would conduct their field work at ICARDA or in countries of West Asia and North Africa.

E.F. Thomson and F.S. Thomson (eds), Increasing Small Ruminant Productivity in Semi-arid Areas
© *1988 ICARDA . ISBN 978-94-010-7086-7*

List of Authors and Participants

Those marked 1 are senior authors and those marked 2 are co-authors.

ABOUL-NAGA, A.M. [1]

Animal Production Research Institute
Ministry of Agriculture
Cairo
EGYPT

AMIR, P. [2]

Winrock International Institute for Agricultural Development
Petit Jean Mountain
Morrilton
ARK 72011
USA

ANKARALI, B. [1]

Tarla Bitkileri
Arastirma Enstitusu
P.K. 453
Ulus/Ankara
TURKEY

BAHHADY, F.A.

International Center for Agricultural Research in the Dry Areas (ICARDA)
PO Box 5466
Aleppo
SYRIA

BEKELE, T. [2]

c/o International Livestock Centre for Africa (ILCA)
PO Box 5689
Addis Ababa
ETHIOPIA

BERGER, Y.M. [2]

Department of Animal Science and Small Ruminant CRSP
University of California, Davis
CA 95616
USA

BIRD, S.H. [2]

Department of Biochemistry, Microbiology and Nutrition
University of New England
Armidale
NSW 2351
AUSTRALIA

BRADFORD, G.E. [1]

Department of Animal Science
University of California
Davis
CA 95616
USA

CABARET, J. [2] Institute Nationale de la Recherche Agronomique (INRA)
Station de Pathologie Avaire et Parasitologie
37380 Monnaie
FRANCE

CAPPER, B.S. Overseas Development Natural Resources Institute (ODNRI)
56-61 Gray's Inn Road
London WC1 8LU
UK

COCKS, P.S. [1] International Center for Agricultural Research in the Dry
Areas (ICARDA)
PO Box 5466
Aleppo
SYRIA

COOPER, P.J.H. International Center for Agricultural Research in the Dry
Areas (ICARDA)
PO Box 5466
Aleppo
SYRIA

DAKKAK, A. [1] Departement de Parasitologie et Maladies Parasitaires
Institut Agronomique et Veterinaire Hassan II
B.P. 6202 Rabat
MOROCCO

EL-HARETH, A.K. Livestock Research Division
Ministry of Agriculture and Agrarian Reform
Hama Station
Hama
SYRIA

EL-KAHRI, A.S. Ministry of Agriculture and Agrarian Reform
Damascus
SYRIA

EL-MASANNAT, E.T. [2] Department of Animal Health and Production
Ministry of Agriculture
PO Box 2395
Amman
JORDAN

EL-SABEH, M.M. Department of Animal Production
Aleppo University
Aleppo
SYRIA

EL-SERAFY, A.M. [2] Department of Animal Production
Ain Shams University
Shoubra Al-Kheima
Cairo
EGYPT

GODDARD, I.G.H. [1] European Economic Community
Jordan Cooperative Organisation
PO Box 1343
Amman
JORDAN

GRUNER, L. [1]

Institute Nationale de la Recherche Agronomique (INRA)
Station de Pathologie Avaire et Parasitologie
37380 Monnaie
FRANCE

HABIB, G. [2]

Department of Biochemistry, Microbiology and Nutrition
University of New England
Armidale
NSW 2351
AUSTRALIA

HOSSAMO, H.E.

The Arab Center for the Study of Arid Zones and Dry Lands
(ACSAD)
PO Box 2440
Damascus
SYRIA

KASALI, O.B. [1]

International Livestock Centre for Africa (ILCA)
PO Box 5689
Addis Ababa
ETHIOPIA

KASSEM, R. [1]

Ministry of Agriculture and Agrarian Reform
El Karaim Station
Salamiyeh, Hama
SYRIA

KING, J.M. [1]

c/o British Embassy
PO Box 87
Third Circle
Jebel Amman
JORDAN

KITCHING, R.P. [1]

Institute of Animal Disease Research
Ash Road
Pirbright
Woking GU24 0NF
UK

KOOPMAN, G.J.

International Center for Agricultural Research in the Dry
Areas (ICARDA)
PO Box 5466
Aleppo
SYRIA

LAND, R.B. [1]

Institute of Animal Physiology and Genetics Research
Edinburgh Research Station
Roslin
Midlothian EH25 9PS
UK

LENG, R.A. [2]

Department of Biochemistry, Microbiology and Nutrition
University of New England
Armidale
NSW 2351
AUSTRALIA

LIGHTFOOT, R.J. [1]

Division of Animal Production
Western Australia Department of Agriculture
South Perth 6151
AUSTRALIA

MAVROGENIS, A.P. [1]   Agricultural Research Institute
                          Ministry of Agriculture and Natural Resources
                          Nicosia
                          CYPRUS

McARTHUR, S.R. [2]   Jordan Australia Dryland Farming Project
                          SAGRIC International
                          PO Box 921374
                          Amman
                          JORDAN

NJAU, B.C. [2]   c/o International Livestock Centre for Africa (ILCA)
                          PO Box 5689
                          Addis Ababa
                          ETHIOPIA

NORDBLOM, T.L.   International Center for Agricultural Research in the Dry
                          Areas (ICARDA)
                          PO Box 5466
                          Aleppo
                          SYRIA

NYGAARD, D.F. [1]   Winrock International Institute for Agricultural Development
                          Petit Jean Mountain
                          Morrilton
                          ARK 72110
                          USA

OUHELLI, H. [2]   Departement de Parasitologie et Maladies Parasitaires
                          Institute Agronomique et Veterinaire Hassan II
                          B.P. 6202 Rabat
                          MOROCCO

ØRSKOV, E.R.   Rowett Research Institute
                          Bucksburn
                          Aberdeen AB2 9SB
                          UK

ORITA, G.   International Center for Agricultural Research in the Dry
                          Areas (ICARDA)
                          Japanese International Cooperation
                          Agency (JICA)
                          PO Box 5466
                          Aleppo
                          SYRIA

OWEN, J.B. [1]   Department of Agriculture
                          University College of North Wales
                          Bangor
                          Gwynedd LL57 2UW
                          UK

PERDOK, H.B. [1]   CAF Farmers' Cooperative
                          PO Box 386
                          Leeuwarden 8901 BD
                          THE NETHERLANDS

PELLET, P.J. [1]   College of Food and Natural Resources
                          University of Massachusetts
                          Amherst
                          MA 01003
                          USA

PIKE, D.J. [2]

Department of Applied Statistics
University of Reading
Reading
UK

RHODES, C.N.

12 Doiranis Street
PO Box 7163
Nicosia
CYPRUS

VAN SCHOONHOVEN, A.

International Center for Agricultural Research in the Dry
Areas (ICARDA)
PO Box 5466
Aleppo
SYRIA

SMITH, W.D. [1]

Moredun Research Institute
408 Gilmerton Road
Edinburgh EH17 7JH
UK

SOMEL, K. [1]

International Center for Agricultural Research in the Dry
Areas (ICARDA)
PO Box 5466
Aleppo
SYRIA

STEINBACH, J. [1]

Wissenschaftliches Zentrum
Tropeninstitut
Justus-Liebig-Universitat Giessen
Ludwigstrasse 21
6300 Giessen
GERMAN FEDERAL REPUBLIC

SUED, A.

Livestock Research Division
Ministry of Agriculture and Agrarian Reform
Douma
SYRIA

THOMSON, E.F. [2]

International Center for Agricultural Research in the Dry
Areas (ICARDA)
PO Box 5466
Aleppo
SYRIA

TLEIMAT, F.

The Arab Center for the Study of Arid Zones and Dry Lands
(ACSAD)
PO Box 2440
Damascus
SYRIA

URQUHART, G.M. [1]

Department of Veterinary Parasitology
University of Glasgow
Bearsden Road
Glasgow G61 1QH
UK

VAN HOUTERT, M. [2]

Department of Biochemistry, Microbiology and Nutrition
University of New England
Armidale
NSW 2351
AUSTRALIA

VAN SOEST, P.J. [1]

Department of Animal Science
Cornell University
Ithaca
NY 14853-4801
USA

WILSMORE, A.J. [1]

Department of Animal Health and Production
The Royal Veterinary College
Bolton Park
Potters Bar
Herts EN6 1NB
UK

WOODS, A.J. [2]

L.T. Consultants
Reading
UK

YASSIN, F.

Department of Agriculture
Aleppo University
Aleppo
SYRIA

YOUNG, V.R. [2]

Department of Applied Biological Sciences
Massachusetts Institute of Technology
Cambridge
MA 02139
USA